# Irritable Bowel Syndrome

*Editor*

WILLIAM D. CHEY

# GASTROENTEROLOGY
# CLINICS OF NORTH AMERICA

www.gastro.theclinics.com

*Consulting Editor*
ALAN L. BUCHMAN

September 2021 • Volume 50 • Number 3

**ELSEVIER**

1600 John F. Kennedy Boulevard • Suite 1800 • Philadelphia, Pennsylvania, 19103-2899
http://www.theclinics.com

**GASTROENTEROLOGY CLINICS OF NORTH AMERICA Volume 50, Number 3**
**September 2021 ISSN 0889-8553, ISBN-13: 978-0-323-80928-3**

Editor: Kerry Holland
Developmental Editor: Hannah Almira Lopez

*Gastroenterology Clinics of North America* (ISSN 0889-8553) is published quarterly by Elsevier Inc., 360 Park Avenue South, New York, NY 10010-1710. Months of issue are March, June, September, and December. Business and Editorial Offices: 1600 John F. Kennedy Blvd., Suite 1800, Philadelphia, PA 19103-2899. Customer Service Office: 6277 Sea Harbor Drive, Orlando, FL 32887-4800. Periodicals postage paid at New York, NY and additional mailing offices. Subscription prices are $365.00 per year (US individuals), $100.00 per year (US students), $945.00 per year (US institutions), $391.00 per year (Canadian individuals), $100.00 per year (Canadian students), $997.00 per year (Canadian institutions), $463.00 per year (international individuals), $220.00 per year (international students), and $997.00 per year (international institutions). Foreign air speed delivery is included in all *Clinics* subscription prices. All prices are subject to change without notice. **POSTMASTER:** Send address changes to *Gastroenterology Clinics of North America*, Elsevier Health Sciences Division, Subscription Customer Service, 3251 Riverport Lane, Maryland Heights, MO 63043. **Telephone: 1-800-654-2452 (U.S. and Canada); 314-447-8871 (outside U.S. and Canada). Fax: 314-447-8029. E-mail: journalscustomerservice-usa@elsevier.com (for print support); journalsonlinesupport-usa@elsevier.com (for online support).**

*Reprints.* For copies of 100 or more, of articles in this publication, please contact the Commercial Reprints Department, Elsevier Inc., 360 Part Avenue South, New York, New York 10010-1710. Tel. 212-633-3874, Fax: 212-633-3820, E-mail: reprints@elsevier.com.

*Gastroenterology Clinics of North America* is also published in Italian by II Pensiero Scientifico Editore, Rome, Italy; and in Portuguese by Interlivros Edicoes Ltda., Rua Commandante Coelho 1085, 21250 Cordovil, Rio de Janeiro, Brazil.

*Gastroenterology Clinics of North America* is covered in *MEDLINE/PubMed (Index Medicus)*, *Excerpta Medica*, *Current Contents/Clinical Medicine*, *Science Citation Index*, *ISI/BIOMED*, and *BIOSIS*.

# Contributors

## CONSULTING EDITOR

### ALAN L. BUCHMAN, MD, MSPH, FACP, FACN, FACG, AGAF
Professor of Clinical Surgery (Gastroenterology), Medical Director, Intestinal Rehabilitation and Transplant Center, The University of Illinois at Chicago/UI Health, Chicago, Illinois, USA

## EDITOR

### WILLIAM D. CHEY, MD, FACG, AGAF, FACP, RFF
Timothy T. Nostrant Collegiate Professor of Gastroenterology, Professor of Nutrition Sciences, Director, Digestive Health Integrated Care Program, Director, GI Physiology Laboratory, Medical Director, Michigan Bowel Control Program, Michigan Medicine, Ann Arbor, Michigan, USA

## AUTHORS

### SAMEER K. BERRY, MD, MBA
Division of Gastroenterology, Michigan Medicine, Ann Arbor, Michigan, USA

### DARREN M. BRENNER, MD
Division of Gastroenterology/Hepatology, Department of Medicine, Associate Professor of Medicine and Surgery, Northwestern University, Chicago, Illinois, USA

### BROOKS D. CASH, MD, AGAF, FACG, FASGE
Chief, Gastroenterology, Hepatology, and Nutrition, The University of Texas Health Science Center at Houston, Houston, Texas, USA

### LIN CHANG, MD
Professor of Medicine and Vice-Chief, Vatche and Tamar Manoukian Division of Digestive Diseases, David Geffen School of Medicine at UCLA, Los Angeles, California, USA

### WILLIAM D. CHEY, MD, FACG, AGAF, FACP, RFF
Timothy T. Nostrant Collegiate Professor of Gastroenterology, Professor of Nutrition Sciences, Director, Digestive Health Integrated Care Program, Director, GI Physiology Laboratory, Medical Director, Michigan Bowel Control Program, Michigan Medicine, Ann Arbor, Michigan, USA

### JILL K. DEUTSCH, MD
Section of Digestive Diseases, Yale School of Medicine - Yale New Haven Health, New Haven, Connecticut, USA

### DOUGLAS A. DROSSMAN, MD
Professor Emeritus of Medicine and Psychiatry, Drossman Center for the Education and Practice of Biopsychosocial Care, UNC Center for Functional GI and Motility Disorders,

The University of North Carolina at Chapel Hill, Chapel Hill, North Carolina, USA; The Rome Foundation and Drossman Gastroenterology PLLC

**RYAN S. GOLDSTEIN, MD**
Gastroenterology, Hepatology, and Nutrition, The University of Texas Health Science Center at Houston, Houston, Texas, USA

**EMILY HALLER, MS, RDN**
Division of Gastroenterology and Hepatology, Michigan Medicine, Ann Arbor, Michigan, USA

**KIMBERLY N. HARER, MD, ScM**
University of Michigan, Division of Gastroenterology, Department of Internal Medicine, Ann Arbor, Michigan, USA

**CHRISTINA H. JAGIELSKI, PhD, MPH**
Clinical Instructor of Medicine, Internal Medicine-Gastroenterology, Michigan Medicine, Ann Arbor, Michigan, USA

**ANTHONY LEMBO, MD**
Professor of Medicine, Division of Gastroenterology and Hepatology, Beth Israel Deaconess Medical Center, Boston, Massachusetts, USA

**JOY J. LIU, MD**
Division of Gastroenterology/Hepatology, Department of Medicine, Fellow, Northwestern University, Chicago, Illinois, USA

**ANDREA MCGOWAN, MPH**
University of Michigan, Division of Gastroenterology, Department of Internal Medicine, Ann Arbor, Michigan, USA

**EDITH PÉREZ DE ARCE, MD**
Assistant Professor, Department of Medicine, Division of Gastroenterology, Hospital Clínico Universidad de Chile, Santiago, Chile

**RODRIGO QUERA, MD**
Adjunct Professor, Division of Gastroenterology, Inflammatory Bowel Disease Program, Clínica Universidad de los Andes, Santiago, Chile

**EAMONN M.M. QUIGLEY, MD, FRCP, FACP, MACG, FRCPI, MWGO**
Professor, Division of Gastroenterology and Hepatology, Lynda K and David M Underwood Center for Digestive Disorders, Houston Methodist Hospital, Weill Cornell Medical College, Houston, Texas, USA

**MEGAN E. RIEHL, PsyD**
Assistant Professor of Medicine, Internal Medicine-Gastroenterology, Michigan Medicine, Ann Arbor, Michigan, USA

**GREGORY S. SAYUK, MD, MPH**
Division of Gastroenterology, Washington University School of Medicine, Department of Psychiatry, Associate Professor of Medicine and Psychiatry, Washington University School of Medicine, St. Louis Veterans Affairs Medical Center, St Louis, Missouri, USA

**KATE SCARLATA, MPH, RDN**
For a Digestive Peace of Mind, LLC Medway, Massachusetts, USA

**JORDAN M. SHAPIRO, MD**
Section of Gastroenterology and Hepatology, Baylor College of Medicine, Houston, Texas, USA

**PRASHANT SINGH, MBBS**
Assistant Professor of Medicine, Division of Gastroenterology and Hepatology, University of Michigan, Ann Arbor, Michigan, USA

**AMI D. SPERBER, MD, MSPH**
Professor Emeritus of Medicine, Faculty of Health Sciences, Ben-Gurion University of the Negev, Beer-Sheva, Israel

**HANS TÖRNBLOM, MD, PhD**
Department of Molecular and Clinical Medicine, Institute of Medicine, Sahlgrenska Academy, University of Gothenburg, Gothenburg, Sweden

**ELIZABETH J. VIDELOCK, MD, PhD**
Assistant Professor of Medicine, Vatche and Tamar Manoukian Division of Digestive Diseases, David Geffen School of Medicine at UCLA, Los Angeles, California, USA

# Contents

> Irritable bowel syndrome (IBS) prevalence rates are based on diagnostic criteria, the basis for case definitions. Diagnostic criteria have a substantial impact on prevalence rates, which are significant for understanding burden of disease, comparing global subpopulations, generating pathophysiologic research, allocation of health care and research resources, and incentivizing and prioritizing new treatments. There are substantial methodological pitfalls in epidemiologic research, so determining regional and global IBS prevalence rates is problematic. The Rome Foundation Global Epidemiology Study was designed to resolve these problems and achieve more valid results. The results of this study are presented in detail; future directions are discussed.

> The pathogenesis of irritable bowel syndrome is multifactorial and complex. Our understanding of its pathophysiology has evolved, but remains incompletely understood. Symptoms result from a dysregulation of brain–gut interactions. Evidence has identified alterations in central and peripheral (gut) mechanisms in irritable bowel syndrome and the bidirectional communication between the brain and the gut. Pertinent mechanisms include disturbed gut motility, visceral hypersensitivity, altered mucosal and immune function, altered gut microbiota, and altered central nervous system processing. This review addresses factors that increase the risk of irritable bowel syndrome and the central and peripheral mechanisms thought to underlie its symptoms.

> Advances in bioinformatics have facilitated investigation of the role of gut microbiota in patients with irritable bowel syndrome (IBS). This article describes the evidence from epidemiologic and clinical observational studies

highlighting the link between IBS and gut microbiome by investigating postinfection IBS, small intestinal bacterial overgrowth, and microbial dysbiosis. It highlights the effects of gut microbiota on mechanisms implicated in the pathophysiology of IBS, including gut-brain axis, visceral hypersensitivity, motility, epithelial barrier, and immune activation. In addition, it summarizes the current evidence on microbiome-guided therapies in IBS, including probiotics, antibiotics, diet, and fecal microbiota transplant.

Irritable bowel syndrome (IBS) is among the most common diagnoses made by medical providers and its symptoms are common causes for health care consultation. IBS is characterized by abdominal pain associated with abnormal stool consistency and/or frequency and is widely considered a diagnosis of exclusion, despite abundant evidence contradicting such an approach. A positive diagnosis is achieved through application of symptom-based clinical criteria, careful history and physical examination, evaluation for alarm sign/symptoms, and judicious use of diagnostic testing. This article reviews the symptom-based criteria for IBS and utility of diagnostic tests commonly included in the evaluation of IBS symptoms.

Patients with irritable bowel syndrome (IBS) frequently perceive eating food as a trigger to their gastrointestinal (GI) distress. Several factors involved in driving GI symptoms include malabsorption and fermentation of food substrates, gut microbiota alterations, nocebo and placebo response, and mast cell activation. Nutritional interventions require individualization based on the heterogeneity of symptoms as well as the risk for maladaptive eating patterns that present in those with IBS. Despite the variety of interventions marketed to individuals with IBS, the low Fermentable, Oligo-, Di-Mono-saccharide, and Polyol diet has the most evidence for efficacy in symptom management.

Irritable bowel syndrome (IBS) is a disorder of gut-brain interaction (DGBI) that is associated with significant physical, emotional, and occupational burden. Factors such as early life stress, sleep disruption, maladaptive coping strategies, symptom hypervigilance, and visceral hypersensitivity negatively affect gut-brain communication and increase the likelihood of developing IBS or worsen IBS severity. Behavioral strategies, such as cognitive behavioral therapy, gut-directed hypnosis, and mindfulness-based treatments, have shown benefit in improving gastrointestinal (GI)-specific quality of life, as well as reducing GI symptoms. Partnering with a GI-specific mental health provider can assist gastroenterologists in providing comprehensive treatment of IBS and other DGBIs.

Irritable bowel syndrome affects 10% to 15% of the population, and up to 90% of patients with irritable bowel syndrome exclude certain foods to improve their gastrointestinal symptoms. Although focused dietary restrictions are a normal, adaptive response, restrictions can spiral out of control and result in maladaptive restriction. Dietary therapies are rapidly becoming first-line treatment of irritable bowel syndrome, and gastroenterologists need to be aware of red flag symptoms of maladaptive eating patterns and the negative effects of prescribing restrictive diets. There is also growing awareness of the association between eating disorders and gastrointestinal symptoms, including irritable bowel syndrome symptoms.

Diarrhea-predominant irritable bowel syndrome is a common functional gastrointestinal disorder that manifests with abdominal pain and diarrheal bowel patterns, without structural explanation. Diarrhea-predominant irritable bowel syndrome is a heterogeneous condition resulting from diverse pathophysiologic processes. Treatment strategies with varied mechanisms of action are beneficial in its management. The clinician must become familiar with a multi-dimensional approach to irritable bowel syndrome. The 3 approved medications are central to disease management. Effective treatment uses off-label medications and emerging therapies and a growing number of over-the-counter and supplemental agents to optimize symptom improvement for the patient with diarrhea-predominant irritable bowel syndrome.

Irritable bowel syndrome with constipation is a common disorder that significantly impairs quality of life. There are now multiple classes of therapeutics that have been shown via rigorous clinical testing to improve the abdominal and bowel symptoms attributed to irritable bowel syndrome with constipation. These include the secretagogues (lubiprostone, linaclotide, plecanatide, tenapenor) and the prokinetic agent tegaserod. This article highlights the pivotal evidence for these agents and most recent treatment guidance from the major North American gastroenterological societies. When pharmaceuticals are used, a patient-specific approach based on efficacy, safety, tolerability, access, and affordability is recommended.

Psychopharmacologic therapies are beneficial in reducing symptoms when treating irritable bowel syndrome (IBS) and other disorders of gut-brain interaction (DGBI). Noradrenaline, serotonin, and dopamine are neurotransmitters of key importance in psychopharmacology and pain-reduction mechanisms. The first-line (tricyclic antidepressants, serotonin noradrenaline reuptake inhibitors, selective serotonin reuptake inhibitors) and second-line (atypical antipsychotics, delta-ligand agents, low-dose naltrexone) neuromodulator treatment options are recommended when IBS-associated abdominal pain is of moderate or severe intensity and is persistent. To understand the implementation strategy, the multidimensional clinical profile as a template is used for presenting 3 case scenarios involving painful IBS and DGBI of varying complexity.

Complementary and alternative medicine (CAM) is a term used to define a broad range of therapies, most commonly grouped into natural products, mind-body medicine, and traditional systems of medicine. Patients with irritable bowel syndrome (IBS) commonly use CAM therapies, although there are many barriers that may keep patients and providers from talking about a patient's CAM use. Despite limited quantity and quality of evidence of CAM for IBS, providers can better counsel patients on CAM use by understanding pitfalls related to CAM use and by learning what is known about CAM.

Irritable bowel syndrome and inflammatory bowel disease differ in their natural evolution, etiopathogenesis, diagnostic criteria, and therapeutic approach. However, recent evidence has suggested some similarities in mechanisms underlying symptom development and progression. There is a relevant role for alterations in the microbiome–brain–gut axis in both diseases. The presence of irritable bowel syndrome symptoms in patients with quiescent inflammatory bowel disease is common in clinical practice. To determine the cause of irritable bowel syndrome symptoms in patients with quiescent inflammatory bowel disease is a clinical challenge. This review aims to illustrate possible causes and solutions for these patients.

Irritable bowel syndrome (IBS) is a common symptom-based condition of heterogeneous pathogenesis and clinical phenotype. This heterogeneity and multidimensional nature creates significant diagnostic and treatment challenges. Recent evidence has documented the benefits of diet and behavioral interventions. These nonmedical strategies are causing a shift from the traditional care model to a multidisciplinary care model. Recent evidence suggests that collaborative, team-based integrated care leads to better clinical outcomes and reduced cost per cure compared with traditional care. Although it is growing increasingly clear that integrated care offers significant benefits to IBS patients, widespread dissemination will require solutions to structural, cultural, and financial barriers.

# GASTROENTEROLOGY
# CLINICS OF NORTH AMERICA

**SERIES OF RELATED INTEREST**

*Gastrointestinal Endoscopy Clinics of North America*
(Available at: https://www.giendo.theclinics.com)
*Clinics in Liver Disease*
(Available at: https://www.liver.theclinics.com)

**THE CLINICS ARE AVAILABLE ONLINE!**
Access your subscription at:
www.theclinics.com

# Foreword

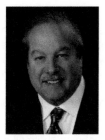

Alan L. Buchman, MD, MSPH
*Consulting Editor*

> *Ultrasound, MIR [MRI], CAT scan [CT], sonogram,*
>
> *Laparoscopy, inoscopy [colonoscopy], I be stressed,*
>
> *The prognosis, diagnosis, IBS*
>
> *And that's irritable bowel child*
> —*I.B.S. by Cam'ron from the Killa Season album (2006)*

Yes, irritable bowel syndrome (IBS) has been written about, sung about, and rapped about. It's only one letter away from IBD, but in reality, actually a world away, although patients with IBS may have IBD and vice versa, and as such, clinicians may sometimes be treating the right problem at the wrong time or the wrong problem at the wrong time.

IBS used to be a wastebasket diagnosis for patients who had abdominal pain of unknown cause, or bloating, or diarrhea, or constipation or alternating diarrhea/constipation, or some combination or permutation of those.

Some people "labeled" with IBS actually had IBD and vice versa. The disease, or perhaps "condition," is not terminal, although there are many patients who seem to feel that it is. Part of that may be born out of frustration with having been thrown into the wastebasket.

Our understanding of IBS has evolved, and perhaps what we still refer to as "IBS" is in reality a plethora of different diseases that range from nondisease to motility disorders, true dietary intolerances, if not allergies, abnormal brain-gut interactions, or an intestinal microbiome that may either cause part of their problems or result from those problems. A new wave of sophistication (to some degree) is being applied in the approach to the diagnosis, understanding, and treatment of IBS.

Regardless of the issues, the reality is patients with "IBS" are uncomfortable, miss work, suffer, and contribute enormous expenditures to the health care system as illustrated in the rap lyrics above.

In this issue of *Gastroenterology Clinics of North America*, Dr Chey has assembled a group of experts who have comprehensively addressed the pathogenesis of IBS,

Gastroenterol Clin N Am 50 (2021) xiii–xiv
https://doi.org/10.1016/j.gtc.2021.04.009
0889-8553/21/© 2021 Published by Elsevier Inc.

**gastro.theclinics.com**

current and emerging therapies (including the potential role of the microbiome and its manipulation), and the psychosocial aspects of the condition and related psychological issues, all with an eye to the future.

Alan L. Buchman, MD, MSPH
Intestinal Rehabilitation and Transplant Center
Department of Surgery/UI Health
University of Illinois at Chicago
840 South Wood Street
Suite 402 (MC958)
Chicago, IL 60612, USA

*E-mail address:*
a.buchman@hotmail.com

# Preface

# Irritable Bowel Syndrome

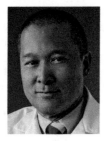

William D. Chey, MD, FACG, AGAF, FACP, RFF
*Editor*

Ten years ago, I eagerly accepted the opportunity to compose and edit an issue of *Gastroenterology Clinics of North America* on Irritable Bowel Syndrome or IBS. A decade later, our world has changed in countless ways, affecting every aspect of our daily lives. From self-driving cars to CRISPR to COVID-19, what a difference a decade has made. Perhaps nowhere is this more apparent than in our understanding of IBS. The way we think about, diagnose, and treat IBS in 2021 is quite different than it was 10 years ago, no doubt related to the explosion of basic, translational, and clinical research addressing this vexing condition. To provide support for this statement, I conducted an unscientific search of *Web of Science* for the term, "Irritable Bowel Syndrome." This search for the dates 2001 to 2010 identified 6890 citations. In comparison, an identical search for the 10 years leading up to the publication of this issue of *Gastroenterology Clinics of North America* (2011-2020) identified 12,977 citations, an increase in citations of almost 90%! If we drill down on this data, we find that for almost any aspect of IBS one can think of, there has been an increase in the number of citations decade over decade. Of course, this expansion in knowledge has been more profound for some areas than others. While "brain-gut" interactions remain relevant and important in a subset of IBS sufferers, the reverse, "gut-brain" interactions, and more specifically, interactions between the luminal microenvironment and the host have thrust issues like diet, bile acids, the gut microbiome, intestinal permeability, and gut immune activation into the limelight.[1] Going back to our unscientific *Web of Science* search, citations addressing IBS and diet have increased by 432% (343 to 1484) from 2001-2010 to 2011-2020. Corresponding growth in citations for IBS and bile acids has been 407% (76 to 309) and IBS and microbiome has been an astounding 6690% (10 to 669).

Amid the dramatic changes in the way we think about IBS, a number of immutable truths remain. The condition remains firmly wedded to characteristic symptoms, including abdominal pain and altered bowel habits.[2] The clinical phenotype, like the

https://doi.org/10.1016/j.gtc.2021.04.007
0889-8553/21/© 2021 Published by Elsevier Inc.
**gastro.theclinics.com**

pathogenesis, remains heterogeneous. With few exceptions, there is a lack of bio-markers that can reliably identify the most effective therapy for an individual patient. As a consequence, in 2021, we are still operating in a world that offers patients empiric treatment based on their clinical phenotype. Patients are left to struggle with the fallout of this archaic, inefficient system in which "effective" treatments typically make fewer than half of patients better and offers a therapeutic gain of 7% to 15% over placebo.[3,4] Cynics would argue that IBS is a "benign" condition, one that does not predispose to the development of cancer or shorten an affected patient's lifespan. While these points are true, they overlook the toll that IBS can take on a patient's ability to carry out their daily professional and personal activities. More severely affected IBS patients truly do suffer. At the end of the day, this is why it is so critically important for health care providers to understand the latest science and how it can help them to make better treatment choices for their IBS patients.

With this as a backdrop, it is indeed timely to provide busy clinicians with focused updates on what is known and what remains unknown regarding IBS. In this issue of *Gastroenterology Clinics of North America*, key opinion leaders will curate, summarize, and put into clinical perspective the most important recent evidence on the epidemiology, pathogenesis, diagnosis, and treatment of IBS. I am eternally grateful to each of the authors for sharing their wisdom with the readers of this outstanding series of reviews. On behalf of this eminent group of experts, friends, and colleagues, I hope that this issue of *Gastroenterology Clinics of North America* shines a light on IBS which helps us to truly see our patients and creates a sense of purpose and optimism for a brighter future in the days to come.

William D. Chey, MD, FACG, AGAF, FACP, RFF
Digestive Health Integrated Care Program
GI Physiology Laboratory
Michigan Bowel Control Program
Michigan Medicine
3912 Taubman Center, SPC 5362
Ann Arbor, MI 48109-5362, USA

*E-mail address:*
wchey@med.umich.edu

Twitter: @umfoodoc (W.D. Chey)

**REFERENCES**

1. Barbara G, Feinle-Bisset C, Ghosal UC, et al. The intestinal microenvironment and functional gastrointestinal disorders. Gastroenterology 2016;150:1305–18.
2. Mearin F, Lacy B, Chang L, et al. Rome IV: the functional bowel disorders. Gastroenterology 2016;150:1393–407.
3. Ford AC, Moayyedi P, Chey WD, et al. American College of Gastroenterology monograph on the management of IBS. Am J Gastroenterol 2018;113:1–18.
4. Lacy BE, Pimentel M, Brenner DM, et al. ACG clinical guideline: management of irritable bowel syndrome. Am J Gastroenterol 2021;116(2):17–44.

# Dedication

This issue of *Gastroenterology Clinics of North America* is dedicated to my parents, Fan and William Y. Chey, who helped me to understand my priorities and potential as a person, physician, investigator, and mentor. I also dedicate the issue to my wife and best friend, Janine, and 3 children, Sam, Russell, and Josie, whose collective unconditional love and support make me whole, keep me grounded, and motivate me to make the most of every day.

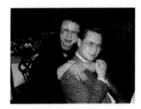

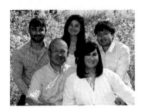

William D. Chey, MD, FACG, AGAF, FACP, RFF
Digestive Health Integrated Care Program
GI Physiology Laboratory
Michigan Bowel Control Program
Michigan Medicine
3912 Taubman Center, SPC 5362
Ann Arbor, MI 48109-5362, USA

*E-mail address:*
wchey@med.umich.edu

Twitter: @umfoodoc (W.D. Chey)

Gastroenterol Clin N Am 50 (2021) xvii
https://doi.org/10.1016/j.gtc.2021.04.008
0889-8553/21/© 2021 Published by Elsevier Inc.

gastro.theclinics.com

# Epidemiology and Burden of Irritable Bowel Syndrome

## An International Perspective

Ami D. Sperber, MD, MSPH

### KEYWORDS

- Irritable bowel syndrome • Disorders of gut-brain interaction • Epidemiology
- Prevalence • Diagnostic criteria • Research methodology • Rome criteria
- Rome Foundation Global Epidemiology Study

### KEY POINTS

- Irritable bowel syndrome (IBS) is the most recognized and researched of the disorders of gut-brain interaction.
- The determination of prevalence rates has real-life effects on the allocation of health care and research resources, drug development, and so on.
- Because of heterogeneous research methods, country, regional, and global prevalence rates for IBS remain elusive.
- The methodology of the Rome Foundation Global Epidemiology Study facilitated a more valid assessment of IBS Rome IV local, regional, and global prevalence rates.
- Prevalence rates by Rome IV are lower than Rome III, reflecting more restrictive diagnostic criteria.

## INTRODUCTION

The disorders of gut-brain interaction (DGBI) are related to any combination of motility disturbance, visceral hypersensitivity, altered mucosal and immune function, altered gut microbiota, and altered central nervous system processing.[1] Irritable bowel syndrome (IBS) is the most recognized and researched of the DGBI. In this article, available data on classical epidemiologic questions, such as the prevalence of IBS and its subtypes, and its distribution by age and sex are presented. However, beyond that, the author endeavors to present and discuss issues related to the validity and reliability of those data, including methodological pitfalls, comparing and/or pooling of data from different studies (**Fig. 1**), the effect of potential regional and cultural differences (diagnostic criteria, normal symptom frequency, symptom experience, interpretation, and reporting), and association with other factors. All these have real-life effects

Faculty of Health Sciences, Ben-Gurion University of the Negev, Beer-Sheva 84105, Israel
*E-mail address:* amiroie@me.com

Gastroenterol Clin N Am 50 (2021) 489–503
https://doi.org/10.1016/j.gtc.2021.04.001
0889-8553/21/© 2021 Elsevier Inc. All rights reserved.

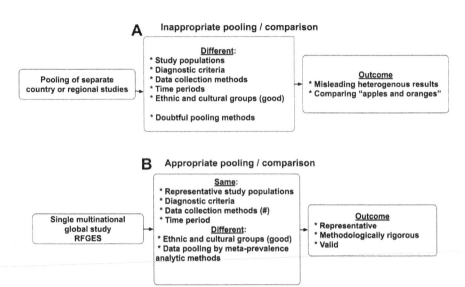

**Fig. 1.** Pitfalls in comparing and/or pooling the results of multiple epidemiologic prevalence studies for IBS: (*A*) individual studies; (*B*) multinational studies.

on the allocation of health care and research resources, drug development, and other matters addressed in later discussion.

There are many definitions and interpretations of the meaning of epidemiology.[2] The Centers for Disease Control and Prevention has defined epidemiology as the scientific, systematic, and data-driven study of the frequency and pattern (distribution) and causes and risk factors (determinants) of health-related conditions in specified populations.[3] In light of this broad range of substantive components, the results of epidemiologic studies can inform, provide guidance, and generate hypotheses for critical fields, including pathophysiology, prevention, and treatment of infectious and noninfectious diseases, including chronic disorders, such as the DGBI. **Box 1** shows the importance and potential benefits of prevalence studies, a central element of epidemiologic research.

## PREVALENCE RATES AND DIAGNOSTIC CRITERIA

Prevalence rates are based on diagnostic criteria, which are the basis for case definitions. Thus, when discussing the epidemiology of the DGBI, it is essential to start with

---

**Box 1**
**What can be gained from assessing prevalence rates of chronic diseases?**

1. Assess and understand the medical, social, and economic burden of disease

2. Enable comparisons across societies, cultures, and ethnic and racial subpopulations

3. Generate hypotheses for pathophysiologic research

4. Allocate health care resources

5. Allocate research funding

6. Determine priorities and provide incentives for the development of new treatment

7. Satisfy scientific and intellectual curiosity

diagnostic criteria, how they are determined, and what their strengths and weaknesses are. This issue is a complex and, often, controversial one. Because there are no diagnostic biomarkers for IBS, the diagnosis is based on symptom reporting and symptom clusters with a minimal diagnostic workup. The first iteration of the Rome Diagnostic criteria (Rome I) was published in 1994, and the last iteration of the Rome Diagnostic criteria (Rome IV) was published in 2016. Rome I was determined through a consensus of experts using the Delphi process with ensuing iterations, including an incrementally greater degree of evidence from dedicated research.[1]

A thorough review of the prevalence rates for IBS in various countries and regions of the world shows significant intracriteria and intercriteria variability, as seen in the results of a meta-regression analysis[4] and a systemic literature review,[5] both conducted before the publication of the Rome IV criteria in 2016. Both reviews found a very broad range of IBS prevalence rates among countries, with extremes ranging from 1.1% in Iran[6] using the Rome III criteria, to 45% in Pakistan[7] using Rome II[4] in 1 study[4] and 1.1% in both France[8] (Rome I) and in Iran[6] (Rome III), to 35.5% in Mexico[5] (Rome II) in the second study.[5]

## METHODOLOGICAL ISSUES

Possible explanations for these strikingly different results are shown in **Fig. 1** and **Box 2**. There is a tendency in the literature to compare the results of individual studies of significantly dissimilar methodology and determine pooled prevalence rates without making appropriate adjustments, resulting in misleading conclusions[5,9,10] (see **Fig. 1**). In light of these shortcomings, a Rome Foundation Working Team on Multinational, Cross-Cultural Research published recommendations for the conduct of this type of study[9] and initiated a global study of DGBI epidemiology (Rome Foundation Global Epidemiology Study [RFGES]), the results of which are discussed in detail here.[11]

IBS is characterized by chronic recurrent abdominal pain, and an irregular bowel habit (texture and frequency). The abdominal pain can improve or worsen with a bowel movement.[12] Symptom-based prevalence studies cannot entirely rule out organic/structural disease as the cause of the symptoms. For example, in the absence of upper endoscopy or anorectal manometry, some individuals diagnosed with a DGBI by survey questionnaire may actually have an organic cause of their symptoms. However, the rate of organic disease in patients who meet symptom-based criteria and have no alarm features is considered low. This issue was addressed in the RFGES whereby participants were asked, in addition to their symptoms, if they had been diagnosed in the past with any of a list of organic gastrointestinal (GI) diagnoses, such as celiac disease, GI cancer, inflammatory bowel disease, peptic ulcer, and so forth, or had undergone GI surgery, such as appendectomy, cholecystectomy, bowel resection, and so forth. The rate of any DGBI diagnosis was 40.3% of all participants. This rate was determined after 7.6% of the overall study population who met the diagnostic criteria for a DGBI was disqualified because they also reported a previous diagnosis of an organic GI disease or GI surgery.[11] Thus, the final prevalence rates did account for other GI diseases, to the degree possible in a questionnaire-based survey, making the final result conservative in comparison with other studies where this adjustment was not made.

### Types of Studies and Methods for Comparing and Pooling Study Results

Can a global prevalence rate for IBS be determined? The 2 reviews mentioned above (meta-analysis and systematic literature review) had slightly different inclusion criteria, but both included general population studies only. Although the inclusion criteria were

---

**Box 2**
**Why is it difficult to determine, compare, and pool prevalence rates?**

1. General issues:
   a. Cultural and geographic differences
   b. Normal frequency values for gastrointestinal symptoms
      i. Basis for frequency criteria for diagnoses
      ii. Discomfort/pain: separate or spectrum of same entity?
      iii. Bloating

2. Methodological issues:
   a. Representativeness of study population
      i. Geographic
      ii. Sex, age, other key variables
   b. Method of data collection
      i. Personal interview
      ii. Telephone
      iii. Mail
      iv. Internet survey
   c. Study population
      i. National representation
      ii. Local/regional representation
      iii. Specific sites: clinic, workplace, shift workers, race/ethnic groups, sex-specific
   d. Translation of study questionnaire into other languages
      i. Professional translators
      ii. Literal translation and cultural adaptation

3. Comparisons of study results
   a. Comparing individual studies: "apples and oranges"
      i. Within countries and regions
      ii. By diagnostic criteria
      iii. Population types
      iv. Data collection methods
   b. Pooling study results: *heterogeneity*
      i. Systematic literature searches
      ii. Meta-regression analyses

4. Protocol to reduce the impact of heterogeneous studies to a minimum
   a. Multinational study, if possible, global
   b. Same time period, methodology, research team, data handling, statistical analyses

---

different as well as the range of years of publication, the final number of publications and participants included in each study was similar at 81 papers and 260,960 participants in the meta-analysis,[4] and 83 papers and 288,103 participants in the systematic literature review,[5] giving greater confidence in the article selection process. In both studies, a pooled global prevalence rate was calculated with a result of 11.2% in the meta-analysis and 8.8% in the literature review. However, an analysis of heterogeneity in the systematic literature review showed that the percentage of residual variation owing to heterogeneity was 99.9%. Thus, the authors of that review concluded that the goal of calculating a global prevalence for IBS was still elusive. Another factor supporting this conclusion was the absence of sufficient data from some areas of the world, notably Africa, Eastern Europe, and Arab countries.

Four studies conducted in the past in Japan, all using the Rome II diagnostic criteria, reported IBS prevalence rates of (a) 6.1%,[13] (b) 10.7%,[14] (c) 14.2%,[15] and (d) 31%.[13] If the results of these 4 studies are compared or pooled, the following would be compared in a study of (a) a community sample, (b) university students, (c) a health screening sample that was close to the average Japanese population, and (d) outpatients in Department of Internal Medicine. Five studies from Mexico, using different diagnostic criteria, reported IBS rates of (a) 4%,[16] (b) 16%,[17] (c) 16.6%,[18] (d) 28.9%,[19] and (e) 35.5%.[20] These Mexican studies also had a great variance in the composition of their study populations. Thus, based on these studies from Japan and Mexico, one would be hard pressed to say what the "actual" prevalence of IBS was in these 2 countries.

To be clear, all types of studies are valid. For example, it is perfectly acceptable to determine IBS rates among university students or outpatients, and the results could be of interest and even generate hypotheses for more general research. However, these results should not be compared or pooled together because the studies are so different in methodology. Furthermore, they cannot be generalized to the overall population or compared with the results of other studies with different study populations, as is done too often.

## THE ROME FOUNDATION GLOBAL EPIDEMIOLOGY STUDY

The RFGES was conducted in the same time period using the same questionnaire and diagnostic criteria (Rome IV) in 33 countries on 6 continents. It was a very complex and challenging project requiring collaboration and support on an unprecedented scale. It took 10 years between the initial idea and establishment of its Executive Committee and the publication of its first paper in 2021 (**Fig. 2**).

The detailed study methodology can be found in the first study paper.[11] The major methodological obstacle was related to data collection methods. In 26 countries where most adults use the Internet, a secured online survey (accessible only to preselected invited participants with a predetermined age and sex distribution and national geographic representation) was conducted using population samples provided by a professional company (Qualtrics, LLC, Provo, UT, USA). There were 7 countries (Bangladesh, India, Indonesia, Iran, Ghana, Malaysia, Nigeria) where an Internet survey was not feasible, so the data were collected by personal household interviews. In 2 countries, China and Turkey, data were collected by both methods for purposes of comparison. Other than data collection, the methods were identical in Internet and

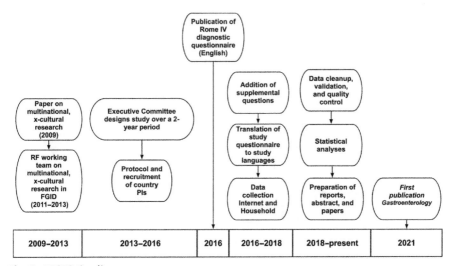

**Fig. 2.** RFGES timeline.

household interview countries. **Fig. 3** shows the global extent of the study and the rates of meeting Rome IV criteria for IBS (inner circle) and for any DGBI (outer circle). For convenience, the Internet survey countries will be referred to as "Internet" countries and the household interview countries will be referred to as "Household" countries in this article.

## PREVALENCE OF IRRITABLE BOWEL SYNDROME IN THE ROME FOUNDATION GLOBAL EPIDEMIOLOGY STUDY
### Irritable Bowel Syndrome Prevalence Rates: Rome IV

Overall, IBS prevalence rates using the Rome IV criteria were consistently lower than in previous studies using earlier iterations of the Rome criteria. This finding was the case for Internet surveys with a pooled prevalence rate in 26 countries of 4.1 (95% confidence interval [CI]: 3.9, 4.2) and in Household countries with a pooled prevalence rate in 9 countries of 1.5% (95% CI: 1.3, 1.7).

The prevalence rates of IBS among Internet survey countries ranged from a low of 1.3% (0.8%–1.8%) in Singapore to 7.6% (6.4%–8.7%) in Egypt (**Fig. 4**A). A striking finding relating to prevalence rates for IBS was the consistency of Rome IV IBS rates among the 26 Internet countries. Nineteen of 26 countries had prevalence rates between 3% and 5%. The outliers other than Singapore and Egypt were Japan (2.2%), China (2.3%), Russia (5.9%), South Africa (5.9%), and the United States (5.3%). Of the 26 countries, 24 countries had rates between 2% and 6% (see **Fig. 4**A).

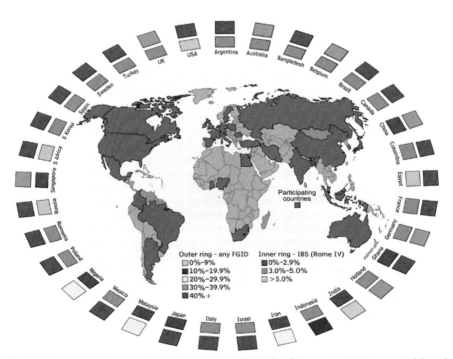

**Fig. 3.** The worldwide prevalence, by country (RFGES), of Rome IV IBS (*inner circle*) and meeting Rome IV diagnostic criteria for any DGBI (*outer circle*). FGID, functional gastrointestinal disorders. (*Courtesy of* the Rome Foundation, Raleigh, NC; with permission.)

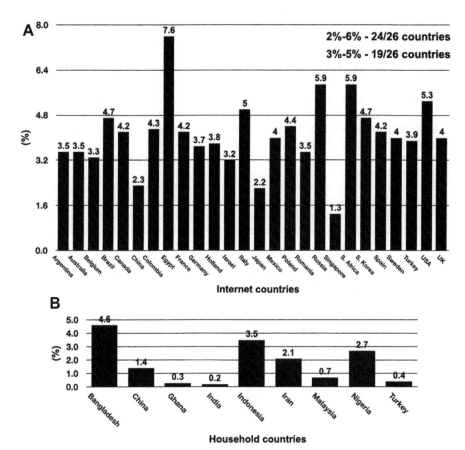

**Fig. 4.** Rome IV prevalence rates in 19 of 26 of the Internet countries; the prevalence rates ranged between 3% and 5% and in 24 of 26 countries between 2% and 6% with Singapore (1.3%) and Egypt (7.6) as outliers (*A*); in the 9 Household countries, 4 countries had prevalence rates less than 1% and only 2 countries were greater than 3% (*B*).

Prevalence rates were more variable in the Household countries with a lower overall range from 0.2% (0.1%–0.3%) [India] to 4.6% (3.7%–5.5%) (Bangladesh). Four of 9 countries had rates less than 1%, and only 2 countries had rates greater than 3% (**Fig. 4**B). The differing results between India and Bangladesh are of particular potential interest for further research because (a) these countries share a common border and similar cultures; and (b) in the case of India, the survey was conducted in 2 geographically separate regions, and the results were the same in both, thus leading further credence to the very low rate of IBS in that country.

### Why Were the Irritable Bowel Syndrome Prevalence Rates Lower in Household Countries Compared with Internet Countries?

The "default" explanation for the differences could be that the differences are real and reflect actual differences between different geographic regions and cultural groups. That hypothesis, based on the study results, could lead to important research into the reasons for these differences. It is possible, for example, that cultural factors lead to a difference in symptom experience, symptom interpretation, and symptom reporting, yielding lower results among some population groups, for example, East and West.[21,22] Other possible explanations include diet and nutrition, early life living conditions and hygiene, and previous GI infections, among others. All these potential factors were assessed in the RFGES.

However, there are other possible explanations related to methodological issues, especially differences between the 2 data collection methods. The Internet survey was anonymous, had full national representation for the study population, and incorporated multiple methods to preclude the risk of incomplete and/or inaccurate data. In contrast, the surveys in the Household countries were based on personal interviews in limited catchment areas. Thus, the survey was not anonymous, and the study population was not nationally representative.

Although the interviewers in the Household countries underwent prior training, including cultural sensitivity, it is reasonable to assume that fewer individuals would acknowledge and share sensitive personal information on GI symptoms, such as their bowel habit, leading to lower case identification and lower prevalence in the Household populations. To speculate further, this effect may be more salient among younger respondents, leading to the finding described in later discussion that prevalence rates in the younger age groups were lower than among the more elderly in the Household countries, whereas the opposite was the case in the anonymous Internet surveys.

### Irritable Bowel Syndrome Prevalence Rates by Sex and Age

In the 2 systematic reviews cited above, the prevalence of IBS was significantly higher in women compared with men,[4,5] showing this to be a global phenomenon. In the RFGES, the pooled prevalence rates for IBS were substantially higher among women in both survey methods, with a female-to-male odds ratio (OR) of 1.8 (1.7–2.0) for the Internet and 2.0 (1.5–2.5) for the Household countries.

Although almost all studies of IBS prevalence included rates by sex, there are much fewer data pieces on prevalence rates by age. In the meta-analysis by Lovell and Ford,[4] prevalence rates were lower with increasing age based on $\geq 50$ years compared with less than 50 years (OR: 0.75; 95% CI: 0.62, 0.92). In the RFGES, IBS prevalence decreased with age in the Internet surveys, from 5.3% (5.0%5.6%) in the 18- to 39-year-old age group to 3.7% (3.5%–4.0%) in the 40- to 64-year-old age group and 1.7% (1.4%–1.9%) in those 65+ years of age, whereas it increased with age in the Household countries from 1.4% (1.1%–1.7%) to 1.5% (1.2%–1.7%) to 1.9% (1.4%–2.4%), respectively, in these age groups.

### COMPARISON OF IRRITABLE BOWEL SYNDROME BY ROME III VERSUS ROME IV DIAGNOSTIC CRITERIA IN ROME FOUNDATION GLOBAL EPIDEMIOLOGY STUDY

The RFGES questionnaire included questions for diagnosis of IBS by the previous Rome III criteria. Because these questions were introduced into the questionnaire after data collection was completed in 12 Internet countries, the results on Rome III are available from 14 of the 26 Internet countries and all 9 Household countries. **Fig. 5** shows data on IBS prevalence by data collection method for both Rome III and Rome IV. The pooled rate by Rome III is higher by a magnitude greater than 2 compared with Rome IV in the entire study population and in both sexes. The prevalence rates were consistently higher among women than men for both diagnostic criteria. Prevalence rates were also higher among women for the 3 age categories (18–39, 40–64, 65+). As was seen in the results for Rome IV, in Rome III, there was a difference in prevalence trends by age with the prevalence decreasing by age in the Internet countries and increasing by age in the Household countries.

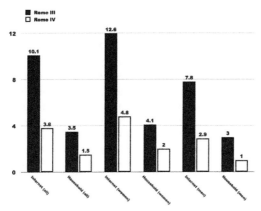

**Fig. 5.** Comparison of pooled prevalence rates between Rome III and Rome IV by data collection type (for 14 Internet countries and 9 Household countries) for total study population and by sex.

In a validation study of the Rome IV questionnaire before its official publication conducted in the United States, United Kingdom, and Canada, the results were very similar with mean Rome III IBS prevalence of 9.0% compared with a mean Rome IV IBS prevalence of 4.6%.[23,24]

### Why Are There Such Large Differences in Irritable Bowel Syndrome Prevalence Between Rome III and Rome IV?

The changes in the Rome IV criteria made them more restrictive, thus leaving out some of the individuals who were diagnosed with IBS by Rome III.[25,26] This finding relates to 2 major changes and 1 more minor change: (a) the removal of the term "discomfort," leaving only "pain" from the question in Rome IV, whereas the Rome III formulation was "pain or discomfort"; (b) the change of symptom frequency for pain (or discomfort) from at least 2 to 3 times monthly (Rome III) to at least weekly (Rome IV); and (c) a change that was less significant in terms of the difference in prevalence rates was the change in the association between pain and bowel habit. In the Rome III criteria, pain had to improve following a bowel movement, whereas in Rome IV, this was changed to either an improvement or a worsening of pain.

Although the prevalence rates for IBS are much lower for Rome IV, the severity of disease is higher in individuals diagnosed with IBS by Rome IV compared with those identified by Rome III, with mean IBS-SSS severity scores of 250 (244–256) and 191 (187–194), respectively, in the 14 Internet countries and 174 (158–190) and 134 (124–144), respectively, in the 9 Household countries. Thus, the Rome IV IBS criteria select out a more restricted group of individuals with more severe symptoms.[27] This selection of more restricted group could have advantages for clinical trials in that the study groups would be more homogeneous but may not identify patients who clinicians would likely diagnose as IBS in clinical practice.

A study of Rome III patients in the Netherlands, using a proxy Rome IV definition, found that Rome IV patients represented a subset of Rome III patients with a more severe clinical disorder.[28] A study from Sweden with a similar methodological approach found that 85% of Rome III patients met the proxy criteria for Rome IV. This subgroup was characterized as female, with poorer quality of life, greater pain severity, bloating, somatization, fatigue, and rectal sensitivity compared with Rome IV–negative individuals.[29]

### Why Was the Term Discomfort Removed from the Diagnostic Criteria?

The case against use of the term discomfort was influenced by the results of a study conducted in the United States by Spiegel and colleagues[30] designed to develop a framework to measure patient symptoms and inform patient-reported outcomes for clinical trials. The investigators concluded that discomfort was a nondiscriminative term that includes symptoms, such as bloating, gas, fullness, flatulence, sensation of incomplete evacuation, and urgency, for which there was a great degree of variance in interpretation and reporting. The participants in this study were all from the United States. It would be reasonable to ask whether similar results would have been obtained had the same study been conducted in Asia, Latin America, Africa, the Middle East, or Europe? It is known that culture and ethnicity affect the way symptoms are interpreted and reported[21,22] and that there are obstacles to translating symptoms in both linguistic and culturally adaptive manners. All the Rome diagnostic questionnaires, as well as almost all other questionnaires on DGBI, were developed in English, primarily in the United States but also in the United Kingdom.[23,31] This finding speaks to the possibility of unintentional ethnocentrism[32] that could make it difficult to compare results in different geographic regions and cultural groups. Compounding these potential confounders is the risk that the questionnaire is translated literally into other languages, in some cases, without cultural adaption and/or cognitive debriefing of representatives of the local population.[33–35]

### Why Was Symptom Frequency for Pain Changed to at Least Weekly Instead of at Least 2 to 3 Times per Week?

This change was based on a survey of a nationally representative sample of US adults to generate data and set thresholds for normal and abnormal symptom frequency based on the participants' responses to questions, such as, "How often did you have discomfort or pain anywhere in your abdomen," with 9 response options between "never" and "greater than 1 time per day."[23] The results of this survey informed the decision as to the threshold for pain for Rome IV IBS. Because this survey was conducted only on US adults, there is a potential problem when extrapolating this result to other countries around the world.

### Which Change, Pain Frequency, Elimination of the Term Discomfort, or the Change in Association of Pain with Bowel Movement Contributed More to the Difference Between Rome III and Rome IV Prevalence Rates?

In a study on the prevalence of functional bowel disorders in 3 English-speaking countries (Canada, United States, United Kingdom),[24] the investigators assessed the relative size effect of the 3 changes on the difference in prevalence rates for IBS by Rome III (9.0%) and Rome IV (4.6%). The relative effect was 80.7% for the change in pain frequency, 16.8% for the removal of the word "discomfort," and 2.5% for the change in association between bowel movements and pain. Thus, the change in pain threshold was by far and away the most important change in the Rome criteria. As such, it will be very important moving forward to determine if this change reflects a global phenomenon in symptom reporting or is more specific for the United States and perhaps other English-speaking countries, such as Canada and the United Kingdom.

### What Else Can Be Learned by Mining the Rome Foundation Global Epidemiology Study Database?

The RFGES database includes close to 90 diagnostic questions to determine all Rome IV DGBI diagnoses. The inclusion of all Rome IV diagnoses is unusual because, to date, few studies, if any, assessed all DGBI; most assessed the major diagnoses, such as IBS, function dyspepsia, functional constipation, and so forth. In addition to facilitating the identification of each and every DGBI individually, it also enabled the determination of 2 other important outcomes: (a) the percentage of individuals with any DGBI diagnosis, which was very high at 40.3% in the RFGES; and (b) the degree of overlap among the DGBI in any individual and the associations between degree of overlap with disease severity, quality of life, and associated risk factors beyond sex and age.

The questionnaire also included close to 90 questions related to multiple variables potentially associated with the prevalence of DGBI and their severity. These details included additional sociodemographic items, questions on living conditions and hygiene at the present time and in childhood (age 7), doctor consultations in general and for bowel problems, medications and abdominal surgeries, known diagnoses of "organic" GI diseases, use of complementary and alternative medical services, history of GI infection and relation to present bowel symptoms, effect of stress on symptoms, degree of concern and embarrassment over bowel function, diet, and embedded questionnaires on quality of life (PROMIS Global-10), somatization, anxiety and depression (Personal Health Questionnaire 4 and 12), IBS severity (IBS-SSS), and so forth. Thus, the database contains a rich source of data for comprehensive future research on DGBI.

### The Example of Postinfection Irritable Bowel Syndrome

The development of IBS following an acute enteric infection in individuals who did not suffer from prior IBS (postinfection irritable bowel syndrome [PI-IBS]) has become a focus of epidemiologic and pathophysiologic research because it is prevalent at about 10% of IBS cases and reflects one of the strongest and most recognizable risk factors for IBS.[36,37] Although there are culture-confirmed pathogens, including bacteria, viruses, and protozoa in some cases, many cases follow an undiagnosed enteric infection and are based on a clear patient history. In PI-IBS cases, where there is culture confirmation, the pathogen is equally likely to be bacterial or viral.[38] Risk factors have been identified for the development of PI-IBS, including female sex, antibiotic treatment of the infection, anxiety, and severity and duration of the initial infection.[39] The RFGES database provides a rich array of associated factors that can be mined to further understand and characterize PI-IBS.

### Where to Go from Here? Future Directions

The Rome Foundation has started the 5-year process of upgrading its diagnostic criteria, which will culminate in publication of the new Rome V diagnostic criteria, expected in 2026. Based on the results of research that have accumulated over the years, this iteration of the Rome diagnostic criteria will be less "eminence based" and more "evidence based."

One important challenge is to gain a firmer global and cross-cultural basis for changes that will be considered from Rome IV to Rome V. Thus, the previous change in pain threshold was based on a study of symptom frequency of GI symptoms in a nationally representative population in the United States. However, it is not clear that these changes are generalizable to other countries and cultural groups, in particular, in Asia, Africa, Latin America, Eastern Europe, and the Middle East. In advance of the finalization of the Rome V criteria, it is essential that parallel symptom frequency norm studies be conducted in at least 5 other geographic regions and cultural groups other than the United States, and that is the plan. The conduct of parallel studies lead to uniform findings confirming that symptom frequency patterns are similar throughout the world and increase confidence in the results of prevalence studies. In contrast, it may turn out that normal and abnormal symptom frequencies are different between, for example, China and the United States. In that case, adjustments would have to be made to "equalize" the diagnostic criteria because it is theoretically possible that at least once a week is the threshold for abnormal symptom presentation in the United States, but a lower or higher threshold would hold for China. Although this process could obviously complicate the conduct of epidemiologic studies on a global level, it would lend credence to comparisons of rates between countries, regions and country groups, because individuals in different populations have different cultural-based interpreting and reporting their symptoms.[21] Another potential obstacle is the translation of the diagnostic questionnaire. This translation of the diagnostic questionnaire must be done with linguistic accuracy, but also with appropriate cultural adaptation. For example, in Brazil and among Israeli Arabs, individuals in different regions and ethnic groups use different terms to describe concepts, such as stool or bowel movement.[40] Another illustration of this issue is the concept of bloating. This term has no equivalent in multiple languages, including Spanish, Italian, Farsi, and others. The most commonly used solution has been a work-around using multiple words to convey the same meaning. These issues will have to be addressed, perhaps by the use of pictograms in order to ensure that individuals in different countries understand the question in the same way.[41,42]

The study of the epidemiology of IBS and the other DGBI goes well beyond dry statistics. It is challenging and complex and can provide vital information. The most important factor is the implementation of well-planned studies using rigorous research methodology and global collaboration. The new age of communication has made achievement of these goals eminently feasible. The outcomes of future studies will inform and facilitate a broad spectrum of endeavors, including clinical practice, basic and clinical research, and the conduct of clinical trials.

## CLINICS CARE POINTS

- The epidemiology of irritable bowel syndrome, especially prevalence rates, has practical importance in clinical practice beyond intellectual curiosity.
- Diagnostic criteria, based on epidemiologic studies, can guide identification of cases and definitions of symptom severity.
- Evidence-based diagnostic criteria can guide the diagnostic process in disorders of gut-brain interaction by enabling a positive diagnosis using a minimum number of diagnostic tests.
- Although diagnostic criteria should be applied strictly in clinical trials and other research, they can be adapted with a flexible approach by clinicians who can add their own clinical experience and intuition in the final diagnostic determination.
- Prevalence rates are also important to clinical practice in that they inform and guide decisions on the development of new treatment modalities.

## DISCLOSURE

There are no conflicts of interest.

## REFERENCES

1. Drossman DA. Functional gastrointestinal disorder and the Rome IV process. In: Drossman DA, Chang L, Chey WD, et al, editors. Functional gastrointestinal

disorders. Disorders of brain-gut interaction, vol. 1, 4th edition. Raleigh (NC): Rome Foundation; 2016. p. 1–32.

2. Frerot M, Lefebvre A, Aho S, et al. What is epidemiology? Changing definitions of epidemiology 1978-2017. PLoS One 2018;13:e0208442.

3. Deputy Director for Public Health Science and Surveillance CfS, Epidemiology, and Laboratory Services, Division of Scientific Education and Professional Development, Principles of epidemiology in public health practice. An introduction to applied epidemiology and biostatistics. Centers for Disease Control and Prevention; 2012. Available at: https://www.cdc.gov/csels/dsepd/ss1978/lesson1/section1.html. Accessed December 9, 2020.

4. Lovell RM, Ford AC. Global prevalence of and risk factors for irritable bowel syndrome: a meta-analysis. Clin Gastroenterol Hepatol 2012;10:712–21.

5. Sperber AD, Dumitrascu D, Fukudo S, et al. The global prevalence of IBS in adults remains elusive due to the heterogeneity of studies: a Rome Foundation working team literature review. Gut 2016;66:1065–72.

6. Khoshkrood-Mansoori B, Pourhoseingholi MA, Safaee A, et al. Irritable bowel syndrome: a population based study. J Gastrointestin Liver Dis 2009;18:413–8.

7. Jafri W, Yakoob J, Jafri N, et al. Irritable bowel syndrome and health seeking behaviour in different communities of Pakistan. J Pak Med Assoc 2007;57:285–7.

8. Bommelaer G, Dorval E, Denis P, et al. Prevalence of irritable bowel syndrome in the French population according to the Rome I criteria. Gastroenterol Clin Biol 2002;26:1118–23.

9. Sperber AD, Gwee K-A, Hungin AP, et al. Conducting multinational, cross-cultural research in the functional gastrointestinal disorders: issues and recommendations. A Rome Foundation working team report. Aliment Pharmacol Ther 2014; 40:1094–102.

10. Sperber AD. The challenge of cross-cultural, multi-national research: potential benefits in the functional gastrointestinal disorders. Neurogastroenterol Motil 2009;21:351–60.

11. Sperber AD, Bangdiwala SI, Drossman DA, et al. Worldwide prevalence and burden of functional gastrointestinal disorders, results of Rome Foundation global study. Gastroenterology 2021;160:99–114.

12. Mearin F, Lacy BE, Chang L, et al. Bowel disorders. Gastroenterology 2016;150: 1393–407.e1395.

13. Shinozaki M, Fukudo S, Hongo M, et al. High prevalence of irritable bowel syndrome in medical outpatients in Japan. J Clin Gastroenterol 2008;42:1010–6.

14. Shiotani A, Miyanishi T, Takahashi T. Sex differences in irritable bowel syndrome in Japanese university students. J Gastroenterol 2006;41:562–8.

15. Kanazawa M, Endo Y, Whitehead WE, et al. Patients and nonconsulters with irritable bowel syndrome reporting a parental history of bowel problems have more impaired psychological distress. Dig Dis Sci 2004;49:1046–53.

16. Schmulson M, Lopez-Colombo A, Mendoza-Gomez A, et al. The Rome III Adult Questionnaire in Spanish-Mexico has a low sensitivity for identifying IBS and higher sensitivity for uninvestigated dyspepsia. Gastroenterology 2012; 143(Suppl. 1):S829.

17. Lopez-Colombo A, Morgan D, Bravo-Gonzalez D, et al. The epidemiology of functional gastrointestinal disorders in Mexico: a population-based study. Gastroenterol Res Pract 2012;2012:606174.

18. Valerio-Ureña J, Vásquez-Fernández F, Jiménez-Pineda A, et al. Prevalencia del síndrome de intestino irritable en población abierta de la ciudad de Veracruz, México. Rev Gastroenterol Mex 2010;75:36–41.

19. Schmulson M, Adeyemo M, Gutierrez-Reyes G, et al. Differences in gastrointestinal symptoms according to gender in Rome II positive IBS and dyspepsia in a Latin American population. Am J Gastroenterol 2010;105:925–32.

20. Schmulson M, Ortiz O, Santiago-Lomeli M, et al. Frequency of functional bowel disorders among healthy volunteers in Mexico City. Dig Dis 2006;24:342–7.

21. Sperber AD, Francisconi C, Fang X, et al. Multicultural aspects of functional gastrointestinal disorders. In: Drossman DA, Chang L, Chey WD, et al, editors. Rome IV functional gastrointestinal disorders – disorders of gut-brain interaction. 4th edition. Raleigh, NC, USA: Rome Foundation; 2016. p. 373–442.

22. Chuah KH, Mahadeva S. Cultural factors influencing functional gastrointestinal disorders in the east. J Neurogastroenterol Motil 2018;24:536–43.

23. Palsson OS, Whitehead WE, van Tilburg MAL, et al. Development and validation of the Rome IV diagnostic questionnaire for adults. Gastroenterology 2016;150: 1481–91.

24. Palsson OS, Whitehead W, Törnblom H, et al. Prevalence of Rome IV functional bowel disorders among adults in the United States, Canada, and the United Kingdom. Gastroenterol 2020;158:1262–73.

25. Longstreth GF, Thompson WG, Chey WD, et al. Functional bowel disorders. In: Drossman SA, Corazziari E, Delvaux M, et al, editors. Rome III. The functional gastrointestinal disorders. McLean, Virginia: Degnon Associates, Inc; 2006. p. 487–555.

26. Mearin F, Lacy BE, Chang L, et al. Bowel disorders. In: Drossman DA, Chang L, Chey WD, et al, editors. Rome IV functional gastrointestinal disorders – disorders of gut-brain interaction. 4th edition. Raleigh NC USA: Rome Foundation; 2016. p. 967–1057.

27. Drossman DA, Chang L, Bellamy N, et al. Severity in irritable bowel syndrome: a Rome Foundation Working Team report. Am J Gastroenterol 2011;106:1749–59.

28. Vork L, Weerts Z, Mujagic Z, et al. Rome III vs Rome IV criteria for irritable bowel syndrome: a comparison of clinical characteristics in a large cohort study. Neurogastroenterol Motil 2018;30.

29. Aziz I, Tornblom H, Palsson OS, et al. How the change in IBS criteria from Rome III to Rome IV impacts on clinical characteristics and key pathophysiological factors. Am J Gastroenterol 2018;113:1017–25.

30. Spiegel BM, Bolus R, Agarwal N, et al. Measuring symptoms in the irritable bowel syndrome: development of a framework for clinical trials. Aliment Pharmacol Ther 2010;32(10):1275–91.

31. Francis CY, Morris J, Whorwell PJ. The irritable bowel severity scoring system: a simple method of monitoring irritable bowel syndrome and its progress. Aliment Pharmacol Ther 1997;11:395–402.

32. Omohundro JT. Thinking like an anthropologist: a practical introduction to cultural anthropology. New York: McGraw Hill; 2008.

33. Kanazawa M, Drossman DA, Shinozaki M, et al. Translation and validation of a Japanese version of the irritable bowel syndrome-quality of life measure (IBS-QOL-J). Biopsychosoc Med 2007;1:6.

34. Sperber AD. Translation and validation of study instruments for cross-cultural research. Gastroenterology 2004;126:S124–8.

35. Conway K, Acquadro C, Patrick DL. Usefulness of translatability assessment: results from a retrospective study. Qual Life Res 2014;23:1199–210.

36. Barbara G, Grover M, Bercik P, et al. Rome Foundation working team report on post-infection irritable bowel syndrome. Gastroenterology 2019;156:46–58 e47.

37. Card T, Enck P, Barbara G, et al. Post-infectious IBS: defining its clinical features and prognosis using an internet-based survey. United Eur Gastroenterol J 2018; 6:1245–53.
38. Donnachie E, Schneider A, Mehring M, et al. Incidence of irritable bowel syndrome and chronic fatigue following GI infection: a population-level study using routinely collected claims data. Gut 2018;67:1078–86.
39. Klem F, Wadhwa A, Prokop LJ, et al. Prevalence, risk factors, and outcomes of irritable bowel syndrome after infectious enteritis: a systematic review and meta-analysis. Gastroenterology 2017;152:1042–1054 e1041.
40. Sperber AD, Friger M, Shvartzman P, et al. Rates of functional bowel disorders among Israeli Bedouins in rural areas compared with those who moved to permanent towns. Clin Gastroenterol Hepatol 2005;3:342–8.
41. Tack J, Carbone F, Holvoet L, et al. The use of pictograms improves symptom evaluation by patients with functional dyspepsia. Aliment Pharmacol Ther 2014; 40:523–30.
42. Carruthers HR, Miller V, Morris J, et al. Using art to help understand the imagery of irritable bowel syndrome and its response to hypnotherapy. Int J Clin Exp Hypn 2009;57:162–73.

# Latest Insights on the Pathogenesis of Irritable Bowel Syndrome

Elizabeth J. Videlock, MD, PhD, Lin Chang, MD*

## KEYWORDS

- Irritable bowel syndrome • IBS • Pathogenesis • Stress • Genetics
- Visceral hypersensitivity

## KEY POINTS

- Irritable bowel syndrome is considered a disorder of gut–brain interaction classified by gastrointestinal symptoms related to any combination of motility disturbance, visceral hypersensitivity, altered mucosal and immune function, altered gut microbiota, and altered central nervous system processing.
- Symptoms of irritable bowel syndrome result from dysregulation of gut–brain interactions, which manifests as enhanced visceral perception and altered bowel habits.
- Factors that increase the risk of developing irritable bowel syndrome include genetic and environmental factors and infection. Common triggers include food and stress.
- Patients with irritable bowel syndrome have enhanced visceral perception owing to peripheral and/or central sensitization.
- Peripheral pathophysiologic mechanisms in irritable bowel syndrome include alterations in neuronal function, luminal and tissue mediators, immune response, intestinal permeability, bile acid processing, serotonin signaling, and gut microbiota.

## INTRODUCTION

The pathogenesis of irritable bowel syndrome (IBS) is complex, and, although it has evolved over the years (**Fig. 1**), it is still not well-understood. A unifying theme is that the symptoms of IBS result from bidirectional dysregulation of brain–gut interactions, which manifests as enhanced visceral perception and altered bowel habits. Growing scientific evidence has led experts to redefine IBS and other functional gastrointestinal (GI) disorders to disorders of gut–brain interaction, which are classified by GI symptoms related to any combination of the following: motility disturbance, visceral hypersensitivity, altered mucosal and immune function, altered gut microbiota, and altered central nervous system processing.[1] There are factors that increase

Vatche and Tamar Manoukian Division of Digestive Diseases, David Geffen School of Medicine at UCLA, Los Angeles, CA, USA
* Corresponding author.
E-mail address: linchang@mednet.ucla.edu

Gastroenterol Clin N Am 50 (2021) 505–522
https://doi.org/10.1016/j.gtc.2021.04.002
0889-8553/21/© 2021 Elsevier Inc. All rights reserved.

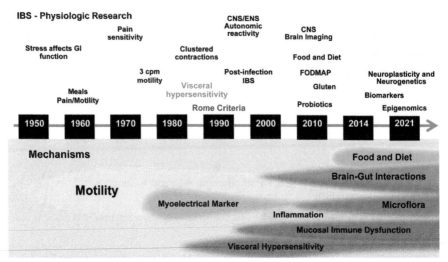

**Fig. 1.** History of physiologic research in IBS and FGIDs. This timeline shows some of the key research studies on the top and the domains of research on the bottom. From 1950 up until 1990, research was primarily focused on motility; however, after 1990 there began new research in the areas of visceral hypersensitivity, brain–gut interactions, immune activation, the microbiota and food and diet. It was the Rome classification system and criteria that allowed for identification of patients with disorders of gut–brain interaction for research in these other domains. CNS, central nervous system; ENS, enteric nervous system. (*Data from* Drossman DA, Chang L, Chey WD, et al. Rome IV Functional Gastrointestinal Disorders – Disorders of Gut-Brain Interaction. 4 ed. Raleigh, NC: Rome Foundation; 2016).

the risk of developing IBS that include genetic predisposition, environmental factors (eg, early adverse life events), and infectious gastroenteritis. Other factors trigger symptoms once IBS manifests and these include food and stress (**Fig. 2**). Thus, IBS may represent a combination of factors involving different pathophysiologic mechanisms. Given the complex pathophysiology of IBS, there is currently no single biomarker that can represent the different pathophysiological mechanisms of IBS.

## FACTORS THAT INCREASE THE RISK OF IRRITABLE BOWEL SYNDROME
### Familial and Genetic Factors

Studies have demonstrated that IBS clusters in families.[2] A case-control study studied 477 patients with IBS and 1492 of their first-degree relatives and 297 controls and 936 of their first-degree relatives. There was a higher proportion of IBS relatives with IBS compared with control relatives (50% vs 27%; odds ratio, 2.75; 95% confidence interval, 2.01–3.76).[3] Another large study used the Swedish Multigeneration Register, which included 60,489 sibling pairs and found an odds ratio of 1.75 (95% confidence interval, 1.63–1.89) for IBS in full siblings.[4]

Most, but not all, twin studies suggest a heritability of IBS,[2] although there also seems to be a strong environmental influence. For example, 1 twin study found that the concordance of having IBS was higher among monozygotic twins than dizygotic twins, but showed that the presence of IBS in the mother was also a strong predictor of having IBS.[5] The role of environmental influences on IBS is further supported by the Swedish Multigeneration Register study, which found that the odds ratio for spouses having IBS was 1.51 (95% confidence interval, 1.24–1.84).[4] These findings suggest

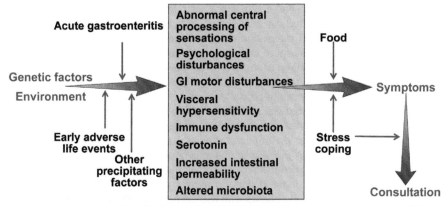

**Fig. 2.** Proposed pathophysiologic model of IBS. There are factors that increase risk of developing IBS, which include genetic factors and environmental factors such as early adverse life events, for example, abuse and infection. The alterations in brain–gut interactions result in multiple central and peripheral mediated pathophysiologic mechanisms (shown in the *blue box*). Once the symptoms of IBS occur, there can be triggers that increase symptom severity, such as food and stressors. The symptom burden and coping behaviors will influence health care seeking. (*Data from* Drossman DA, Chang L, Chey WD, et al. Rome IV Functional Gastrointestinal Disorders – Disorders of Gut-Brain Interaction. 4 ed. Raleigh, NC: Rome Foundation; 2016).

that environmental factors, including learned behavior, can contribute to the development of IBS symptoms.

In addition to familial clustering and twin studies in IBS,[4,6] genetic association studies support that there is a genetic predisposition to developing IBS. The first large genome-wide association study in IBS consisted of 534 patients with IBS and 4932 controls without recurrent abdominal problems.[7] No single nucleotide polymorphisms (SNPs) met the significance threshold for genome-wide association ($P < 5 \times 10^{-8}$). However, there were 14 genes with a $P$ value of less than $10^{-4}$ that selected for validation in several population-based case-control cohorts (n = 3511). One locus (7p22.1) was found to be significant and includes the genes KDEL endoplasmic reticulum protein retention receptor 2 (*KDELR2*) and glutamate receptor, ionotropic, delta 2 (*Grid2*) interacting protein (*GRID2IP*).[7]

A subsequent, larger genome-wide association study used a population-based cohort in the United Kingdom that included 9576 cases with self-reported IBS and 336,499 controls.[8] One locus, rs10512344 on chromosome 9q31.2, was significantly different in IBS and controls. This finding was also replicated in a multinational cohort of patients with 2045 and 7955 controls. Interestingly, the 9q31.2 SNP was entirely accounted for by the female group and had strongest genetic risk effects in age at menarche. Age at menarche is thought to be an indicator of possible health complications and disease in later life. This study also found that IBS risk genes were enriched for intracellular calcium activated chloride channel activity, ion-gated channel activity, and anion channel activity, and for targets of the miR-15 family of microRNAs.[8]

Other genetic studies found that 2% to 3% of patients with IBS have rare functional variants of the voltage-gated channel $Na_v1.5$ (*SCN5A*), causing a channelopathy or the sucrose isomaltase (*SI*) gene causing carbohydrate malabsorption.[9,10]

There are multiple studies that have evaluated the association of the serotonin (5-HT) transporter gene, known as 5-HTTLPR, with IBS. Although high-quality studies and a meta-analysis failed to find a significant association of 5-HTTLPR with IBS,[11,12] several other studies did find an association.[13,14] In one study, a higher colonic mucosal expression of SERT messenger RNA and protein was seen for the L/L geno-type of this SNP, which was more common in constipation-predominant IBS (IBS-C).[13] Other SNPs that have been associated with IBS are found in the genes for corti-cotropin releasing factor receptor 1 (CRF-1R),[15] catechol-O-methyltransferase (COMT), interleukins, and tumor necrosis factor-$\alpha$.[6,14]

In addition to genetic risk factors, researchers have identified alterations in a variety of epigenetic factors in IBS that were recently reviewed (Fig. 3).[16] Epigenetics refers to modifications in gene expression that can change the phenotype without changing the genetic sequence (genotype). Epigenetic changes described in IBS include alterations in gene methylation[17] and expression of noncoding microRNAs.[16,18] These epigenetic changes may be owing, at least in part, to early adverse life events, for example, abuse, which are increased in patients with IBS compared with healthy controls (dis-cussed elsewhere in this article).[19,20] Animal[21] and human[22,23] studies have demon-strated that early adverse life events are associated with epigenetic modifications, which can result in long-term effects. Future studies are needed to validate some of these genetic and epigenetic findings and to determine their functional relevance in IBS.

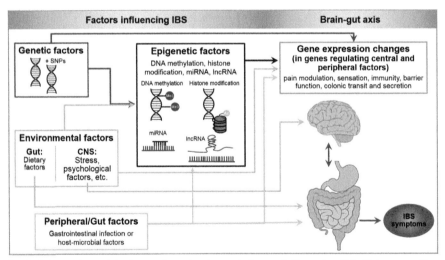

Fig. 3. Schematic model of genetic and epigenetic factors influencing IBS. *Pink arrows* illus-trate that genetic factors including single genetic polymorphisms (SNPs) can influence the gene expression either directly or mediated by epigenetic factors including DNA methyl-ation, histone modifications, microRNA (miRNA) and long noncoding RNA (lncRNA) expres-sion (*purple arrow*). Environmental factors including stress and psychological factors at the central nervous system (CNS) level and dietary factors at the GI level can induce changes in gene expression mediated by epigenetic or nongenetic/epigenetic factors, and can have a direct influence on CNS and gut function (*blue arrows*). Peripheral or gut factors including GI infection or other host or microbial factors, can potentially modify the function of genes mediated by epigenetic or nonepigenetic factors, and influence the CNS and gut function (*green arrows*) such as, pain modulation, sensation, immunity, barrier function, colonic transit and secretion to manifest the symptoms of IBS (*orange-red arrow*). (*From* Mahurkar-Joshi S, Chang L. Epigenetic Mechanisms in Irritable Bowel Syndrome. Front Psy-chiatry. 2020 Aug 14;11:805. doi: 10.3389/fpsyt.2020.00805).

## Prior Gastrointestinal Infection

Postinfection IBS (PI-IBS) is the new onset of IBS symptoms after the resolution of an acute infectious gastroenteritis. Acute gastroenteritis is characterized by 2 or more of the following symptoms: fever, vomiting, diarrhea, or a positive bacterial stool culture.[24] GI infection is the strongest risk factor for IBS and increases the risk of IBS at 12 months by about 4-fold.[25] Individuals who are particularly at risk for PI-IBS are those with a history of gastroesophageal reflux disease or dyspepsia, more severe diarrheal illness, younger age, female sex, anxiety or depression, or chronic stressful life events at the time of the infection.[24] The bowel habit subtypes most often seen in PI-IBS are diarrhea or mixed bowel habit.[24] With regard to type of pathogen causing PI-IBS, pooled incidence rates were: bacterial, 13.8%, protozoal/parasitic, 41.9%, and viral, 6.4%.[25] The highest incidence of PI-IBS was 35% to 45%, which occurred with a drinking water outbreak with both *Campylobacter jejuni* and *Escherichia coli* O157: H7.[26]

## Stressful Life Events

Studies have demonstrated an association between current stressful life events in childhood and/or adulthood and IBS.[19,20] The association of stress and IBS is further supported by the finding that stressful life events increased the risk of developing PI-IBS.[27] Patients with IBS have a higher prevalence of early adverse life events during childhood that include physical, sexual, or emotional abuse; severe illness or death of a parent; an incarcerated individual in the household; perinatal gastric suctioning; and exposure to wartime conditions.[28–32]

In a recently published study, we found that stressful life events experienced in adulthood is also associated with IBS.[20,33] Patients with IBS perceive life events as more negative than healthy controls. The presence of adulthood life events that are perceived more negatively was associated with worse IBS symptom severity and poorer IBS-related quality of life. Negatively perceived adulthood life events were also associated with a dysregulated stress response to hormone challenge in patients with IBS compared with controls.

Deployment during wartime is a significant stressor associated with IBS. IBS has been recognized as a part of the "Gulf War Syndrome." In a study of US Navy Seabees, who are known to be among the most symptomatic Gulf War veterans, those who were deployed to the Persian Gulf were more than 3 times more likely to have IBS compared with Seabees deployed to other locations or not deployed.[34] Another study found that Persian Gulf veterans with chronic GI symptoms showed evidence of visceral and somatic hypersensitivity.[35] It would be helpful to know if these individuals developed new-onset symptoms after deployment or if their symptoms were present before deployment and were exacerbated by wartime stress.

It is important to understand the stressors that trigger the onset and exacerbations of IBS symptoms to help guide disease management, including the development of preventive strategies.

## PATHOPHYSIOLOGIC MECHANISMS OF IRRITABLE BOWEL SYNDROME
### Increased Visceral Perception

Gut sensation and function is influenced by activity of the gut lumen, mucosa and submucosa, enteric nervous system, and central nervous system, and the communication between these entities (**Fig. 4**). Stimuli within the gut, for example, mechanical or chemical stimuli, are detected by primary afferent nerves, which are extrinsic, intrinsic, or intestinofugal. Spinal afferent nerves project to the dorsal horn of the spinal cord

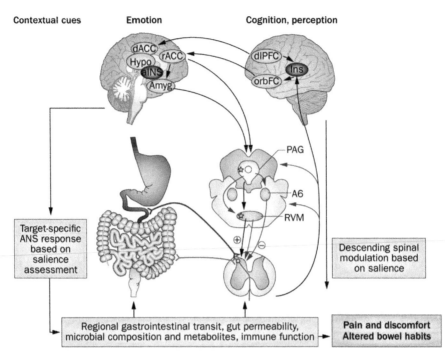

**Fig. 4.** Integrated bidirectional brain–gut model of IBS pathophysiology. This figure is a proposed model for involvement of the brain–gut axis in the generation of IBS symptoms (chronic abdominal pain associated with altered bowel habits). Under normal circumstances, visceral and external signals are evaluated by the salience network, which generates brain outputs in terms of targeted ANS responses (regulating GI and immune function) and descending pain modulatory activity (regulating pain sensitivity at the dorsal horn level). Target organ alterations (either peripherally or ANS stimulated) are signaled back to the brain via neural, endocrine or immune-related channels. These signals are processed within subregions of the INS, and depending on their subjective salience, are consciously perceived (associated with activation of anterior INS) as normal gut sensations, discomfort or pain. IBS symptoms can arise from several primary peripheral or central mechanisms. Amyg, amygdala; ANS, autonomic nervous system; dACC, dorsal anterior cingulate cortex; dlPFC, dorsolateral prefrontal cortex; Hypo, hypothalamus; INS, insula; orbFC, orbitofrontal cortex; PAG, periaqueductal gray; rACC, rostral anterior cingulate cortex; RVM, rostral ventromedial medulla. (*From* Mayer EA, Labus JS, Tillisch K, Cole SW, Baldi P. Toward a systems view of IBS. Nat Rev Gastroenterol Hepatol. 2015 Oct;12(10):592-605. doi: 10.1038/nrgastro.2015.121. Epub 2015 Aug 25).

with cells bodies located in the dorsal root ganglia. The sensory input ascends along the dorsal column and then to the contralateral ventroposterolateral nucleus of the thalamus and to various cortical regions. Brain networks, including the sensorimotor, salience, central autonomic, emotional arousal, and central executive networks, process and modulate visceral input.[36] Under normal circumstances, visceral signals are evaluated by the salience network and insula, which assesses the importance of these signals and whether they are perceived as normal gut sensations, discomfort, or pain. Brain outputs include autonomic nervous system responses, which regulate gut and immune function, and descending pain modulatory pathways, which regulate pain sensitivity at the dorsal horn level of the spinal cord.

Increased perception of visceral stimuli and IBS symptoms develops from either greater sensitivity of visceral afferent pathways (peripheral sensitization) or central amplification of visceral afferent input at the brain and spinal cord level (central sensitization).[36] Peripheral sensitization of sensory nerves occurs when nerves are activated by mediators released from immune cells and epithelial cells, or via alterations in second messenger systems or gene expression.[36] Increased visceral stimulation, for example, owing to injury or inflammation, can lead to increased central nervous system responsiveness, or central sensitization, which results in decreased sensory thresholds (ie, increased sensitivity).

Enhanced visceral perception as measured by increased perception of rectal or colonic balloon distension has been demonstrated in a significant subset of patients with IBS by multiple research centers.[37–39] Patients with IBS demonstrate decreased pressure thresholds to pain and discomfort and/or increased perceptual ratings and viscerosomatic referral areas to balloon distension in the intestine. The fact that enhanced visceral perception is not present in all patients with IBS and that sensory thresholds only modestly correlate with symptoms limits sensory thresholds to distension as a diagnostic and therapeutic biomarker.[37,38]

### Altered Central Nervous System Processing and Modulation

Brain imaging studies have demonstrated both structural and functional alterations in task-related brain networks in patients with IBS compared with healthy controls, with some of the findings correlating with IBS symptom severity.[36,40] In addition, studies suggest that emotional factors can influence visceral perception and contribute to the differences between patients with IBS and healthy controls.[41] A comprehensive review on the role of brain imaging in IBS and other disorders of gut–brain interaction summarized the alterations in the functional, structural, and anatomic networks in the resting state and in response to task related functions reported in these conditions. These networks include the default mode, emotional arousal, central autonomic control, central executive control, sensorimotor processing, and salience. Neuroimaging findings in patients with IBS include (1) greater cortical thickness and volume of sensorimotor cortex that correlates with symptom severity, particularly in women, (2) alterations in the functional connectivity of the anterior insula and amygdala, (3) greater engagement of the salience detection and emotional arousal networks in response to actual and expected rectal distension, (4) decreased corticolimbic inhibitory feedback, and (5) increased activation of the central autonomic network that regulates the autonomic nervous system response.[42] Alterations in these networks provide conceivable explanations for increased anticipatory anxiety and hyperattentiveness to GI sensations, catastrophizing behavior, autonomic hyperarousal, and expectancy of outcomes in IBS.[42]

### Gastrointestinal Transit and Motility

Multiple studies have reported alterations in small intestinal and colonic motility in patients with IBS. Findings in patients with IBS include increased motility in fasting states and in response to meals and cholecystokinin,[43] increased number of rapid contractions in response to balloon distention,[44] accelerated transit time in a subset of patients with diarrhea-predominant IBS (IBS-D),[45] and that changes in motility can be induced by psychological and physical stress.[46] Although transit differs between bowel habit subtypes, abnormal transit is more likely to be present in patients with IBS-D (accelerated in up to 48%), and less so in patients with IBS-C (delayed in 21%).[47]

### Peripheral Factors Involved in Irritable Bowel Syndrome Pathogenesis

The interplay of multiple luminal and peripheral factors can contribute to changes in GI function and ultimately symptoms of IBS (**Fig. 5**). In the gut, the network of multiple cells including epithelial, immune, neuronal, and microbiota comprise the "gut connectome," which communicates with the brain via neural, endocrine, and inflammatory pathways. The brain to gut communication is mainly mediated via the autonomic nervous system pathways to the gut.[42]

#### Nerve fibers

An increase in nerve fibers, for example, those expressing receptors for substance P and transient receptor potential vanilloid type 1 (TRPV1), cannabinoid receptors,[48] and protease-activated receptors[49] have been reported in patients with IBS compared with controls.[50] Further support of the significance of neuronal mechanisms in IBS is demonstrated by a study where colonic mucosal gene expression profiling was conducted in patients with IBS-C and IBS-D and healthy controls and compared with publicly available profiling data from additional cohorts.[51] Gene profiling and network analyses revealed pathways and genes related to neurally mediated pain in IBS, particularly IBS-C.

#### Luminal and tissue mediators

Several studies have demonstrated that luminal or tissue mediators can sensitize primary afferent nerves and contribute to increased visceral sensitivity in IBS.

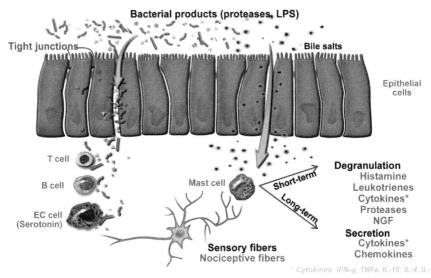

**Fig. 5.** Cross-talk at the mucosal border. Cellular and molecular factors involved in epithelial barrier alterations in patients with IBS. Mucosal immune cells including B cells, T cells, other local cells such as enteroendocrine (EC) cells and mast cells (MC) can release several soluble mediators that can alter tight junction (TJ) function, thus increasing paracellular permeability. In the lumen of the gut, bacterial products including serine and cysteine proteases and bile salts are also able to increase paracellular permeability. These epithelial barrier defects allow the perpetuation of a mucosal low-grade immune activation associated with the stimulation of afferent nerves fibers. (*Modified from* Piche T. Tight junctions and IBS–the link between epithelial permeability, low-grade inflammation, and symptom generation? Neurogastroenterol Motil. 2014 Mar;26(3):296-302. doi: 10.1111/nmo.12315. PMID: 24548256; with permission).

Supernatants from mucosal biopsies from patients with IBS increase the firing of afferent neurons in animal models[52,53] and submucosal neurons in human biopsies.[54] A class of mediators that is thought to increase neuronal activity is proteases, which are increased in IBS supernatants. Furthermore, protease inhibitors decrease the heightened visceral sensitivity that occurs from intracolonic administration of IBS biopsy supernatants in mice.[52] Histamine is another mediator that has been shown to increase excitation of TRPV1 neurons via the histamine 1 receptor.[55]

### Altered mucosal barrier function
Based on different methods of measuring intestinal permeability, there is evidence that a subset of patients with IBS (particularly PI-IBS and IBS-D) have increased intestinal permeability. There is decreased expression of tight junction proteins in the colon and jejunum of patients with IBS-D.[56] Increased permeability has been associated with greater abdominal pain severity and visceral hyperalgesia.[57,58] Alterations in mucosal barrier function seems to play a role in the interaction between stress, visceral hypersensitivity, and altered immune function and gut microbiota in IBS. Intestinal permeability has also become a target for emerging IBS treatments.

### Altered immune function
Increased immune activation is thought to play a role in the pathophysiology of IBS. This role is best demonstrated in PI-IBS, where increased numbers of T lymphocytes and levels of proinflammatory cytokine IL-1$\beta$ in the rectal mucosa were present compared with that in controls.[27,59] Interestingly, sensitization of TRPV1 neurons persisted 2 years after the gastroenteritis, but differences in lymphocytes or mucosal cytokine messenger RNA expression were no longer present.[60] These findings suggest that immune changes may be transient and could explain the inconsistent and conflicting results in unselected patients with IBS.

A systematic review and meta-analysis of 22 studies found increased mast cells and CD3+ cells in the left colonic mucosa in patients with IBS compared with controls.[61] There has been much interest in the role of mast cells in increasing peripheral sensitization and intestinal permeability in patients with IBS through the release of histamine.[50,62] One study demonstrated an increased number of mast cells in close proximity to sensory neurons in patients with IBS compared with controls and this finding correlated with increased abdominal pain severity and frequency.[62] Increased mast cells have also been associated with increased colonic permeability and diarrhea symptoms.[63] However, other studies have found comparable or even lower numbers of mucosal immune cells in patients with IBS and controls.[52,64,65]

There have been studies showing increased proinflammatory cytokine and/or lower anti-inflammatory cytokine profiles in patients with IBS, but this has been mainly in blood samples and not in the colonic mucosa.[66] Increased tumor necrosis factor alpha-$\alpha$ and IL-6 levels were present in IBS compared with controls,[67,68] although other studies contradict these findings.[64,69] Furthermore, SNPs in genes encoding proinflammatory cytokines such as IL-6 and TNFSF15 increase risk of IBS and an SNP for the anti-inflammatory cytokine IL-10 decreases the risk of IBS.[14,70,71] Colonic mucosal cytokine levels are more variable; however, a few studies have shown decreased levels of the anti-inflammatory cytokine, IL-10.[64,72] Most studies have failed to show a significant association between cytokine levels or cell counts with symptoms.[64,67–69]

### Bile acid processing
Bile acid diarrhea is reportedly present in approximately 25% of patients with IBS-D.[73–75] Bile acids increase secretion, motility, and visceral sensitivity to rectal

distention. Bile acid-related visceral hypersensitivity is thought to be due to activation of the farnesoid X receptor on mast cells resulting in increased expression of nerve growth factor and subsequent increased TRPV1 expression on dorsal root ganglion neurons.[76] Bile acids may also be clinically relevant in some patients with IBS-C who have decreased total bile acids and decreased fecal deoxycholic acid.[77,78]

### Serotonin signaling mechanisms

About 95% of 5-HT is present in the GI tract. It is stored in enterochromaffin cells (ECCs) and in enteric serotonergic neurons.[79] ECCs release 5-HT in response to a variety of stimuli. 5-HT is a neurotransmitter and binds to receptors on enteric neurons and vagal and spinal afferent nerves, which modulate gut motility, secretion, and sensation. 5-HT is taken up into cells via reuptake transporter proteins, such as the 5-HT reuptake transporter, SERT. Gut microbiota and their metabolites, including short-chain fatty acids and secondary bile acids, can influence 5-HT signaling and GI function by activating receptors on ECCs to increase 5-HT production and on enteric neurons to regulate gut motility.[80,81]

A number of studies support that 5-HT is involved in the altered motility and transit present in patients with IBS. Postprandial platelet depleted plasma 5-HT levels are elevated in patients with IBS-D and correlate with more rapid colonic transit times.[82,83] In patients with IBS-C, the mechanisms responsible for 5-HT release are thought to be impaired because ECCs have increased 5-HT content but postprandial 5-HT levels are low.[82] The significant role of 5-HT in IBS is supported by the efficacy of several approved serotonergic agents in the treatment of patients with IBS-D and IBS-C.

### Gut microbiota

There is growing evidence that the gut microbiota may play a role in IBS. However, studies comparing the fecal microbiome in patients with IBS and healthy controls have produced variable findings. A recent meta-analysis of 24 studies found that microbial diversity was decreased in IBS and that the microbiome of patients with IBS had an increased abundance of family Enterobacteriaceae, family Lactobacillaceae, and genus *Bacteroides*, and decreased abundance of *Clostridiales* I, genus *Faecalibacterium*, and genus *Bifidobacterium*.[84] The gut microbiota has been associated with gut motility and transit in animal models. It is thought that these effects relate to neuroactive microbial metabolites, but direct evidence supporting this hypothesis is lacking.[85,86]

Microbes also contribute to the bidirectional communication within the brain–gut axis. The brain receives complex afferent input from the gut and microbial metabolites, and in turn sends modulatory signals back to the gut primarily via the autonomic nervous system, which in turn influence intestinal and gut microbial function. Altered gut microbial metabolites can also feed back to the brain, influencing pontine arousal systems and brain networks.[85]

### Dysregulated Stress Responsiveness

IBS is considered a stress-sensitive disorder. The stress response is an integrated and coordinated physiologic process that can result in physiologic adaptation or pathologic maladaptation. The main central stress response output systems are the hypothalamic–pituitary–adrenal (HPA) axis and the locus coeruleus–noradrenergic system. Stress is a state of perceived or actual threat to homeostasis.[87] "Allostasis" refers to the active process of adapting to stressors via mediators such as cortisol and the autonomic, metabolic and immune systems that act together to maintain homeostasis. Chronic wear and tear on the body can lead to disease or reaching one's "allostatic load or overload," which refers to the cumulative effect of multiple stressors as well as the dysregulation of allostasis (eg, too much or too little cortisol, or adrenaline or inflammation in response to a challenge). The allostatic load results from either too much stress or not efficiently responding to the stress.[87]

Activation of the HPA axis results in synthesis and release of corticotropin-releasing factor in the paraventricular nucleus of the hypothalamus. Corticotropin-releasing factor stimulates the release of adrenocorticotropin hormone from the anterior pituitary gland, which leads to the release of cortisol from the adrenal glands. Cortisol levels are regulated by negative feedback at the level of the hypothalamus and the pituitary. Corticotropin-releasing factor also acts as a neurotransmitter and activates the autonomic nervous system, resulting in an integrated response to stress.

Experimental stress increases visceral sensitivity, gut motility and permeability, and immune response (**Fig. 6**).[39,88,89] The HPA axis has also been associated with visceral sensitivity via central sensitization at the level of the dorsal root ganglia and brain.[90,91] Altered HPA axis responses have been demonstrated in patients with IBS compared with controls.[92] These alterations have been shown to be associated with an increased number of early adverse life events, negatively perceived stressful life events in adulthood and decreased resilience, which have all been demonstrated in IBS.[20,33,93,94] An enhanced HPA axis response in early life stress models has been linked to decreased negative feedback owing to increased DNA methylation of the glucocorticoid receptor promoter, which results in decreased glucocorticoid receptor expression.[21]

Patients with IBS show changes in autonomic nervous system tone, specifically a greater sympathetic/parasympathetic (vagal) balance[95] with differences occurring

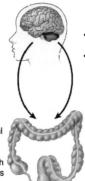

**GI Motility**
•Suppressed gastric and small bowel motor activity
•↑ colonic motor activity

**Intestinal Permeability and Secretion**
• ↑ small intestinal permeability to mental stressor in controls
• ↓ stress-induced net water flux and chloride secretion in healthy women with moderate stress vs those with low stress

**HPA axis**
• ↑ basal and stimulated ACTH and/or cortisol in IBS vs controls
• Lack of response to meal and/or mental stressor vs. controls

**Visceral Perception**
• ↓ nonpainful & pain thresholds during psychological stress in IBS but not controls
• Higher stress, anxiety, and anger ratings in IBS vs controls

**Autonomic Tone**
• ↑ blood pressure and heart rate after mental stress in IBS and controls (no group differences)

Fig. 6. Stress-induced physiologic changes in IBS. Experimental stress has been shown to be associated with physiologic changes involved in bidirectional brain–gut interactions that are relevant in IBS pathogenesis. Stress can alter GI motility, intestinal permeability and secretion, the hypothalamic–pituitary–adrenal (HPA) axis, visceral perception thresholds, and ratings to balloon distention of the rectum and colon, and autonomic nervous system tone. (*Data from* Chang L. Invited review: The role of stress on physiologic responses and clinical symptoms in IBS. Gastroenterology 2011;140(3):761-765; and Vanuytsel T, van Wanrooy S, Vanheel H, Vanormelingen C, Verschueren S, Houben E, Salim Rasoel S, Tóth J, Holvoet L, Farré R, Van Oudenhove L, Boeckxstaens G, Verbeke K, Tack J. Psychological stress and corticotropin-releasing hormone increase intestinal permeability in humans by a mast cell-dependent mechanism. Gut. 2014 Aug;63(8):1293-9).

between bowel habit subtypes[96] and men and women.[97,98] Autonomic nervous system changes are also seen in patients with more severe symptoms. The autonomic nervous system's effect on pain sensitivity, immune response and gut motility are particularly relevant in the pathogenesis of IBS.

## SUMMARY

Valuable scientific advances have been made over the past few decades, which have improved our understanding of the pathogenesis of IBS. Although there is not a consensus on the exact, underlying mechanisms to explain the symptoms of IBS, this condition is now well-recognized as a disorder of gut–brain interactions. Evidence suggests that, although IBS is characterized by the presence of abdominal pain associated with altered bowel habits, it remains a heterogenous disorder where the cluster of IBS symptoms may arise from several etiologies that can differ within subgroups of patients. IBS symptoms can arise from various primary peripheral or central mechanisms, but once brain–gut interactions become altered, it is more challenging to identify causality.[36] Future efforts to integrate multiple levels of data (eg, symptoms, gene and protein expression, neuroimaging measures, microbial-related measures) to identify phenotypic subgroups with specific pathophysiologic mechanisms that may serve as diagnostic and/or therapeutic targets are needed.

## CLINICS CARE POINTS

- In IBS, there are abdominal symptoms that are sensory symptoms, i.e. are associated with visceral hypersensitivity, which are abdominal pain, discomfort and bloating. There are also bowel habit symptoms which include stool form and frequency. There is only a modest correlation between abdominal and bowel habit symptoms. Therefore, some patients can report persistent abdominal pain, discomfort and bloating even when bowel habits are normalized with treatment.
- It is important to identify factors associated with the onset of symptoms and also the exacerbation of symptoms, which can be targets for treatment.
- Once IBS symptoms develop, it can be difficult to determine if symptoms are due to peripheral vs central factors since there is dynamic bidirectional communication between the brain and gut. However, central factors are likely predominant in driving symptoms in patients with more severe symptoms and those with overlapping conditions, e.g. fibromyalgia, anxiety, depression, interstitial cystitis, etc.
- Describing the pathophysiologic mechanisms of IBS that explain the patient's symptoms help to validate the symptoms and avoid ordering multiple diagnostic tests to exclude other gastrointestinal conditions.

## DISCLOSURE

Dr E.J. Videlock does not have anything to disclose. Dr L. Chang has served on scientific advisory boards or consulted with Ironwood Pharmaceuticals, Arena Pharmaceuticals, Allergan and Cosmo. She has research grants from the National Institute of Health (NIH) and Arena and Vanda Pharmaceuticals. She serves on the Rome Foundation Board of Directors.

## REFERENCES

1. Drossman DA, Chang L, Chey WD, et al. Rome IV functional gastrointestinal disorders – disorders of gut-brain interaction. 4th edition. Raleigh, NC: Rome Foundation; 2016.
2. Saito YA, Mitra N, Mayer EA. Genetic approaches to functional gastrointestinal disorders. Gastroenterology 2010;138(4):1276.
3. Saito YA, Petersen GM, Larson JJ, et al. Familial aggregation of irritable bowel syndrome: a family case-control study. Am J Gastroenterol 2010;105(4):833.
4. Waehrens R, Ohlsson H, Sundquist J, et al. Risk of irritable bowel syndrome in first-degree, second-degree and third-degree relatives of affected individuals: a nationwide family study in Sweden. Gut 2015;64(2):215.
5. Levy RL, Jones KR, Whitehead WE, et al. Irritable bowel syndrome in twins: heredity and social learning both contribute to etiology. Gastroenterology 2001;121(4):799.
6. Saito YA. The role of genetics in IBS. Gastroenterol Clin North Am 2011;40(1):45.
7. Ek WE, Reznichenko A, Ripke S, et al. Exploring the genetics of irritable bowel syndrome: a GWA study in the general population and replication in multinational case-control cohorts. Gut 2015;64(11):1774.
8. Bonfiglio F, Zheng T, Garcia-Etxebarria K, et al. Female-specific association between variants on chromosome 9 and self-reported diagnosis of irritable bowel syndrome. Gastroenterology 2018;155(1):168.
9. Henstrom M, Diekmann L, Bonfiglio F, et al. Functional variants in the sucrase-isomaltase gene associate with increased risk of irritable bowel syndrome. Gut 2018;67(2):263.
10. Beyder A, Mazzone A, Strege PR, et al. Loss-of-function of the voltage-gated sodium channel NaV1.5 (channelopathies) in patients with irritable bowel syndrome. Gastroenterology 2014;146(7):1659.
11. Saito YA, Larson JJ, Atkinson EJ, et al. The role of 5-HTT LPR and GNbeta3 825C>T polymorphisms and gene-environment interactions in irritable bowel syndrome (IBS). Dig Dis Sci 2012;57(10):2650.
12. Van Kerkhoven LA, Laheij RJ, Jansen JB. Meta-analysis: a functional polymorphism in the gene encoding for activity of the serotonin transporter protein is not associated with the irritable bowel syndrome. Aliment Pharmacol Ther 2007;26(7):979.
13. Wang YM, Chang Y, Chang YY, et al. Serotonin transporter gene promoter region polymorphisms and serotonin transporter expression in the colonic mucosa of irritable bowel syndrome patients. Neurogastroenterol Motil 2012;24(6):560.
14. Zhu S, Wang B, Jia Q, et al. Candidate single nucleotide polymorphisms of irritable bowel syndrome: a systemic review and meta-analysis. BMC Gastroenterol 2019;19(1):165.
15. Orand A, Naliboff B, Gadd M, et al. Corticotropin-releasing hormone receptor 1 (CRH-R1) polymorphisms are associated with irritable bowel syndrome and acoustic startle response. Psychoneuroendocrinology 2016;73:133.
16. Mahurkar-Joshi S, Chang L. Epigenetic mechanisms in irritable bowel syndrome. Front Psychiatry 2020;11:805.
17. Mahurkar S, Polytarchou C, Iliopoulos D, et al. Genome-wide DNA methylation profiling of peripheral blood mononuclear cells in irritable bowel syndrome. Neurogastroenterol Motil 2016;28(3):410.
18. Mahurkar-Joshi S, Rankin CR, Videlock EJ, et al. The Colonic Mucosal MicroRNAs, MicroRNA-219a-5p and MicroRNA-338-3p, are Downregulated in Irritable

Bowel Syndrome and Are Associated With Barrier Function and MAPK Signaling. Gastroenterology 2021;160:2409–22. https://doi.org/10.1053/j.gastro.2021.02. 040. Epub 2021 Feb 20.

19. Whitehead WE, Crowell MD, Robinson JC, et al. Effects of stressful life events on bowel symptoms: subjects with irritable bowel syndrome compared with subjects without bowel dysfunction. Gut 1992;33(6):825.

20. Parker CH, Naliboff BD, Shih W, et al. Negative events during adulthood are associated with symptom severity and altered stress response in patients with irritable bowel syndrome. Clin Gastroenterol Hepatol 2019;17:2245–52.

21. Rinne T, de Kloet ER, Wouters L, et al. Hyperresponsiveness of hypothalamic-pituitary-adrenal axis to combined dexamethasone/corticotropin-releasing hormone challenge in female borderline personality disorder subjects with a history of sustained childhood abuse. Biol Psychiatry 2002;52(11):1102.

22. Carpenter LL, Carvalho JP, Tyrka AR, et al. Decreased adrenocorticotropic hormone and cortisol responses to stress in healthy adults reporting significant childhood maltreatment. Biol Psychiatry 2007;62(10):1080.

23. McGowan PO, Sasaki A, D'Alessio AC, et al. Epigenetic regulation of the glucocorticoid receptor in human brain associates with childhood abuse. Nat Neurosci 2009;12(3):342.

24. Barbara G, Grover M, Bercik P, et al. Rome foundation working team report on post-infection irritable bowel syndrome. Gastroenterology 2019;156(1):46.

25. Klem F, Wadhwa A, Prokop LJ, et al. Prevalence, risk factors, and outcomes of irritable bowel syndrome after infectious enteritis: a systematic review and meta-analysis. Gastroenterology 2017;152(5):1042.

26. Marshall JK, Thabane M, Garg AX, et al. Incidence and epidemiology of irritable bowel syndrome after a large waterborne outbreak of bacterial dysentery. Gastroenterology 2006;131(2):445.

27. Dunlop SP, Jenkins D, Neal KR, et al. Relative importance of enterochromaffin cell hyperplasia, anxiety, and depression in postinfectious IBS. Gastroenterology 2003;125(6):1651.

28. Chitkara DK, van Tilburg MA, Blois-Martin N, et al. Early life risk factors that contribute to irritable bowel syndrome in adults: a systematic review. Am J Gastroenterol 2008;103(3):765.

29. Bradford K, Shih W, Videlock EJ, et al. Association between early adverse life events and irritable bowel syndrome. Clin Gastroenterol Hepatol 2012;10(4):385.

30. Park SH, Videlock EJ, Shih W, et al. Adverse childhood experiences are associated with irritable bowel syndrome and gastrointestinal symptom severity. Neurogastroenterol Motil 2016;28(8):1252.

31. Drossman DA, Leserman J, Nachman G, et al. Sexual and physical abuse in women with functional or organic gastrointestinal disorders. Ann Intern Med 1990;113(11):828.

32. Klooker TK, Braak B, Painter RC, et al. Exposure to severe wartime conditions in early life is associated with an increased risk of irritable bowel syndrome: a population-based cohort study. Am J Gastroenterol 2009;104(9):2250.

33. Bennett EJ, Tennant CC, Piesse C, et al. Level of chronic life stress predicts clinical outcome in irritable bowel syndrome. Gut 1998;43(2):256.

34. Gray GC, Reed RJ, Kaiser KS, et al. Self-reported symptoms and medical conditions among 11,868 Gulf War-era veterans: the Seabee Health Study. Am J Epidemiol 2002;155(11):1033.

35. Dunphy RC, Bridgewater L, Price DD, et al. Visceral and cutaneous hypersensitivity in Persian Gulf war veterans with chronic gastrointestinal symptoms. Pain 2003;102(1–2):79.
36. Mayer EA, Labus JS, Tillisch K, et al. Towards a systems view of IBS. Nat Rev Gastroenterol Hepatol 2015;12(10):592.
37. Bouin M, Plourde V, Boivin M, et al. Rectal distention testing in patients with irritable bowel syndrome: sensitivity, specificity, and predictive values of pain sensory thresholds. Gastroenterology 2002;122(7):1771.
38. Ludidi S, Conchillo JM, Keszthelyi D, et al. Rectal hypersensitivity as hallmark for irritable bowel syndrome: defining the optimal cutoff. Neurogastroenterol Motil 2012;24(8):729.
39. Posserud I, Agerforz P, Ekman R, et al. Altered visceral perceptual and neuroendocrine response in patients with irritable bowel syndrome during mental stress. Gut 2004;53(8):1102.
40. Tillisch K, Mayer EA, Labus JS. Quantitative meta-analysis identifies brain regions activated during rectal distension in irritable bowel syndrome. Gastroenterology 2011;140(1):91.
41. Elsenbruch S, Rosenberger C, Enck P, et al. Affective disturbances modulate the neural processing of visceral pain stimuli in irritable bowel syndrome: an fMRI study. Gut 2010;59(4):489.
42. Mayer EA, Labus J, Aziz Q, et al. Role of brain imaging in disorders of brain-gut interaction: a Rome Working Team Report. Gut 2019;68(9):1701.
43. Chey WY, Jin HO, Lee MH, et al. Colonic motility abnormality in patients with irritable bowel syndrome exhibiting abdominal pain and diarrhea. Am J Gastroenterol 2001;96(5):1499.
44. Ritchie J. Pain from distension of the pelvic colon by inflating a balloon in the irritable colon syndrome. Gut 1973;14(2):125.
45. Vassallo M, Camilleri M, Phillips SF, et al. Transit through the proximal colon influences stool weight in the irritable bowel syndrome. Gastroenterology 1992;102(1):102.
46. Almy TP. Experimental studies on the irritable bowel syndrome. Am J Med 1951;10:60.
47. Camilleri M, McKinzie S, Busciglio I, et al. Prospective study of motor, sensory, psychologic, and autonomic functions in patients with irritable bowel syndrome. Clin Gastroenterol Hepatol 2008;6(7):772.
48. Cenac N, Altier C, Motta JP, et al. Potentiation of TRPV4 signalling by histamine and serotonin: an important mechanism for visceral hypersensitivity. Gut 2010;59(4):481.
49. Zhao JH, Dong L, Shi HT, et al. The expression of protease-activated receptor 2 and 4 in the colon of irritable bowel syndrome patients. Dig Dis Sci 2012;57(1):58.
50. Akbar A, Yiangou Y, Facer P, et al. Increased capsaicin receptor TRPV1-expressing sensory fibres in irritable bowel syndrome and their correlation with abdominal pain. Gut 2008;57(7):923.
51. Videlock EJ, Mahurkar-Joshi S, Hoffman JM, et al. Sigmoid colon mucosal gene expression supports alterations of neuronal signaling in irritable bowel syndrome with constipation. Am J Physiol Gastrointest Liver Physiol 2018;315(1):G140.
52. Cenac N, Andrews CN, Holzhausen M, et al. Role for protease activity in visceral pain in irritable bowel syndrome. J Clin Invest 2007;117(3):636.
53. Barbara G, Wang B, Stanghellini V, et al. Mast cell-dependent excitation of visceral-nociceptive sensory neurons in irritable bowel syndrome. Gastroenterology 2007;132(1):26.

54. Buhner S, Li Q, Berger T, et al. Submucous rather than myenteric neurons are activated by mucosal biopsy supernatants from irritable bowel syndrome patients. Neurogastroenterol Motil 2012;24(12):1134.

55. Wouters MM, Balemans D, Van Wanrooy S, et al. Histamine receptor H1-mediated sensitization of TRPV1 mediates visceral hypersensitivity and symptoms in patients with irritable bowel syndrome. Gastroenterology 2016; 150(4):875.

56. Martinez C, Vicario M, Ramos L, et al. The jejunum of diarrhea-predominant irritable bowel syndrome shows molecular alterations in the tight junction signaling pathway that are associated with mucosal pathobiology and clinical manifestations. Am J Gastroenterol 2012;107(5):736.

57. Piche T, Barbara G, Aubert P, et al. Impaired intestinal barrier integrity in the colon of patients with irritable bowel syndrome: involvement of soluble mediators. Gut 2009;58(2):196.

58. Zhou Q, Zhang B, Verne GN. Intestinal membrane permeability and hypersensitivity in the irritable bowel syndrome. Pain 2009;146(1–2):41.

59. Gwee KA, Collins SM, Read NW, et al. Increased rectal mucosal expression of interleukin 1beta in recently acquired post-infectious irritable bowel syndrome. Gut 2003;52(4):523.

60. Balemans D, Mondelaers SU, Cibert-Goton V, et al. Evidence for long-term sensitization of the bowel in patients with post-infectious-IBS. Sci Rep 2017;7(1): 13606.

61. Bashashati M, Moossavi S, Cremon C, et al. Colonic immune cells in irritable bowel syndrome: a systematic review and meta-analysis. Neurogastroenterol Motil 2018;30(1).

62. Barbara G, Stanghellini V, De Giorgio R, et al. Activated mast cells in proximity to colonic nerves correlate with abdominal pain in irritable bowel syndrome. Gastroenterology 2004;126(3):693.

63. Vivinus-Nebot M, Dainese R, Anty R, et al. Combination of allergic factors can worsen diarrheic irritable bowel syndrome: role of barrier defects and mast cells. Am J Gastroenterol 2012;107(1):75.

64. Chang L, Adeyemo M, Karagiannides I, et al. Serum and colonic mucosal immune markers in irritable bowel syndrome. Am J Gastroenterol 2012;107(2):262.

65. Braak B, Klooker TK, Wouters MM, et al. Mucosal immune cell numbers and visceral sensitivity in patients with irritable bowel syndrome: is there any relationship? Am J Gastroenterol 2012;107(5):715.

66. Ohman L, Isaksson S, Lindmark AC, et al. T-cell activation in patients with irritable bowel syndrome. Am J Gastroenterol 2009;104(5):1205.

67. Bennet SMP, Palsson O, Whitehead WE, et al. Systemic cytokines are elevated in a subset of patients with irritable bowel syndrome but largely unrelated to symptom characteristics. Neurogastroenterol Motil 2018;30(10):e13378.

68. Vara EJ, Brokstad KA, Hausken T, et al. Altered levels of cytokines in patients with irritable bowel syndrome are not correlated with fatigue. Int J Gen Med 2018; 11:285.

69. Nasser Y, Petes C, Simmers C, et al. Activation of peripheral blood CD4+ T-Cells in IBS is not associated with gastrointestinal or psychological symptoms. Sci Rep 2019;9(1):3710.

70. Barkhordari E, Rezaei N, Ansaripour B, et al. Proinflammatory cytokine gene polymorphisms in irritable bowel syndrome. J Clin Immunol 2010;30(1):74.

71. Barkhordari E, Rezaei N, Mahmoudi M, et al. T-helper 1, T-helper 2, and T-regulatory cytokines gene polymorphisms in irritable bowel syndrome. Inflammation 2010;33(5):281.
72. Macsharry J, O'Mahony L, Fanning A, et al. Mucosal cytokine imbalance in irritable bowel syndrome. Scand J Gastroenterol 2008;43(12):1467.
73. Valentin N, Camilleri M, Altayar O, et al. Biomarkers for bile acid diarrhoea in functional bowel disorder with diarrhoea: a systematic review and meta-analysis. Gut 2016;65(12):1951.
74. Aziz I, Mumtaz S, Bholah H, et al. High prevalence of idiopathic bile acid diarrhea among patients with diarrhea-predominant irritable bowel syndrome based on Rome III criteria. Clin Gastroenterol Hepatol 2015;13(9):1650.
75. Slattery SA, Niaz O, Aziz Q, et al. Systematic review with meta-analysis: the prevalence of bile acid malabsorption in the irritable bowel syndrome with diarrhoea. Aliment Pharmacol Ther 2015;42(1):3.
76. Li WT, Luo QQ, Wang B, et al. Bile acids induce visceral hypersensitivity via mucosal mast cell-to-nociceptor signaling that involves the farnesoid X receptor/nerve growth factor/transient receptor potential vanilloid 1 axis. FASEB J 2019;33(2):2435.
77. Vijayvargiya P, Camilleri M, Burton D, et al. Bile and fat excretion are biomarkers of clinically significant diarrhoea and constipation in irritable bowel syndrome. Aliment Pharmacol Ther 2019;49(6):744.
78. Vijayvargiya P, Busciglio I, Burton D, et al. Bile acid deficiency in a subgroup of patients with irritable bowel syndrome with constipation based on biomarkers in serum and fecal samples. Clin Gastroenterol Hepatol 2018;16(4):522.
79. Gershon MD, Tack J. The serotonin signaling system: from basic understanding to drug development for functional GI disorders. Gastroenterology 2007; 132(1):397.
80. Spohn SN, Mawe GM. Non-conventional features of peripheral serotonin signalling - the gut and beyond. Nat Rev Gastroenterol Hepatol 2017;14(7):412.
81. Yano JM, Yu K, Donaldson GP, et al. Indigenous bacteria from the gut microbiota regulate host serotonin biosynthesis. Cell 2015;161(2):264.
82. Atkinson W, Lockhart S, Whorwell PJ, et al. Altered 5-hydroxytryptamine signaling in patients with constipation- and diarrhea-predominant irritable bowel syndrome. Gastroenterology 2006;130(1):34.
83. Houghton LA, Atkinson W, Lockhart C, et al. Sigmoid-colonic motility in health and irritable bowel syndrome: a role for 5-hydroxytryptamine. Neurogastroenterol Motil 2007;19(9):724.
84. Pittayanon R, Lau JT, Yuan Y, et al. Gut microbiota in patients with irritable bowel syndrome-a systematic review. Gastroenterology 2019;157(1):97–108.
85. Martin CR, Osadchiy V, Kalani A, et al. The brain-gut-microbiome axis. Cell Mol Gastroenterol Hepatol 2018;6(2):133.
86. Foster JA, Rinaman L, Cryan JF. Stress & the gut-brain axis: regulation by the microbiome. Neurobiol Stress 2017;7:124.
87. McEwen BS. Protective and damaging effects of stress mediators: central role of the brain. Dialogues Clin Neurosci 2006;8(4):367.
88. Dickhaus B, Mayer EA, Firooz N, et al. Irritable bowel syndrome patients show enhanced modulation of visceral perception by auditory stress. Am J Gastroenterol 2003;98(1):135.
89. Welgan P, Meshkinpour H, Hoehler F. The effect of stress on colon motor and electrical activity in irritable bowel syndrome. Psychosom Med 1985;47(2):139.

90. Myers B, Greenwood-Van Meerveld B. Elevated corticosterone in the amygdala leads to persistent increases in anxiety-like behavior and pain sensitivity. Behav Brain Res 2010;214(2):465.

91. Ibeakanma C, Ochoa-Cortes F, Miranda-Morales M, et al. Brain-gut interactions increase peripheral nociceptive signaling in mice with postinfectious irritable bowel syndrome. Gastroenterology 2011;141(6):2098.

92. Videlock EJ, Shih W, Adeyemo M, et al. The effect of sex and irritable bowel syndrome on HPA axis response and peripheral glucocorticoid receptor expression. Psychoneuroendocrinology 2016;69:67.

93. Videlock EJ, Adeyemo M, Licudine A, et al. Childhood trauma is associated with hypothalamic-pituitary-adrenal axis responsiveness in irritable bowel syndrome. Gastroenterology 2009;137(6):1954.

94. Park SH, Naliboff BD, Shih W, et al. Resilience is decreased in irritable bowel syndrome and associated with symptoms and cortisol response. Neurogastroenterol Motil 2018;30(1).

95. Aggarwal A, Cutts TF, Abell TL, et al. Predominant symptoms in irritable bowel syndrome correlate with specific autonomic nervous system abnormalities. Gastroenterology 1994;106(4):945.

96. Jarrett ME, Burr RL, Cain KC, et al. Autonomic nervous system function during sleep among women with irritable bowel syndrome. Dig Dis Sci 2008;53(3):694.

97. Tillisch K, Mayer EA, Labus JS, et al. Sex specific alterations in autonomic function among patients with irritable bowel syndrome. Gut 2005;54(10):1396.

98. Cheng P, Shih W, Alberto M, et al. Autonomic response to a visceral stressor is dysregulated in irritable bowel syndrome and correlates with duration of disease. Neurogastroenterol Motil 2013;25(10):e650.

# Emerging Role of the Gut Microbiome in Irritable Bowel Syndrome

Prashant Singh, MBBS[a],*, Anthony Lembo, MD[b]

## KEYWORDS

- Microbial dysbiosis • Breath test • Abdominal pain • Diarrhea • Constipation

## KEY POINTS

- Epidemiologic studies suggest acute gastroenteritis can trigger the onset of irritable bowel syndrome (IBS), leading to development of postinfection IBS.
- Small intestinal bacterial overgrowth is associated with diarrhea-predominant IBS, whereas increased levels of methanogenic Archaea, specifically *Methanobrevibacter smithii*, are associated with constipation-predominant IBS.
- Fecal and/or gut mucosal microbiome are altered in at least a subset of patients with IBS.
- Alterations in gut microbiome can affect the gut-brain axis, visceral sensitivity, intestinal barrier, intestinal secretion, gut motility. and immune activation, which in turn can cause IBS symptoms.
- Therapies targeting the microbiome, such as probiotics, antibiotics, diet, and fecal microbiota transplant, can improve symptoms in subsets of patients with IBS.

## INTRODUCTION

Microorganisms, including bacteria, Archaea, fungi, eukaryotic viruses, and bacteriophages, residing in the human gut are collectively referred to as the gut microbiome. Most of these organisms are commensal. The collection of all gut microbiome genes in an individual represents a genetic repertoire that is significantly more abundant than the human genome. The gut microbiome is influenced by factors related to birth (ie, vaginal delivery vs cesarean section) and early infancy (ie, infant feeding, infections, and antibiotics). The gut microbiome is further modulated in adult life by lifestyle (ie, exercise and diet), gastrointestinal (GI) infections, and antibiotics.

Conflicts of interest: None.
[a] Division of Gastroenterology and Hepatology, University of Michigan, MSBR1, Room 6520 B, 1150 West Medical Center Drive, Ann Arbor, MI 48109, USA; [b] Division of Gastroenterology and Hepatology, Beth Israel Deaconess Medical Center, Rabb/Rose 1, 330 Brookline Avenue, Boston, MA 02215, USA
* Corresponding author.
*E-mail address:* singhpr@med.umich.edu

Gastroenterol Clin N Am 50 (2021) 523–545
https://doi.org/10.1016/j.gtc.2021.03.003
0889-8553/21/© 2021 Elsevier Inc. All rights reserved.

Recent omics-based epidemiologic, clinical, and translational human studies, along with in vitro and in vivo studies in animals, have shown that gut microbial communities play a key role in the pathogenesis of several GI, as well as non-GI diseases. Despite significant interindividual variation, around 90% of all taxa in the human gut microbiome belong to just 2 phyla: Bacteroidetes and Firmicutes. Other phyla consistently found in the human distal gut are Proteobacteria, Actinobacteria, Fusobacteria, and Verrucomicrobia. Few species of Archaea (mostly *Methanobrevibacter smithii*) are represented. There are important differences between fecal and mucosa-associated communities within the same individual.[1] Bacterial composition in the lumen varies from cecum to rectum with pronounced variability in the microbial composition in the same individual when measured across months, weeks, and even days.[2] Factors such as diet, drug intake, traveling, or colonic transit time can affect microbial composition of fecal samples over time. Fluctuations in the gut microbiome among individuals can be significant, although the microbial pattern tends to return to its baseline over time.[2]

This article focuses on the role of microbiome in irritable bowel syndrome (IBS). IBS is a multifactorial disorder characterized by alterations in gut motility, barrier function, low-grade immune activation, visceral hypersensitivity (VH), and hypervigilance toward gut symptoms.[3] It summarizes the current evidence of microbial dysbiosis in IBS, discusses the literature on the role of microbiome in mediating central and peripheral dysfunctions summarized earlier, and discusses potential microbial components and products leading to these dysfunctions. In addition, it discusses the current state of evidence on therapies targeting microbiome in the management of IBS.

## POSTINFECTION IRRITABLE BOWEL SYNDROME

Even before McKendrick and Read[4] reported the first case of IBS following outbreaks of *Salmonella* in the United Kingdom, there were reports in the literature of chronic GI symptoms following gastroenteritis.[4,5] Subsequently, multiple studies have reported what is now known as postinfection IBS, with incidence ranging from 3% to 31%.[6] A recent meta-analysis of 45 studies that prospectively followed infectious outbreaks found that the pooled incidence of IBS was 14.5% at more than 12 months after acute gastroenteritis.[7] Several host-related factors increased the likelihood of developing IBS, including female gender, psychosomatic comorbidities such as presence of anxiety, depression, somatization, and neuroticism.[7] In addition, severity of the infectious gastroenteritis (such as presence of bloody stool, episode lasting >7 days) was also associated with development of postinfection IBS.[7] Various types of infectious gastroenteritis have been implicated, such as bacterial, protozoal, and viral infections.

## SMALL INTESTINAL BACTERIAL OVERGROWTH AND IRRITABLE BOWEL SYNDROME

Several studies have reported increased prevalence of small intestinal bacterial overgrowth (SIBO) in patients with IBS compared with healthy controls based on either glucose or lactulose breath testing. Patients with IBS have a 3.5 to 4.7 times higher odds of having an abnormal breath test compared with healthy controls, depending on the criteria used to define a positive test.[8,9] As expected, because of the invasive nature, difficulty in performing, and lack of a clear threshold to define SIBO, few studies have used small bowel cultures to diagnosis SIBO in IBS. Initial studies showed patients with IBS are more likely to have small intestinal bacterial counts of greater than $10^3$ colony-forming units (CFU) per milliliter compared with healthy controls.[10] These findings have been validated using newer technologies such as quantitative polymerase chain reaction (PCR).[11]

The predominant archaeon and methane producer in human gut is *M smithii*.[12] Methane has been shown to slow down small bowel transit in animal studies (discussed later), and has been associated with constipation-predominant IBS (IBS-C).[13] Similarly, increased methane excretion on breath testing has been associated with decreases in stool consistency and transit time and an increase in constipation severity.[14–16] However, more recent studies have failed to confirm these associations.[17] In a recent study, Parthasarathy and colleagues[18] found that the fecal microbiota correlated with colonic transit and breath methane production but methane levels did not correlate with colonic transit, going against a link between breath methane levels and slow transit constipation. In this study, constipated patients had a unique profile of colonic mucosal microbiota that discriminated between constipation and health with an accuracy of 94% independent of diet and colonic transit.[18] In addition, treating constipated patients with increased breath methane levels with targeted antibiotics has been shown to improve constipation symptoms.[19] However, it is unclear whether this effect is caused by reduction in methane levels or some other mechanism related or unrelated to microbiome perturbation. Therefore, it is not clear whether methane is caused by constipation or is the cause of constipation.

## MICROBIOME ALTERATIONS IN IRRITABLE BOWEL SYNDROME

There are several studies assessing microbiome alterations in patients with IBS (**Table 1**). Most of these studies assessed fecal microbiome, whereas a few have investigated both mucosal and fecal microbiome. Only a few of these studies have shown an IBS-specific microbial signature, whereas others have failed to replicate these findings in larger studies.[20,21] Several, but not all, studies have shown that microbial diversity is reduced in patients with IBS compared with healthy controls.[22] Although there is significant heterogeneity in the findings of these studies, a recent meta-analysis showed an overabundance of the phylum Bacteroidetes and the families of Lactobacillaceae and Enterobacteriaceae in patients with IBS compared with healthy controls.[22] There also seems to be a decreased abundance of genus *Faecalibacterium* and *Bifidobacterium*.[22] Only a few studies have focused solely on diarrhea-predominant IBS (IBS-D), showing an overabundance of phylum Bacteroidetes and a decrease in genus *Bifidobacterium*.[22] Although a few studies have found an association between specific bacteria groups and disease severity, these findings have not been consistently replicated by additional studies,[23] likely because of significant limitations of these studies: heterogeneity of patients with IBS (including subtypes), single-center studies with small sample size, and lack of demographic details on healthy controls (ie, whether they were age or gender matched).

## GUT MICROBIOTA AND THE GUT-BRAIN AXIS

The gut-brain axis is a bidirectional communication network involving neural, endocrine, and immune pathways between the central nervous system (CNS) and enteric nervous system (ENS).[24] Studies in germ-free (GF) mice have shown that gut bacterial colonization with commensals is central to development and maturation of both the ENS and CNS.[25,26] Moreover, the gut microbiota also seems to influence stress reactivity, anxietylike behavior, and the development of the hypothalamus-pituitary axis, which regulates stress response.[27–31] In addition, the gut microbiota also modulates the serotoninergic system, because an increase in serotonin turnover and altered levels of related metabolites have been reported in the limbic system of GF animals.[28] Engevik and colleagues[32] found that *Bifidobacterium dentium* and its metabolite, acetate, increased intestinal serotonin concentrations along with expression of serotonin

**Table 1**
Microbiome analysis in irritable bowel syndrome[a]

| Study | Subjects | Sample and Techniques | Findings |
|---|---|---|---|
| Kerckhoffs et al,[96] 2009 | 41 IBS and 26 healthy controls | Fecal and duodenal mucosa brush samples, FISH analyses for microbiome composition, qPCR for *Bifidobacterium* spp | Lower *Bifidobacterium* counts in duodenum and fecal samples in IBS |
| Kerckhoffs et al,[97] 2011 | 37 IBS and 20 healthy controls | Fecal and duodenal mucosa brush samples; bacterial 16S rRNA using DGGE and qPCR | Higher levels of *Pseudomonas aeruginosa* in duodenal mucosa and feces of patients with IBS |
| Codling et al[98] 2010 | 47 IBS and 33 healthy controls | Fecal samples using 16S rRNA DGGE | Lower microbial diversity in patients with IBS |
| Ponnusamy et al,[99] 2011 | 11 IBS and 8 non-IBS | Fecal samples using 16S rRNA DGGE and qPCR | Higher diversity of total bacteria, Bacteroidetes and *Lactobacillus* in IBS<br>Lower diversity of *Bifidobacterium* and *Clostridium coccoides* in IBS |
| Rajilić-Stojanović et al,[100] 2011 | 62 IBS and 46 healthy controls | Fecal samples using phylogenetic microarray and qPCR | 2-fold increased ratio of the Firmicutes to Bacteroidetes This resulted from an approximately 1.5-fold increase in numbers of *Dorea*, *Ruminococcus*, and *Clostridium* spp (P<.005); a 2-fold decrease in the number of Bacteroidetes (P<.0001); a 1.5-fold decrease in numbers of *Bifidobacterium* and *Faecalibacterium* spp (P<.05) |
| Saulnier et al,[60] 2011 | 22 pediatric IBS and 22 healthy controls | Fecal samples using 16S gene sequencing | Higher levels of Gammaproteobacteria in IBS, including more *Haemophilus parainfluenzae* |

| Carroll et al,[101] 2012 | 23 IBS-D and 23 healthy controls | Fecal samples using 16S gene sequencing | Reduced microbial richness in IBS-D Increased levels of Enterobacteriaceae in IBS-D Decreased levels of *Faecalibacterium* in IBS-D |
|---|---|---|---|
| Jeffery et al,[20] 2020 | 37 IBS and 20 healthy controls | Fecal samples using 16S rRNA gene sequencing | Lower microbial diversity in IBS A subset of patients with IBS with microbial composition different from healthy controls characterized by increased Firmicutes and decreased Bacteroidetes among other findings |
| Rangel et al,[102] 2015 | 33 IBS and 16 healthy controls | Fecal and colonic mucosal biopsies using phylogenetic microarray | A significantly lower abundance of the bacterial group uncultured Clostridiales I in the mucosal-associated microbiota in IBS. Many differences in IBS in fecal samples. Notable findings include increases in Actinobacteria, Bacilli, several *Clostridium* clusters, and Proteobacteria, and a decrease in Bacteroidetes |
| Tap et al,[23] 2017 | Cohort 1: 110 IBS, 39 healthy controls Cohort 2: 29 IBS, 17 healthy controls | Fecal samples and mucosal biopsies using 16S rRNA gene sequencing | By using classic approaches, no differences in fecal microbiota abundance or composition Using machine learning approach, signature for severe IBS included presence of methanogens, and enterotypes enriched with Clostridiales or *Prevotella* spp |
| Maharshak et al,[103] 2018 | 23 IBS-D and 24 healthy subjects | Fecal samples and mucosal biopsies using 16S rRNA gene sequencing | Decreased richness in IBS fecal samples only *Faecalibacterium* lower in IBS-D. *Dorea* higher in IBS-D |

(continued on next page)

**Table 1**
*(continued)*

| Study | Subjects | Sample and Techniques | Findings |
|---|---|---|---|
| Vich Vila et al,[104] 2018 | 181 patients with IBS. The control group were recruited from LifeLine Deep cohort (n = 893) and Maastricht IBS case-control cohort (n = 132) without GI complaints | Metagenomic shotgun sequencing using fecal samples | Increase in several species of phylum Actinobacteria. Decrease in species of Bacteroidetes, Increase in species of Streptococcaceae and Lachnospiraceae families |
| Dior et al,[89,105] 2016 | 16 IBS-D, 15 IBS-C and 15 healthy controls | Fecal samples analyzed using RT-PCR | Increase in *Escherichia coli* in patients with IBS-D, and an increase in *Bacteroides* and *Bifidobacterium* in patients with IBS-C |
| Chung et al,[106] 2016 | 28 IBS and 19 healthy controls | Fecal and jejunal mucosal samples analyzed using 16s rRNA gene sequencing | Patients with IBS had a higher proportion of Veillonellaceae in stool than controls. Prevotellaceae was more abundant in jejunal mucosa of patients with IBS than in controls |
| Chassard et al,[107] 2012 | 14 IBS-C women and 12 sex-matched healthy subject | Feces analyzed using FISH and anaerobic bacterial culture | Butyrate-producing *Roseburia–Eubacterium rectale* group reduced in IBS-C vs controls |
| Duboc et al,[108] 2012 | 14 IBS-D and 18 healthy controls | Fecal microbiota composition was assessed by quantitative PCR | There was a significant increase of *E coli* and a significant decrease of *Clostridium leptum* and *Bifidobacterium* in patients with IBS-D |
| Jalanka-Tuovinen et al,[63] 2014 | 11 postinfection IBS, 11 postinfection bowel dysfunction, 12 postinfection without bowel dysfunction, 12 IBS-D, and 11 healthy controls | 16S rRNA gene phylogenetic microarray analysis with HITChip, 16S rRNA gene qPCR with group and species-specific primers | 12-fold increase in Bacteroidetes phylum in IBS, whereas healthy controls had 35-fold more uncultured Clostridia |

| Study | Subjects | Method | Findings |
|---|---|---|---|
| Pozuelo et al,[109] 2015 | 113 IBS and 66 healthy controls | Fecal samples using 16S rRNA gene sequencing | Patients with IBS-M and IBS-D had lower relative abundance of butyrate-producing bacteria |
| Ringel-Kulka et al,[110] 2016 | 60 IBS and 20 healthy controls | Fecal samples using 16S rRNA gene sequencing | Subjects with IBS showed significantly higher levels of species of *Lactobacillus* and *Streptococcus* with the most significant increase being observed in IBS subjects without bloating. Members of the Firmicutes phylum (*Oscillibacter, Anaerovorax, incertae sedis XIII, Streptococcus,* and Eubacteriaceae) were significantly decreased in IBS-D and M-IBS compared with healthy controls |
| Shukla et al,[111] 2015 | 47 IBS and 30 healthy controls | qPCR with group-specific primers in fecal samples | Lower abundance of *Bifidobacterium* and increased abundance of *Ruminococcus, Ruminococcus productus–C coccoides, Veillonella, Bacteroides thetaiotaomicron, P aeruginosa,* and gram-negative bacteria in patients with IBS |
| Tana et al,[112] 2010 | 26 IBS and 26 healthy controls | 16S rRNA gene qPCR with group-specific and species-specific primers, culture, microscopy | Higher counts of *Veillonella* and *Lactobacillus* in subjects with IBS compared with controls |

*Abbreviations:* DGGE, denaturing gradient gel electrophoresis; FISH, fluorescence in situ hybridization; HITChip, human intestinal tract chip; IBS-C, constipation-predominant IBS; IBS-D, diarrhea-predominant IBS; IBS-M, IBS with mixed bowel habits; qPCR, quantitative PCR; rRNA, ribosomal RNA; RT-PCR, reverse transcription PCR.

[a] Modified from Pimentel et al.[113]

receptors, and serotonin transporter in in vivo and/or in vitro models. Moreover, *B dentium*–treated GF mice had higher hippocampal expression of serotonin receptor and showed less repetitive and anxietylike behaviors relative to GF controls. Similarly, modulation of brain regions controlling central processing of emotion and sensation have also been shown in response to ingestion of fermented milk with probiotics (Bifidobacterium, Lactobacillus, and *Streptococcus thermophiles*) in healthy controls.[33] In a landmark study, De Palma and colleagues[34] showed GF mice inoculated with the fecal microbiota from patients with IBS-D, but not the fecal microbiota from healthy controls, showed rapid GI transit, alterations in the intestinal barrier, and anxietylike behavior. Similarly, in a double-blind randomized controlled trial, the probiotic *Bifidobacterium longum* improved depression scores and quality of life in patients with IBS compared with placebo.[35] Interestingly, brain functional MRI studies performed before and after the intervention showed that *B longum* reduced responses to negative emotional stimuli in multiple brain areas, including the amygdala and frontolimbic regions, compared with placebo.[35] One way by which the gut microbiota could alter brain function and behavior is via short-chain fatty acids (SCFAs).[36] As an example, propionic acid produced by gut bacteria readily crosses the blood-brain barrier and influences brain function and behavior in animals.[36] Besides SCFAs, gut microbes such as *Lactobacillus* and *Bifidobacterium* can also generate γ-amino butyric acid (GABA), an inhibitory neurotransmitter in the human brain.[37] These studies highlight the important role of the gut microbiota and its metabolites in modulating the gut-brain axis.

## GUT MICROBIOTA AND VISCERAL HYPERSENSITIVITY

VH is defined as enhanced perception of mechanical triggers applied to the bowel, which is reflected clinically as pain and discomfort.[38] Using visceral distension models, the prevalence of VH in patients with IBS varies from 33% to 50%.[38] Evidence to suggest that the gut microbiome plays a key role in mediating VH includes the observation that probiotics and antibiotics alter VH. Verdu and colleagues[39] showed that antibiotics induce VH in mice, whereas *Lactobacillus paracasei* NCC2461 reduces VH. Similar effects of other probiotics, such as *L paracasei* and *Lactobacillus acidophilus* NCFM in normalizing stress-induced VH has also been shown.[40,41] Similarly, the poorly absorbed oral antibiotic rifaximin has been shown to normalize VH in chronic psychological stress rodent models by altering the composition of the ileal microbiota.[42] Furthermore, Crouzet and colleagues[43] recently showed that inoculation of GF mice with the fecal microbiota from patients with IBS induced VH to colorectal distention, whereas microbiota inoculation from healthy volunteers did not. The mechanisms by which the gut microbiome modulates VH in IBS are not well understood but might involve bacterial components such as lipopolysaccharide (LPS), bacterial products such as SCFAs, or gases such as hydrogen sulfide.[44–47]

## GUT MICROBIOTA AND GASTROINTESTINAL MOTILITY

GI motility requires complex coordination among neurons, interstitial cells of Cajal, and smooth muscle. Recent studies suggest an interdependent relationship between the gut microbiome and transit. Kashyap and colleagues[48] recently showed that introducing fecal microbiota from a healthy human into GF mice (humanized mice) altered GI transit and colonic contractility. The magnitude and directionality of this effect depended on the type of carbohydrates in the diet, suggesting that the diet plays a significant role in the microbial influence on the GI tract.[48] In contrast, the abundance of gut microbial communities was altered by changes in GI transit.[48] Accelerating or decelerating GI transit using polyethylene glycol or loperamide, respectively, led to differences in the gut microbiome that were reversed on return to a normal GI transit.[48] Gut microbiota and its metabolites can influence GI motility by either direct effects on enteric neurons or indirect effects on immune cells causing release of bioactive molecules. Bacterial metabolites such as SCFAs and deconjugated bile salts are known to generate potent motor responses in both animals and humans.[49,50] Similar to SCFAs, secondary metabolites from aromatic amino acids such as tryptamine have also been shown to increase contractility in ex vivo preparations of guinea pig ileum by stimulating serotonin release.[51] In contrast, methane produced by bacterial fermentation has been shown to reduce small intestinal transit.[13] Likewise, hydrogen sulfide, which is derived from sulfate-reducing bacteria, has also been shown to inhibit small intestinal and colonic contractility via potassium channels.[52] However, it is unclear whether luminal hydrogen sulfide overcomes the detoxification process present in colonic mucosa and what role (if any) it has in IBS. In addition to bacterial metabolites, bacterial components can also modulate gut motility. This process is best exemplified by LPS derived from gram-negative bacteria, which has been suggested to promote the survival of enteric nitrergic neurons that promote gut motility through Toll-like receptor (TLR) 4 signaling.[53]

## GUT MICROBIOTA AND INTESTINAL PERMEABILITY

The GI tract is a semipermeable barrier that allows the absorption of nutrients and immune sensing, while limiting the transport of potentially harmful antigens and microorganisms into the body. The gut barrier is impaired in several GI and non-GI diseases, including IBS. Gut barrier function has been shown to be impaired in about 40% of patients with IBS-D and those with postinfection IBS and seems to correlate with severity of IBS symptoms.[54–56] A recent study showed that up to 40% of patients with postinfection IBS have high fecal proteolytic activity, which in turn increases paracellular permeability by decreasing expression of the tight junction protein occludin, and redistributing occludin from tight junctions to cytosol, decreasing microbial diversity.[57]

The gut microbiome also plays a key role in the pathophysiology of diet-induced IBS symptoms. A diet high in fermentable oligosaccharides, disaccharides, monosaccharides, and polyols (FODMAPs) has been shown to cause intestinal barrier loss in rodent models through an LPS-TLR4 pathway that decreases colonic epithelial tight junction proteins.[44] Interestingly, patients with IBS have higher fecal LPS levels compared with heathy controls and studies have reported increased colonocyte expression of TLR4 receptor in biopsies from patients with IBS.[44] Another possible mechanism by which gut microbiota modulates gut barrier function is via SCFAs. Butyrate, a microbial-derived SCFA, helps maintain gut barrier function by increasing expression of tight junction proteins.[58] However, the role of butyrate or other SCFAs in IBS pathophysiology is not clear because most of the studies are descriptive, have conflicting data on SCFA levels in patients with IBS, have not accounted for confounding factors such as colon transit, and rely on fecal SCFA levels rather than luminal SCFAs (discussed later).

In addition to affecting tight junction proteins, the gut microbiota also regulates mucus production in the intestines. Intestinal mucus forms a barrier between the lumen and the epithelial cells, thereby protecting the epithelial surface from pathogens. Constituents of the microbiota that degrade mucin, such as *Ruminococcus torques*, *Ruminococcus gnavus*, and *Akkermansia muciniphila*, have been reported to be increased and their levels associated with severity of bowel symptoms in patients with IBS.[59,60]

## GUT MICROBIOME AND IMMUNE ACTIVATION

Mucosal immune activation underlying IBS has been an important area of investigation, with several studies showing low-grade inflammation and infiltration of inflammatory cells, notably mast cells, in the intestinal mucosa of patients with IBS. Mast cells express pattern recognition receptors, including TLR2 and TLR4. Increased levels of fecal LPS, serum LPS, and increased mucosal TLR4 expression have been observed in patients with IBS.[44,61,62] Increased levels of fecal and serum LPS in IBS can activate mast cells through TLR4, which in turn causes release of inflammatory mediators such as histamine, tryptase, and prostaglandin $E_2$. These mast cell mediators are increased in mucosa of patients with IBS and lead to barrier loss and VH, and thus may lead to symptom generation in IBS.

Studies have shown that the fecal microbiome of patients with postinfection IBS significantly differs from healthy controls, with increased Bacteroidetes phylum and decreased uncultured Clostridiales.[63] These microbiome changes were associated with mucosal expression of inflammatory cytokines such as interleukin (IL) 1β and IL-6.[63] Moreover, compared with healthy controls, patients with postinfection IBS have been found to have increased mucosal enteroendocrine cells, intraepithelial lymphocytes, and T lymphocytes in the lamina propria.[64,65] Taken together, these findings suggest that low-grade mucosal immune activation in response to microbiome perturbation plays a significant role in the pathophysiology of postinfection IBS.

Besides increased number of mucosal innate immune cells, levels of proinflammatory and antiinflammatory cytokines are also altered in patients with IBS. Several studies have shown an increase in proinflammatory cytokines (tumor necrosis factor-α, IL-1β, IL-6, IL-8) and a decrease in antiinflammatory cytokines such as IL-10.[59] Probiotics have been investigated given their ability to restore cytokine balance in rodent models.[59] In a randomized, double-blind, placebo-controlled, crossover study in older adults without GI symptoms, a probiotic containing *Lactobacillus gasseri* KS-13, *Bifidobacterium bifidum* G9-1, and *B longum* MM2 increased the levels of ex vivo antiinflammatory IL-10 production, possibly via increasing the levels of fecal *Bifidobacterium* and *Lactobacillus* and reducing the levels of *Escherichia coli*.[66] Similarly, a placebo-controlled, randomized controlled trial in patients with IBS showed that a 12-week course of *Bifidobacterium infantis* normalized the abnormal IL-10/IL-12 ratio seen in patients with IBS.[67] In addition to probiotics, bacterial metabolites of dietary nutrients have also been shown to be antiinflammatory. Butyrate produced by dietary fiber fermentation has an antiinflammatory effect, via inhibition of nuclear factor kappa-B and downstream proinflammatory cytokine production from colonic epithelial cells as well as inflammatory cells (such as mast cells).[68,69]

## ALTERATION OF MICROBIOME MEDIATORS AFFECTING GUT PHYSIOLOGY IN IRRITABLE BOWEL SYNDROME
### Tryptamine

Tryptamine is a tryptophan-derived monoamine that is abundant in human feces. Tryptamine concentrations increase nearly 200-fold in feces following colonization of GF mice with human gut microbiota, suggesting that bacterial metabolism of tryptophan generates luminal tryptamine.[70] Using in vitro and in vivo models, Bhattarai and colleagues[70] showed that tryptamine increases ionic flux across the colonic epithelium and increases fluid via 5-hydroxytryptamine receptor 4 (5-HT$_4$R) activation, which in turn accelerates colonic transit in mice. In another study, patients with IBS-D were found to have increased tryptamine levels compared with healthy controls.[71] Baseline colonic secretion was also increased in patients with IBS-D, suggesting either an inherent change in epithelial transport or an increase in metabolites that promote fluid secretion.[71] Application of tryptamine to colonic mucosal biopsies from healthy controls and patients with IBS-D also increased secretion in both groups to similar extents.[71] This finding indicates that the colonic epithelium of patients with IBS and healthy controls is capable of tryptamine-induced fluid secretion, and observed changes could thus be caused by changes in tryptamine abundance. Overall, it is possible that increased fecal tryptamine abundance leads to increased mucosal secretion in a subset of patients with IBS-D; however, this needs to be validated in larger studies.

### Short-Chain Fatty Acids

Several studies, including a meta-analysis, have shown decreased fecal levels of butyrate and propionate in the feces of patients with IBS-C and increased levels of butyrate in IBS-D.[72] However, the functional significance of these in vivo changes in fecal SCFA levels are not clear because most of these studies are observational. Moreover, the fermentation and production of SCFAs occur in the proximal colon and most of the SCFAs are absorbed rapidly by the colon epithelial cells, which means that the intestinal transit time affects the fecal SCFA levels.[73] The differences in the fecal levels of different SCFAs between the IBS subtypes may therefore be caused by differences in the intestinal transit time between these subtypes.[73]

### Lipopolysaccharide

In rodent models, a high-FODMAP diet led to the development of gram-negative dysbiosis and associated increased levels of fecal LPS. These changes were further shown to cause colonic barrier dysfunction, mast cell recruitment, and VH, findings seen in patients with IBS-D.[44] Translating these findings into human disease, patients with IBS-D had significantly increased fecal LPS levels compared with healthy controls, and LPS levels significantly decreased after introduction of a low-FODMAP diet.[44] In addition, intracolonic administration of fecal supernatants from patients with IBS-D induced VH in rodent models, which was reversed after a low-FODMAP diet or in the presence of an LPS antagonist.[44] This finding suggests fecal LPS plays a key role in VH induced by a high-FODMAP diet in patients with IBS-D. However, it is not clear whether this effect by LPS is mediated via direct stimulation of TLR4 receptor on enteric neurons or indirectly via activation of TLR4 receptors on mast cells (or other immune cells).

### Proteases

Fecal as well as mucosal proteolytic activity has been shown to be increased in patients with IBS-D.[74] However, it is not clear whether this increased proteolytic activity is derived from host and/or the microbiome. In a recent study, transplant of GF mice with feces from patients with IBS-D with high fecal proteolytic activity led to ineffective inhibition or, in some cases, an increase in fecal proteolytic activity compared with GF state.[57] This finding suggests either microbial production of proteases or decreased production of protease inhibitors such as siropins, miropins, or elafins in a subset of patients with IBS-D.[57] However, this needs to be further investigated in future studies.

## MICROBIOME-DIRECTED THERAPIES
### Prebiotics and Probiotics

Prebiotic are nondigestible food ingredients that stimulate the growth and/or activity of health-promoting bacteria (ie, *Lactobacillus* and *Bifidobacterium*). Most prebiotics are carbohydrates (eg, galacto-oligosaccharides, pyrodextrins, lactulose). A recent meta-analysis of prebiotics in IBS identified only 3 trials that met criteria for inclusion.[75] Two of the trials included in this meta-analysis assessed fructo-oligosaccharides and the third assessed trans-galacto-oligosaccharide.[76–78] Both of the fructo-oligosaccharide trials found no significant improvement compared with placebo, although there seemed to be a trend toward benefit with short-chain fructo-oligosaccharide in 1 of the trials.[76,77] In the third trial, 2 doses of trans-galacto-oligosaccharide were assessed for 4 weeks in 60 patients with IBS using a crossover design.[78] Both doses of trans-galacto-oligosaccharides showed significant improvement in global IBS symptoms but no effect on mean abdominal pain scores.[78] Given the paucity of data, a definitive conclusion on the efficacy of prebiotics in IBS cannot be made at this time.

Probiotics are organisms that confer a health benefit on the host. The popularity of probiotics has increased recently because of the interest in the role of the gut microbiome in health. However, data supporting the use of probiotics in IBS remain controversial because of the lack of large, multicenter, high-quality studies using rigorous end points and clinical outcomes. Although there are many trials with probiotics in IBS, few use the same strain of probiotic or the same combination of probiotics, thereby limiting the ability to pool the data from these studies and make definitive conclusions regarding their efficacy. A recent meta-analysis identified 37 trials using probiotics in IBS that met their entry criteria, which included 4403 subjects.[75] In this meta-analysis, trials that used combination probiotics (n = 21 trials) resulted in a significant pooled effect (relative risk, 0.79; confidence interval, 0.68–0.91) for global symptom improvement. Significant heterogeneity ($I^2$ = 72%) and publication bias were present in these trials, limiting the confidence in any recommendations that could be offered. In contrast, trials that used single probiotics (n = 16 trials) found no significant pooled effect, with the exception of *Escherichia* spp and *Streptococcus* spp, which did show a significant pooled effect. However, because there were few trials (2 trials with *Escherichia* spp and 1 with *Streptococcus faecium*), with small numbers of subjects (the trial with *Streptococcus* included only 34 subjects), no definitive conclusions could be made as to their efficacy.

A few of the larger, higher-quality trials with probiotics in patients with IBS are worth reviewing in detail. In 1 trial, 362 women with IBS were randomized to 3 different doses of B infantis 35624 ($10^6$, $10^8$, $10^{10}$ CFU/mL) or placebo for 4 weeks.[79] Only patients receiving the $10^8$-CFU/mL dose had significant improvement in the primary end point, which was abdominal pain or discomfort.[79] B infantis 35624 also improved bloating and bowel-related symptoms (eg, bowel dysfunction, straining). All subtypes of IBS seemed to benefit, although there was a trend toward greater efficacy in IBS-D.

In the second study, 379 patients with IBS were randomized to *Saccharomyces cerevisiae* I-3856 or placebo for 12 weeks.[80] A small numerical, but not statistically significant, improvement was present for the primary end point (32% vs 27%; P>.05), which was a greater than 50% reduction in intestinal pain/discomfort for at least 4 out of the last 8 weeks of the study.[80] There was a significant improvement in patients with IBS-C, which may be worth exploring further in the future.[80]

In the third trial, 298 patients with IBS were randomized to receive E coli DSM 17252 or placebo for 8 weeks.[81] A greater percentage of patients receiving E coli DSM 17252 reported improvement compared with placebo in the primary end points of abdominal pain score (19% vs 7% P<.05) and general symptom score (19% vs 5%; P<.05).[81]

Probiotics are a potentially important treatment; however, current data are limited and do not conclusively support their general use for IBS at this time. Recent guidelines by both the American College of Gastroenterology and the American Gastrointestinal Association recommend against the use of probiotics for treatment of

IBS.[82,83] Large, multicenter trials with rigorous end points, of at least 12 weeks' duration, are needed to make conclusions on efficacy of specific strains of probiotics.

## Antibiotics

Antibiotics, particularly nonabsorbable antibiotics, seem to improve symptoms in some patients with IBS. One of the first trials with antibiotics randomized 111 patients with IBS (Rome I criteria) with varying subtypes to receive neomycin or placebo.[84] Neomycin resulted in a 35% improvement in a composite score of IBS symptoms compared with 11.4% for placebo ($P<.05$).[84] Patients whose lactulose breath test for SIBO normalized following treatment with neomycin were significantly more likely to have improvement in symptoms compared with patients whose breath test did not normalize.

Rifaximin, a nonsystemic derivative of rifamycin, is by far the best studied and only US Food and Drug Administration (FDA)–approved antibiotic for the treatment of IBS.[85] Two identically designed phase III trials (TARGET 1 and 2, N = 1260) randomized patients with IBS without constipation according to ROME II criteria to receive rifaximin 550 mg 3 times a day for 2 weeks or placebo.[85] Patients were followed for an additional 10 weeks, although the primary end point was assessed during the 4 weeks after completion of the treatment. A significantly greater proportion of patients receiving rifaximin reported adequate relief of global IBS symptoms for at least 2 of the first 4 weeks after treatment (40.7% vs 31.7% for placebo, pooled; $P<.001$). In addition, a greater proportion of patients reported relief of IBS-related bloating (40.2% vs 30.3% for placebo, pooled; $P<.001$). Improvement compared with placebo persisted during the 10-week follow-up period, although overall efficacy decreased in both groups and was no longer statistically significantly different at the end of the follow-up period.

To answer questions of whether repeat treatment with rifaximin is effective and safe, a third phase III trial (TARGET 3) was conducted.[86] In this trial, 636 patients with IBS-D according to Rome III who responded to open-label rifaximin and developed recurrence of symptoms during an 18-week follow-up period were randomized to receive 2 courses of rifaximin 550 mg 3 times a day for 2 weeks or placebo separated by 6 weeks.[86] The primary end point was assessed during the 4 weeks after completion of the first retreatment. In total, 1074 patients with IBS-D were enrolled and received open-label rifaximin 550 mg 3 times a day for 2 weeks. Of these patients, 44% had a response to rifaximin; however, 64% (n = 692) of responders had a relapse of symptoms during the 18-week follow-up period and were randomized to receive double-blind rifaximin or placebo. A greater percentage of patients randomized to receive double-blind rifaximin were responders compared with those who received placebo (38% vs 32%; $P = .03$). Abdominal pain, but not stool consistency, was significantly improved with rifaximin versus placebo. Similar results were seen with the second retreatment. The results of this trial support repeat treatment with rifaximin after initial response to treatment, although it should be noted that the improvement compared with placebo was small, which may have been caused, at least in part, by the patients entering into the double-blind phase having lower symptom severity compared with their baseline before receiving open-label rifaximin.

In an effort to better understand the mechanism of action of rifaximin, a subset of patients (N = 93) in the TARGET 3 trial underwent lactulose hydrogen breath testing before and 4 weeks after completion of the initial, open-label treatment with rifaximin.[87] Among patients with a positive breath test at baseline, a greater percentage were responders to rifaximin than those with a negative test (60% vs 26%; $P = .002$). Moreover, patients whose breath test normalized after treatment had a response rate of nearly 77%. These results support the role of rifaximin in altering the microbiome potentially within the small intestine.

Importantly rifaximin seems to be well tolerated, with an adverse event rate in trials similar between rifaximin and placebo. Patients in the TARGET 3 trial showed no evidence of developing on-going bacterial resistance, nor did there seem to be significant alterations in the microbiome.[88] Likewise, side effects such as diarrhea or *Clostridium difficile* colitis were rare.[89] One case of *C difficile* colitis was reported in the TARGET 3 trial in a patient who was off rifaximin and had used interceding antibiotics. The American College of Gastroenterology guidelines on IBS supports the use of rifaximin to treat global symptoms in patients with IBS-D (strong recommendation; moderate level of evidence).

### Diet Modification

The microbiome is heavily influenced by the types of food that is eaten. Further, most patients with IBS report food to be a trigger of their symptoms.[90] Foods such as dairy, wheat, cabbage, caffeine, alcohol, onion, garlic, beans, spices, and fried food are commonly reported as triggers for symptoms in patients with IBS.[90] Not surprisingly, several diets have been studied in IBS. Two of the diets in particular, the low-FODMAP diet and, to a lesser extent, a gluten-free diet, have been studied in randomized controlled trials.[90] These studies are reviewed in detail in the Emily Haller and Kate Scarlata's article, "Diet Interventions for Irritable Bowel Syndrome (IBS): Separating the Wheat from the Chafe," in this issue.

### Fecal Microbiota Transplant

Fecal microbiota transplant (FMT) has been proved to be an effective treatment of recurrent *C difficile* colitis. In IBS, the data has been more mixed. Studies have used a variety of routes of administration (eg, oral capsule, nasojejunal infusion, and colonoscopy), formulations (eg, frozen, dried, and fresh), and number and type of donors. A recent meta-analysis of 5 randomized trials that included 267 patients with IBS found colonoscopy delivery of FMT to be effective, whereas nasojejunal tube delivery showed only a trend toward benefit, and oral capsules offered no benefit.[91] Subsequently, a large, single-center trial by El-Salhy and colleagues,[92] which included patients with IBS of all subtypes, assessed the efficacy of FMT (30 g and 60 g) delivered via a gastroscope into the distal duodenum versus placebo (autologous FMT). All FMT was acquired from a single so-called superdonor who was in excellent health (normal body mass index, on no medications, breastfed, healthy diet, and so forth) and had limited lifetime exposure to antibiotics. After 3 months, 76% in the 30-g FMT group and 89% in the 60-g FMT group were responders (as defined as a $\geq 50$ decrease in the IBS-symptom severity score) compared with 24% in patients receiving autologous FMT. Similar differences were present using the FDA and European Medicines Agency responder end points. The donor's microbiota profile was particularly richer than average in *Lactobacillus*, Lachnospiraceae, and Verrucomicrobia, and lower in *Shigella* and *Escherichia* spp. Whether this microbiota profile is important for response remains to be determined.

Another recent randomized placebo-controlled trial assessed the efficacy of FMT via nasojejunal infusion in 62 patients with refractory IBS (defined as failure of $\geq 3$ conventional therapies) of all subtypes with predominant bloating.[93] After 12 weeks, 56% of patients who received FMT reported improvement in both IBS symptoms scores and quality of life compared with 26% of patients receiving placebo ($P = .03$). No specific taxa were found in the stool of patients who responded to FMT, although responders had higher diversity of microbiomes before receiving FMT than

**Table 2**
Evidence supporting the role of microbiome in irritable bowel syndrome[a]

| Epidemiology | Several Studies Support IBS Can Be Precipitated by Acute Gastroenteritis |
|---|---|
| Diagnostics | Hydrogen breath tests are more commonly abnormal in IBS suggesting SIBO<br>Duodenal cultures more commonly grow coliforms in IBS suggesting SIBO<br>Stool microbiome analyses in several studies different from healthy controls<br>*M smithii* (and breath methane) increased in IBS-C |
| Translational studies | Gut-brain axis dysfunction, VH, barrier dysfunction can be transplanted in rodent models using feces from patients with IBS |
| Probiotics | Conflicting data on its efficacy in IBS. Available data are of low methodological quality and larger, multicenter, well-designed studies of at least 12-wk duration with rigorous end points are needed |
| Antibiotics | Nonabsorbable antibiotics show short-term benefit in patients with IBS without constipation. A higher proportion of initial responders to rifaximin have symptom improvement with retreatment compared with placebo |
| Diet | Restricting fermentable carbohydrates (known to modulate microbiome) causes symptomatic improvement in IBS |

[a] Modified from Pimentel et al.[113]

nonresponders. Importantly, 21% of patients who received FMT reported improvement in symptoms for longer than 1 year, compared with only 5% of patients who received placebo. A second FMT improved symptoms in 67% of patients who had an initial response but not in patients who did not respond initially to the FMT.

The potential risks of FMT need to be carefully examined in IBS. The study by El-Salhy and colleagues[92] reported adverse effects in 20% of the FMT group versus 2% in the autologous FMT group, including 2 patients who developed diverticulitis in the FMT group and none with diverticulitis in the autologous FMT group. Most side effects associated with FMT are mild and self-limiting. Severe side effects seem to be rare.[94] A recent report of antibiotic-resistant *E coli* bacteremia in 2 immunosuppressed patients, 1 of whom died, highlights the potential for serious complications with FMT.[95]

## SUMMARY

There is growing evidence supporting the role of the microbiome in the pathophysiology of IBS (**Table 2**). Studies show that an episode of gastroenteritis can trigger development of postinfection IBS. Observational studies have found that a significant proportion of patients with IBS have SIBO, as shown by abnormal breath test and/or small intestinal culture. Furthermore, studies show that a significant proportion of patients (if not all) with IBS show alterations in mucosal and fecal microbiome compared with healthy controls. Moreover, basic and translational studies suggest that microbial components/products can cause dysfunction of the gut-brain axis, visceral sensitivity, intestinal barrier, motility, intestinal secretion, and mucosal immune activation. In addition, several interventions targeting the gut microbiome, including prebiotics, probiotics, antibiotics, diet modification, and FMT, have opened up the potential for new treatments for patients with IBS that target the underlying cause rather than focusing only on improving symptoms. This article supports the concept that IBS is, at least in some patients, a microbiome-associated condition. If this is true, it opens the door to the development of novel therapies designed to modulate the gut microbiome. Future research is needed to identify the underlying mechanisms responsible for the link between the gut microbiome and IBS symptoms, develop biomarkers to identify the subset of patients with IBS with a microbiome-based cause of their gut symptoms, and develop and properly validate novel, efficacious therapies targeting the gut microbiome.

## CLINICS CARE POINTS

- A subset of patients with diarrhea-predominant IBS have small intestinal bacterial overgrowth and treatment often leads to symptom improvement.
- Constipation-predominant IBS can be associated with methanogenic Archaea and there is some evidence that treating constipated patients with increased breath methane levels with targeted antibiotics can improve constipation symptoms.
- Therapies targeting the microbiome such as prebiotics, probiotics, antibiotics, diet and fecal microbiota transplant can improve symptoms in subset of patients with IBS. Among these therapies, the best evidence is for gut-specific antibiotics such as Rifaximin and dietary interventions such as low FODMAP diet.

## REFERENCES

1. Eckburg PB, Bik EM, Bernstein CN, et al. Diversity of the human intestinal microbial flora. Science 2005;308(5728):1635–8.
2. Caporaso JG, Lauber CL, Costello EK, et al. Moving pictures of the human microbiome. Genome Biol 2011;12(5):R50.
3. Enck P, Aziz Q, Barbara G, et al. Irritable bowel syndrome. Nat Rev Dis Primers 2016;2:16014.
4. McKendrick MW, Read NW. Irritable bowel syndrome–post salmonella infection. J Infect 1994;29(1):1–3.
5. Chaudhary NA, Truelove SC. The irritable colon syndrome. A study of the clinical features, predisposing causes, and prognosis in 130 cases. Q J Med 1962;31:307–22.
6. Ghoshal UC, Gwee K-A. Post-infectious IBS, tropical sprue and small intestinal bacterial overgrowth: the missing link. Nat Rev Gastroenterol Hepatol 2017;14(7):435–41.
7. Klem F, Wadhwa A, Prokop LJ, et al. Prevalence, risk factors, and outcomes of irritable bowel syndrome after infectious enteritis: a systematic review and meta-analysis. Gastroenterology 2017;152(5):1042–54.e1.
8. Shah ED, Basseri RJ, Chong K, et al. Abnormal breath testing in IBS: a meta-analysis. Dig Dis Sci 2010;55(9):2441–9.
9. Ford AC, Spiegel BMR, Talley NJ, et al. Small intestinal bacterial overgrowth in irritable bowel syndrome: systematic review and meta-analysis. Clin Gastroenterol Hepatol 2009;7(12):1279–86.
10. Posserud I, Stotzer P-O, Björnsson ES, et al. Small intestinal bacterial overgrowth in patients with irritable bowel syndrome. Gut 2007;56(6):802–8.

11. Giamarellos-Bourboulis E, Tang J, Pyleris E, et al. Molecular assessment of differences in the duodenal microbiome in subjects with irritable bowel syndrome. Scand J Gastroenterol 2015;50(9):1076–87.

12. Gaci N, Borrel G, Tottey W, et al. Archaea and the human gut: new beginning of an old story. World J Gastroenterol 2014;20(43):16062–78.

13. Pimentel M, Lin HC, Enayati P, et al. Methane, a gas produced by enteric bacteria, slows intestinal transit and augments small intestinal contractile activity. Am J Physiol Gastrointest Liver Physiol 2006;290(6):G1089–95.

14. Konstantinos Triantafyllou CC, Pimentel M. Methanogens, methane and gastrointestinal motility. J Neurogastroenterol Motil 2014;20(1):31–40.

15. Suri J, Kataria R, Malik Z, et al. Elevated methane levels in small intestinal bacterial overgrowth suggests delayed small bowel and colonic transit. Medicine (Baltimore) 2018;97(21):e10554.

16. Chatterjee S, Park S, Low K, et al. The degree of breath methane production in IBS correlates with the severity of constipation. Am J Gastroenterol 2007;102(4):837–41.

17. Singh P, Duehren S, Katon J, et al. Breath methane does not correlate with constipation severity or bloating in patients with constipation. J Clin Gastroenterol 2019. https://doi.org/10.1097/MCG.0000000000001239.

18. Parthasarathy G, Chen J, Chen X, et al. Relationship between microbiota of the colonic mucosa vs feces and symptoms, colonic transit, and methane production in female patients with chronic constipation. Gastroenterology 2016;150(2):367–79.e1.

19. Pimentel M, Chang C, Chua KS, et al. Antibiotic treatment of constipation-predominant irritable bowel syndrome. Dig Dis Sci 2014;59(6):1278–85.

20. Jeffery IB, Das A, O'Herlihy E, et al. Differences in fecal microbiomes and metabolomes of people with vs without irritable bowel syndrome and bile acid malabsorption. Gastroenterology 2020;158(4):1016–28.e8.

21. Hugerth LW, Andreasson A, Talley NJ, et al. No distinct microbiome signature of irritable bowel syndrome found in a Swedish random population. Gut 2020;69(6):1076–84.

22. Pittayanon R, Lau JT, Yuan Y, et al. Gut microbiota in patients with irritable bowel syndrome-A systematic review. Gastroenterology 2019;157(1):97–108.

23. Tap J, Derrien M, Törnblom H, et al. Identification of an intestinal microbiota signature associated with severity of irritable bowel syndrome. Gastroenterology 2017;152(1):111–23.e8.

24. Carabotti M, Scirocco A, Maselli MA, et al. The gut-brain axis: interactions between enteric microbiota, central and enteric nervous systems. Ann Gastroenterol 2015;28(2):203–9.

25. Stilling RM, Dinan TG, Cryan JF. Microbial genes, brain & behaviour - epigenetic regulation of the gut-brain axis. Genes Brain Behav 2014;13(1):69–86.

26. Barbara G, Stanghellini V, Brandi G, et al. Interactions between commensal bacteria and gut sensorimotor function in health and disease. Am J Gastroenterol 2005;100(11):2560–8.

27. Clarke G, Grenham S, Scully P, et al. The microbiome-gut-brain axis during early life regulates the hippocampal serotonergic system in a sex-dependent manner. Mol Psychiatry 2013;18(6):666–73.

28. Diaz Heijtz R, Wang S, Anuar F, et al. Normal gut microbiota modulates brain development and behavior. Proc Natl Acad Sci U S A 2011;108(7):3047–52.

29. Neufeld KM, Kang N, Bienenstock J, et al. Reduced anxiety-like behavior and central neurochemical change in germ-free mice. Neurogastroenterol Motil 2011;23(3):255–64, e119.

30. Nishino R, Mikami K, Takahashi H, et al. Commensal microbiota modulate murine behaviors in a strictly contamination-free environment confirmed by culture-based methods. Neurogastroenterol Motil 2013;25(6):521–8.

31. Sudo N, Chida Y, Aiba Y, et al. Postnatal microbial colonization programs the hypothalamic–pituitary–adrenal system for stress response in mice. J Physiol 2004;558(Pt 1):263–75.

32. Engevik MA, Luck B, Visuthranukul C, et al. Human-derived bifidobacterium dentium modulates the mammalian serotonergic system and gut–brain axis. Cell Mol Gastroenterol Hepatol 2020;11(1):221–48.

33. Tillisch K, Labus J, Kilpatrick L, et al. Consumption of fermented milk product with probiotic modulates brain activity. Gastroenterology 2013;144(7): 1394–401, 1401.e1-4.

34. De Palma G, Lynch MDJ, Lu J, et al. Transplantation of fecal microbiota from patients with irritable bowel syndrome alters gut function and behavior in recipient mice. Sci Transl Med 2017;9(379).

35. Pinto-Sanchez MI, Hall GB, Ghajar K, et al. Probiotic bifidobacterium longum NCC3001 reduces depression scores and alters brain activity: a pilot study in patients with irritable bowel syndrome. Gastroenterology 2017;153(2): 448–59.e8.

36. Silva YP, Bernardi A, Frozza RL. The role of short-chain fatty acids from gut microbiota in gut-brain communication. Front Endocrinol (Lausanne) 2020;11:25.

37. Duranti S, Ruiz L, Lugli GA, et al. Bifidobacterium adolescentis as a key member of the human gut microbiota in the production of GABA. Sci Rep 2020;10(1): 14112.

38. Farzaei MH, Bahramsoltani R, Abdollahi M, et al. The role of visceral hypersensitivity in irritable bowel syndrome: pharmacological targets and novel treatments. J Neurogastroenterol Motil 2016;22(4):558–74.

39. Verdú EF, Bercik P, Verma-Gandhu M, et al. Specific probiotic therapy attenuates antibiotic induced visceral hypersensitivity in mice. Gut 2006;55(2):182–90.

40. Rousseaux C, Thuru X, Gelot A, et al. Lactobacillus acidophilus modulates intestinal pain and induces opioid and cannabinoid receptors. Nat Med 2007; 13(1):35–7.

41. Eutamene H, Lamine F, Chabo C, et al. Synergy between Lactobacillus paracasei and its bacterial products to counteract stress-induced gut permeability and sensitivity increase in rats. J Nutr 2007;137(8):1901–7.

42. Xu D, Gao J, Gillilland M, et al. Rifaximin alters intestinal bacteria and prevents stress-induced gut inflammation and visceral hyperalgesia in rats. Gastroenterology 2014;146(2):484–96.e4.

43. Crouzet L, Gaultier E, Del'Homme C, et al. The hypersensitivity to colonic distension of IBS patients can be transferred to rats through their fecal microbiota. Neurogastroenterol Motil 2013;25(4):e272–82.

44. Zhou S-Y, Gillilland M, Wu X, et al. FODMAP diet modulates visceral nociception by lipopolysaccharide-mediated intestinal inflammation and barrier dysfunction. J Clin Invest 2018;128(1):267–80.

45. Xu D, Wu X, Grabauskas G, et al. Butyrate-induced colonic hypersensitivity is mediated by mitogen-activated protein kinase activation in rat dorsal root ganglia. Gut 2013;62(10):1466–74.

46. Tsubota-Matsunami M, Noguchi Y, Okawa Y, et al. Colonic hydrogen sulfide-induced visceral pain and referred hyperalgesia involve activation of both Ca(v)3.2 and TRPA1 channels in mice. J Pharmacol Sci 2012;119(3):293–6.

47. Xu G-Y, Winston JH, Shenoy M, et al. The endogenous hydrogen sulfide producing enzyme cystathionine-beta synthase contributes to visceral hypersensitivity in a rat model of irritable bowel syndrome. Mol Pain 2009;5:44.

48. Kashyap PC, Marcobal A, Ursell LK, et al. Complex interactions among diet, gastrointestinal transit, and gut microbiota in humanized mice. Gastroenterology 2013;144(5):967–77.

49. Kamath PS, Phillips SF, Zinsmeister AR. Short-chain fatty acids stimulate ileal motility in humans. Gastroenterology 1988;95(6):1496–502.

50. Quigley EMM. Microflora modulation of motility. J Neurogastroenterol Motil 2011; 17(2):140–7.

51. Takaki M, Mawe GM, Barasch JM, et al. Physiological responses of guinea-pig myenteric neurons secondary to the release of endogenous serotonin by tryptamine. Neuroscience 1985;16(1):223–40.

52. Gallego D, Clavé P, Donovan J, et al. The gaseous mediator, hydrogen sulphide, inhibits in vitro motor patterns in the human, rat and mouse colon and jejunum. Neurogastroenterol Motil 2008;20(12):1306–16.

53. Anitha M, Vijay-Kumar M, Sitaraman SV, et al. Gut microbial products regulate murine gastrointestinal motility via Toll-like receptor 4 signaling. Gastroenterology 2012;143(4):1006–16.e4.

54. Singh P, Silvester J, Chen X, et al. Serum zonulin is elevated in IBS and correlates with stool frequency in IBS-D. United Eur Gastroenterol J 2019;7(5): 709–15.

55. Zhou Q, Zhang B, Verne GN. Intestinal membrane permeability and hypersensitivity in the irritable bowel syndrome. Pain 2009;146(1–2):41–6.

56. Mujagic Z, Ludidi S, Keszthelyi D, et al. Small intestinal permeability is increased in diarrhoea predominant IBS, while alterations in gastroduodenal permeability in all IBS subtypes are largely attributable to confounders. Aliment Pharmacol Ther 2014;40(3):288–97.

57. Edogawa S, Edwinson AL, Peters SA, et al. Serine proteases as luminal mediators of intestinal barrier dysfunction and symptom severity in IBS. Gut 2020; 69(1):62–73.

58. Peng L, Li Z-R, Green RS, et al. Butyrate enhances the intestinal barrier by facilitating tight junction assembly via activation of AMP-Activated Protein Kinase in Caco-2 Cell Monolayers. J Nutr 2009;139(9):1619–25.

59. Bhattarai Y, Muniz Pedrogo DA, Kashyap PC. Irritable bowel syndrome: a gut microbiota-related disorder? Am J Physiol Gastrointest Liver Physiol 2017; 312(1):G52–62.

60. Saulnier DM, Riehle K, Mistretta T-A, et al. Gastrointestinal microbiome signatures of pediatric patients with irritable bowel syndrome. Gastroenterology 2011;141(5):1782–91.

61. Belmonte L, Beutheu Youmba S, Bertiaux-Vandaële N, et al. Role of toll like receptors in irritable bowel syndrome: differential mucosal immune activation according to the disease subtype. PLoS One 2012;7(8):e42777.

62. Dlugosz A, Nowak P, D'Amato M, et al. Increased serum levels of lipopolysaccharide and antiflagellin antibodies in patients with diarrhea-predominant irritable bowel syndrome. Neurogastroenterol Motil 2015;27(12):1747–54.

63. Jalanka-Tuovinen J, Salojärvi J, Salonen A, et al. Faecal microbiota composition and host-microbe cross-talk following gastroenteritis and in postinfectious irritable bowel syndrome. Gut 2014;63(11):1737–45.

64. Spiller RC, Jenkins D, Thornley JP, et al. Increased rectal mucosal enteroendocrine cells, T lymphocytes, and increased gut permeability following acute Campylobacter enteritis and in post-dysenteric irritable bowel syndrome. Gut 2000;47(6):804–11.

65. Dunlop SP, Jenkins D, Neal KR, et al. Relative importance of enterochromaffin cell hyperplasia, anxiety, and depression in postinfectious IBS. Gastroenterology 2003;125(6):1651–9.

66. Spaiser SJ, Culpepper T, Nieves C, et al. Lactobacillus gasseri KS-13, Bifidobacterium bifidum G9-1, and Bifidobacterium longum MM-2 ingestion induces a less inflammatory cytokine profile and a potentially beneficial shift in gut microbiota in older adults: a randomized, double-blind, placebo-controlled, crossover study. J Am Coll Nutr 2015;34(6):459–69.

67. O'Mahony L, McCarthy J, Kelly P, et al. Lactobacillus and bifidobacterium in irritable bowel syndrome: symptom responses and relationship to cytokine profiles. Gastroenterology 2005;128(3):541–51.

68. Canani RB, Costanzo MD, Leone L, et al. Potential beneficial effects of butyrate in intestinal and extraintestinal diseases. World J Gastroenterol 2011;17(12): 1519–28.

69. Folkerts J, Stadhouders R, Redegeld FA, et al. Effect of dietary fiber and metabolites on mast cell activation and mast cell-associated diseases. Front Immunol 2018;9:1067.

70. Bhattarai Y, Williams BB, Battaglioli EJ, et al. Gut microbiota produced tryptamine activates an epithelial g-protein coupled receptor to increase colonic secretion. Cell Host Microbe 2018;23(6):775–85.e5.

71. Mars RAT, Yang Y, Ward T, et al. Longitudinal multi-omics reveals subset-specific mechanisms underlying irritable bowel syndrome. Cell 2020;182(6): 1460–73.e17.

72. Sun Q, Jia Q, Song L, et al. Alterations in fecal short-chain fatty acids in patients with irritable bowel syndrome: a systematic review and meta-analysis. Medicine (Baltimore) 2019;98(7):e14513.

73. Lewis SJ, Heaton KW. Increasing butyrate concentration in the distal colon by accelerating intestinal transit. Gut 1997;41(2):245–51.

74. Barbara G. Proteases in irritable bowel syndrome: a lot more than just digestive enzymes. Clin Gastroenterol Hepatol 2007;5(5):548–9.

75. Ford AC, Harris LA, Lacy BE, et al. Systematic review with meta-analysis: the efficacy of prebiotics, probiotics, synbiotics and antibiotics in irritable bowel syndrome. Aliment Pharmacol Ther 2018;48(10):1044–60.

76. Olesen M, Gudmand-Hoyer E. Efficacy, safety, and tolerability of fructooligosaccharides in the treatment of irritable bowel syndrome. Am J Clin Nutr 2000;72(6): 1570–5.

77. Azpiroz F, Dubray C, Bernalier-Donadille A, et al. Effects of scFOS on the composition of fecal microbiota and anxiety in patients with irritable bowel syndrome: a randomized, double blind, placebo controlled study. Neurogastroenterol Motil 2017;29(2).

78. Silk DBA, Davis A, Vulevic J, et al. Clinical trial: the effects of a trans-galactooligosaccharide prebiotic on faecal microbiota and symptoms in irritable bowel syndrome. Aliment Pharmacol Ther 2009;29(5):508–18.

79. Whorwell PJ, Altringer L, Morel J, et al. Efficacy of an encapsulated probiotic Bifidobacterium infantis 35624 in women with irritable bowel syndrome. Am J Gastroenterol 2006;101(7):1581–90.
80. Spiller R, Pélerin F, Cayzeele Decherf A, et al. Randomized double blind placebo-controlled trial of Saccharomyces cerevisiae CNCM I-3856 in irritable bowel syndrome: improvement in abdominal pain and bloating in those with predominant constipation. United Eur Gastroenterol J 2016;4(3):353–62.
81. Enck P, Zimmermann K, Menke G, et al. Randomized controlled treatment trial of irritable bowel syndrome with a probiotic E.-coli preparation (DSM17252) compared to placebo. Z Gastroenterol 2009;47(2):209–14.
82. Su GL, Ko CW, Bercik P, et al. AGA clinical practice guidelines on the role of probiotics in the management of gastrointestinal disorders. Gastroenterology 2020; 159(2):697–705.
83. Lacy BE, Pimentel M, Brenner DM, et al. ACG clinical guideline: management of irritable bowel syndrome. Am J Gastroenterol 2021;116(1):17–44.
84. Pimentel M, Chow EJ, Lin HC. Normalization of lactulose breath testing correlates with symptom improvement in irritable bowel syndrome. a double-blind, randomized, placebo-controlled study. Am J Gastroenterol 2003;98(2):412–9.
85. Pimentel M, Lembo A, Chey WD, et al. Rifaximin therapy for patients with irritable bowel syndrome without constipation. N Engl J Med 2011;364(1):22–32.
86. Lembo A, Pimentel M, Rao SS, et al. Repeat treatment with rifaximin is safe and effective in patients with diarrhea-predominant irritable bowel syndrome. Gastroenterology 2016;151(6):1113–21.
87. Rezaie A, Heimanson Z, McCallum R, et al. Lactulose breath testing as a predictor of response to rifaximin in patients with irritable bowel syndrome with Diarrhea. Am J Gastroenterol 2019;114(12):1886–93.
88. Fodor AA, Pimentel M, Chey WD, et al. Rifaximin is associated with modest, transient decreases in multiple taxa in the gut microbiota of patients with diarrhoea-predominant irritable bowel syndrome. Gut Microbes 2019;10(1): 22–33.
89. Schoenfeld P, Pimentel M, Chang L, et al. Safety and tolerability of rifaximin for the treatment of irritable bowel syndrome without constipation: a pooled analysis of randomised, double-blind, placebo-controlled trials. Aliment Pharmacol Ther 2014;39(10):1161–8.
90. Singh P, Nee J. Role of diet in diarrhea-predominant irritable bowel syndrome. J Clin Gastroenterol 2021;55(1):25–9.
91. Ianiro G, Eusebi LH, Black CJ, et al. Systematic review with meta-analysis: efficacy of faecal microbiota transplantation for the treatment of irritable bowel syndrome. Aliment Pharmacol Ther 2019;50(3):240–8.
92. El-Salhy M, Hatlebakk JG, Gilja OH, et al. Efficacy of faecal microbiota transplantation for patients with irritable bowel syndrome in a randomised, double-blind, placebo-controlled study. Gut 2020;69(5):859–67.
93. Holvoet T, Joossens M, Vázquez-Castellanos JF, et al. Fecal microbiota transplantation reduces symptoms in some patients with irritable bowel syndrome with predominant abdominal bloating: short- and long-term results from a placebo-controlled randomized trial. Gastroenterology 2020. https://doi.org/10.1053/j.gastro.2020.07.013.
94. Dailey FE, Turse EP, Daglilar E, et al. The dirty aspects of fecal microbiota transplantation: a review of its adverse effects and complications. Curr Opin Pharmacol 2019;49:29–33.

95. DeFilipp Z, Bloom PP, Torres Soto M, et al. Drug-Resistant E. coli Bacteremia Transmitted by Fecal Microbiota Transplant. N Engl J Med 2019;381(21): 2043–50.

96. Kerckhoffs APM, Samsom M, van der Rest ME, et al. Lower Bifidobacteria counts in both duodenal mucosa-associated and fecal microbiota in irritable bowel syndrome patients. World J Gastroenterol 2009;15(23):2887–92.

97. Kerckhoffs APM, Ben-Amor K, Samsom M, et al. Molecular analysis of faecal and duodenal samples reveals significantly higher prevalence and numbers of Pseudomonas aeruginosa in irritable bowel syndrome. J Med Microbiol 2011;60(Pt 2):236–45.

98. Codling C, O'Mahony L, Shanahan F, et al. A molecular analysis of fecal and mucosal bacterial communities in irritable bowel syndrome. Dig Dis Sci 2010; 55(2):392–7.

99. Ponnusamy K, Choi JN, Kim J, et al. Microbial community and metabolomic comparison of irritable bowel syndrome faeces. J Med Microbiol 2011;60(Pt 6):817–27.

100. Rajilić-Stojanović M, Biagi E, Heilig HGHJ, et al. Global and deep molecular analysis of microbiota signatures in fecal samples from patients with irritable bowel syndrome. Gastroenterology 2011;141(5):1792–801.

101. Carroll IM, Ringel-Kulka T, Siddle JP, et al. Alterations in composition and diversity of the intestinal microbiota in patients with diarrhea-predominant irritable bowel syndrome. Neurogastroenterol Motil 2012;24(6):521–30, e248.

102. Rangel I, Sundin J, Fuentes S, et al. The relationship between faecal-associated and mucosal-associated microbiota in irritable bowel syndrome patients and healthy subjects. Aliment Pharmacol Ther 2015;42(10):1211–21.

103. Maharshak N, Ringel Y, Katibian D, et al. Fecal and mucosa-associated intestinal microbiota in patients with diarrhea-predominant irritable bowel syndrome. Dig Dis Sci 2018;63(7):1890–9.

104. Vich Vila A, Imhann F, Collij V, et al. Gut microbiota composition and functional changes in inflammatory bowel disease and irritable bowel syndrome. Sci Transl Med 2018;10(472):eaap8914.

105. Dior M, Delagrèverie H, Duboc H, et al. Interplay between bile acid metabolism and microbiota in irritable bowel syndrome. Neurogastroenterol Motil 2016; 28(9):1330–40.

106. Chung C-S, Chang P-F, Liao C-H, et al. Differences of microbiota in small bowel and faeces between irritable bowel syndrome patients and healthy subjects. Scand J Gastroenterol 2016;51(4):410–9.

107. Chassard C, Dapoigny M, Scott KP, et al. Functional dysbiosis within the gut microbiota of patients with constipated-irritable bowel syndrome. Aliment Pharmacol Ther 2012;35(7):828–38.

108. Duboc H, Rainteau D, Rajca S, et al. Increase in fecal primary bile acids and dysbiosis in patients with diarrhea-predominant irritable bowel syndrome. Neurogastroenterol Motil 2012;24(6):513–20, e246-247.

109. Pozuelo M, Panda S, Santiago A, et al. Reduction of butyrate- and methane-producing microorganisms in patients with Irritable Bowel Syndrome. Sci Rep 2015;5:12693.

110. Ringel-Kulka T, Benson AK, Carroll IM, et al. Molecular characterization of the intestinal microbiota in patients with and without abdominal bloating. Am J Physiol Gastrointest Liver Physiol 2016;310(6):G417–26.

111. Shukla R, Ghoshal U, Dhole TN, et al. Fecal microbiota in patients with irritable bowel syndrome compared with healthy controls using real-time polymerase chain reaction: an evidence of dysbiosis. Dig Dis Sci 2015;60(10):2953–62.
112. Tana C, Umesaki Y, Imaoka A, et al. Altered profiles of intestinal microbiota and organic acids may be the origin of symptoms in irritable bowel syndrome. Neurogastroenterol Motil 2010;22(5):512–9, e114-115.
113. Pimentel M, Lembo A. Microbiome and its role in irritable bowel syndrome. Dig Dis Sci 2020;65(3):829–39.

# Making a Confident Diagnosis of Irritable Bowel Syndrome

Ryan S. Goldstein, MD, Brooks D. Cash, MD*

## KEYWORDS

• Irritable bowel syndrome • Diagnosis • Rome criteria • Alarm symptoms

## KEY POINTS

• Symptom-based criteria can facilitate the diagnosis and characterization of irritable bowel syndrome subtypes.
• Minimal laboratory or endoscopic testing is required to establish the diagnosis of irritable bowel syndrome.
• Alarm signs or symptoms, such as hematochezia or weight loss, in patients with irritable bowel syndrome symptoms should dictate appropriately directed diagnostic evaluation.

## INTRODUCTION

Irritable bowel syndrome (IBS) is a chronic functional gastrointestinal (GI) disorder with an incompletely understood etiology. IBS is not a condition that is limited to specialty gastroenterology practice. The prevalence of IBS in a typical primary care practices has been estimated to be 12% compared with 28% in a typical ambulatory gastroenterology setting.[1] A similar population prevalence of 11.2% was observed globally in a systematic review and meta-analysis of 80 population-based cross-sectional surveys.[2] Because there is no specific biomarker for IBS, the diagnosis of the condition can be confusing for clinicians. As a result, many practitioners consider a diagnosis of IBS one that requires exclusion of organic GI diseases. This exclusionary approach to the diagnosis of IBS contributes to the significant burden attributable to IBS on patients, health services, and payers.[3] Annual estimates of per-patient expenditures due to IBS in the United States range from $742 to $7547.[4] In a comprehensive assessment of the burden for GI illnesses in the United States, IBS was associated with $1.6 billion in direct and $19.2 billion in indirect costs.[5] IBS has such a negative impact

Gastroenterology, Hepatology and Nutrition, UT Health Science Center at Houston, 6431 Fannin Street, MSB 4.234, Houston, TX 77030, USA
* Corresponding author.
*E-mail address:* Brooks.D.Cash@uth.tmc.edu

Gastroenterol Clin N Am 50 (2021) 547–563
https://doi.org/10.1016/j.gtc.2021.03.004
0889-8553/21/© 2021 Elsevier Inc. All rights reserved.

on patient quality of life that many patients with IBS indicated that they would sacrifice 10 years to 15 years of their remaining life expectancy for an expeditious and effective remedy.[6] This article explores current recommendations for the diagnostic assessment of patients with suggestive IBS.

## DIAGNOSTIC CRITERIA FOR IRRITABLE BOWEL SYNDROME

The differential diagnosis in patients with symptoms of IBS is wide-ranging, and no reliable laboratory or radiographic biomarker exists for IBS. Over the past 50 years, there have been multiple attempts to simplify and standardize diagnostic criteria for IBS, including the Manning criteria and Rome criteria[7–11] (**Table 1**). The primary purpose for developing and validating symptom-based diagnostic criteria is to facilitate the achievement of a positive diagnosis of IBS and to minimize expensive and unnecessary diagnostic tests. The Manning criteria, proposed in 1978, had a positive predictive value for the diagnosis of IBS between 65% and 75%, depending on the number of symptoms present and the number of symptoms included.[7] The Manning criteria have been validated in several clinical studies[12,13] but are not used as widely as the Rome criteria.

In 1988, the Working Committee for the 13th International Congress of Gastroenterology meeting, held in Rome, Italy, created clinical criteria for IBS, ostensibly to guide patient selection for clinical research.[8] Over the past 3 decades, there have been numerous versions of the Rome criteria that have been refined through updated reviews of available literature and consensus among experts in the field. Since their inception, the Rome criteria have provided a standardized clinical definition for IBS and a consistent framework for selecting patients for clinical research. In 2006, the Rome III criteria were introduced and contained 2 notable changes compared with previous versions of the Rome criteria.[10] The first was the recommendation to classify IBS subtypes based on stool consistency rather than stool frequency. The second was the removal of bloating as a primary symptom of IBS, although bloating is a commonly reported symptom by patients ultimately diagnosed with IBS. A validation study of patients with IBS symptoms according to the Rome III criteria found them to have 68.8% sensitivity and 79.5% specificity for the diagnosis of IBS.[14]

The Rome IV criteria were published in June 2016 and were designed to represent a multicultural symptom-based diagnostic approach to IBS, reflecting the increasing agreement with, and influence of, the criteria in non-Western countries.[15] There are several notable changes from Rome III to Rome IV. The term, *abdominal discomfort*, was removed from the diagnostic criteria for Rome IV, because some languages do not have an English-equivalent word for discomfort and because of the vagueness of the word discomfort.[16] In addition, because of the frequently intermittent nature and severity of IBS symptoms for individual patients, the required frequency of abdominal pain was increased from 3 days per month to 1 day per week, on average. This change was based on a sizable population study performed to enhance the sensitivity and specificity of the Rome III criteria.[17] The Rome IV criteria also explicitly categorized IBS subtypes based on predominant bowel habits on days with abnormal bowel movements and not the percentage of total stools. The changes introduced in the Rome IV criteria increased the specificity of the symptom-based criteria and decreased the prevalence of IBS, when assessed through a multinational Internet survey, compared to the Rome III criteria.[18] Conversely, the prevalence of functional diarrhea and functional constipation increased with the Rome IV criteria, highlighting the importance and impact of the symptoms included in IBS diagnostic criteria.

**Table 1**
Symptom-based criteria for the diagnosis of irritable bowel syndrome

| Manning (1978)[7] | Rome I (1989)[8] | Rome II (1999)[9] | Rome III (2006)[10] | Rome IV (2016)[11] |
|---|---|---|---|---|
| Chronic or recurrent abdominal pain for at least 6 mo | >12 wk of continuous or recurrent symptoms of abdominal pain or discomfort: | >12 wk, which need not be consecutive, in the preceding 12 mo, of abdominal discomfort or pain with 2 or more of the following: | Recurrent abdominal pain or discomfort at least 3 d/mo in the last 3 mo associated with 2 or more of the following: | Recurrent abdominal pain, on average, at least 1 d/wk in the last 3 mo, associated with 2 or more of the following: |
| Abdominal pain with 2 or more of the following: | 1. Relieved with defecation | • Relieved with defecation | • Improvement with defecation | • Related to defecation |
| • Abdominal pain relieved by defecation | 2. Associated with change in frequency of stool or | • Onset associated with change in stool frequency | • Onset associated with a change in frequency of stool | • Associated with a change (in frequency of stool |
| • Looser stools with the onset of pain | 3. Associated with a change in consistency of stool | • Onset associated with a change in form (appearance) of stool | • Onset associated with a change in stool form (appearance) | • Associated with a change in stool form (appearance) |
| • More frequent stools with the onset of pain | Two or more of the following, at least on one-fourth of occasions or days: | | Criteria fulfilled for the last 3 mo with symptom onset at least 6 mo prior to diagnosis | Criteria fulfilled for the last 3 mo with symptom onset at least 6 mo prior to diagnosis |
| • Visible Abdominal distention | 1. Altered stool frequency | | | |
| • Passage of mucus in stools | 2. Altered stool form | | | |
| • Sensation of incomplete evacuation | 3. Passage of mucus | | | |
| | 4. Bloating or feeling of abdominal distention | | | |

According to the Rome III criteria, IBS patients can be classified as having predominant diarrhea (IBS-D), constipation (IBS-C), mixed diarrhea and constipation (IBS-M), and unsubtyped IBS (IBS-U) to facilitate the choice of symptomatic treatment.[10] In the Rome IV criteria, the IBS-C subtype applies when abnormal stools are hard/lumpy greater than or equal to 25% of the time and loose/watery less than 25% of the time. The criteria for the IBS-D subtype requires loose/watery stool greater than or equal to 25% of the time and hard/lumpy stool less than 25% of the time. For IBS-M, loose/watery stool and hard/lumpy stool are both present in greater than or equal to 25% abnormal stools. The IBS-U subtype is not widely encountered in clinical practice, but patients classified as IBS-U do not fulfill any of these stool form criteria.[15] These classifications, however, are subject to recall bias and reflect symptoms over a relatively fixed historical period, and switching from one IBS subtype to another over time has been widely reported.[19] In a prospective assessment of abnormal bowel habits of women with IBS, Drossman and colleagues[20] found that more than 75% moved to 1 of the other subtypes at least once over a 1-year period. Further complicating the extrapolation of the Rome criteria to routine primary care and GI clinical practice is the fact that IBS exists on a continuum with other disorders of gut-brain interaction, such as chronic idiopathic constipation, functional diarrhea, and functional bloating.[21]

## DIAGNOSTIC APPROACH TO IRRITABLE BOWEL SYNDROME

The diagnosis of IBS relies on a strong physician-patient relationship to serve as the foundation for an effective diagnosis and communication of realistic treatment expectations. During the clinical interview, it is important for the clinician to be an attentive listener and to offer an explanation of the pathophysiology and positive diagnosis of IBS as well as subsequent therapeutic strategies.[22] In 2009, the American College of Gastroenterology (ACG) IBS task force issued a position statement highlighting that no single symptom-based criteria offered perfect accuracy for the diagnosis of IBS.[23] Therefore, a diagnosis of IBS requires a thoughtful approach, using limited and appropriate diagnostic tests, and attentive follow-up to ensure the correct diagnosis. Diagnosis of IBS relies on 4 fundamental elements: (1) clinical history; (2) physical examination; (3) judicious laboratory testing involving stool, blood, tissue, or breath sampling; and (4) endoscopic evaluation when clinically indicated.

### Clinical History

In order to achieve a positive diagnosis of IBS, a detailed history is necessary to exclude alarm sign/symptoms suggestive of organic GI disease and to determine the subtype of IBS using the Bristol Stool Form Scale (BSFS).[24] The BSFS is a reliable marker for colonic transit time/water content and is the basis of the Rome IV criteria IBS subtypes.[24,25] For greatest BSFS accuracy, patients should be taken off medications that can alter their bowel habits and BSFS assessments should be done on those days. In addition to questioning patients about previous and current medication usage (antibiotics, proton pump inhibitors, nonsteroidal anti-inflammatory drugs, opiates, and angiotensin-converting enzyme inhibitors), special attention also should be directed to diet because many patients with IBS attribute their symptoms, especially diarrhea and abdominal pain, to food intolerances.[26] Diagnostic accuracy also can be enhanced by a psychosocial review, recognizing the frequent comorbidities of anxiety, depression, somatization, and physical or sexual abuse.[27]

Screening patients with IBS symptoms for the presence or absence of alarm signs/symptoms is recommended to identify patients at greatest risk for harboring organic disease as a cause for their abdominal symptoms and minimize delays in diagnosis. The ACG IBS task force specifies alarm signs/symptoms as follows: age greater than or equal to 50, unintentional weight loss, iron deficiency anemia, family history of inflammatory bowel disease (IBD), family history of colorectal cancer (CRC), family history of celiac disease (CD), hematochezia, or nocturnal diarrhea[23] (**Box 1**). In one study, Hammer and colleagues[28] investigated the significance of alarm signs/symptoms to predict organic diseases in patients with suspected IBS and found that IBS was identified correctly in 93% of cases with an absence of alarm signs/symptoms. When additional nonalarm symptoms and the Manning criteria were added, the diagnostic accuracy increased slightly to 96%.[28] More recently, Patel and colleagues[25] conducted a cross-sectional survey of patients with IBS symptoms undergoing colonoscopy and found a significantly higher prevalence of organic GI disease among those reporting alarm signs/symptoms (27.7%), compared with those not reporting alarm signs/symptoms (15.4%; $P = .002$). Therefore, when alarm signs/symptoms are reported, appropriately targeted diagnostic evaluations should be pursued.

## Physical Examination

A physical examination should be performed in every patient presenting with suspected IBS to exclude physical manifestations of organic diseases. A benign physical examination supports the symptom-based diagnosis of IBS, especially when accompanied by an absence of alarm signs/symptoms. Abnormal physical examination findings, such as an abdominal mass, lymphadenopathy, arthropathy, hepatosplenomegaly, or ascites, warrant additional evaluation.[29] The Carnett test can be a useful physical examination maneuver to identify patients with abdominal wall pain due to myofascial pain, cutaneous nerve entrapment, or radiculopathy.[30] Due to the potential for coexistence of disorders of rectal evacuation with IBS, digital rectal examination should be considered a crucial part of the physical examination of patients with IBS symptoms.[15] Patients with diarrhea admitting to episodes of fecal incontinence or patents with suspected pelvic floor dysfunction may require additional testing with endoscopic ultrasound, anorectal manometric examination, and/or specialized imaging.[29,31,32]

## Blood Testing

Blood tests, such as complete blood cell count (CBC), complete metabolic panel (CMP), and thyroid function test (TFT), and inflammatory markers, such as erythrocyte sedimentation rate (ESR) and C-reactive protein (CRP), are frequently obtained as part

---

**Box 1**
**Classic alarm signs/symptoms**

Age $\geq$ 50

Unintentional weight loss

Iron deficiency anemia

Family history of IBD

Family history of CRC

Family history of CD

Hematochezia

Nocturnal diarrhea

of the initial evaluation of patients with suspected IBS. Although these tests are relatively inexpensive and noninvasive, there is little evidence to suggest that their performance results in meaningful identification of organic disease and management changes in patients with suspected IBS who do not endorse alarm signs/symptoms. In a trial by Tolliver and colleagues,[33] CBC and serum chemistries performed in 196 patients with suspected IBS failed to identify organic disease in any patient. They did identify 1 out of 171 (0.6%) patients with suspected IBS who had an abnormal TSH, although it is unclear if the identified thyroid abnormality was found to be responsible for the IBS symptoms. Similarly, Cash and colleagues conducted one of the largest studies to date of the diagnostic yield of commonly obtained screening tests in patients with IBS symptoms and also found no significant increased yield of organic disease diagnoses based on the results of routine blood tests (CBC, CMP, TFT, ESR, and CRP) between a cohort of approximately 500 patients with nonconstipated IBS and 500 healthy controls.[34]

Many patients with IBS identify specific foods as the primary triggers for their symptoms and a significant proportion point to gluten-containing foods as their perceived source of their symptoms. Celiac disease is a chronic multisystem autoimmune disorder that induces a small bowel enteropathy due to an immune-mediated response to deamidated gliadin found in wheat, rye, and barley in genetically susceptible individuals.[35] The estimated global prevalence of CD based on serologic studies is approximately 1%[36,37] and in the United States the prevalence ranges from 0.40% to 0.95%.[38] There are disparate results from studies that have investigated the prevalence of CD among patients with IBS. Sanders and colleagues screened 300 consecutive new patients in the United Kingdom who met the Rome II IBS criteria versus a matched control group.[39] Using anti-endomysial antibodies (anti-EMAs) and serum IgA and IgG antigliadin antibodies with confirmational duodenal biopsies in serologically positive subjects, they identified CD in 14 (4.6%) patients with IBS symptoms, compared with only 2 (0.7%) among controls (odds ratio [OR] 7.0; $P$ = .004). In contrast, studies from North America have not identified an increased prevalence of CD among patients with IBS symptoms.[40] Cash and colleagues[41] found the same prevalence of biopsy-proven CD among patients with nonconstipated IBS compared with controls in a prospective study, although the patients with IBS symptoms were more likely than controls to have abnormal antigliadin antibodies. A 2017 meta-analysis of 36 studies found the prevalence of a positive serologic test for CD among patients with suspected IBS between 2.6% and 5.7%, whereas the biopsy-proved prevalence of CD was 3.3%.[42] This finding was comparable to a previous estimate from a 2009 meta-analysis, including 14 studies and 4202 patients, which found a 4-fold greater prevalence of CD among individuals with suspected IBS than controls.[43]

The recently updated ACG guidelines recommend serologic testing for CD with an IgA anti–tissue transglutaminase (anti-tTG) and quantitative serum IgA level (to exclude selective IgA deficiency) in patients with IBS symptoms and diarrhea.[44] Other guidelines recommend anti-tTG testing or anti-EMA testing be obtained for the diagnosis of CD, due to the high sensitivity and specificity of these tests.[45,46] The sensitivity of anti-tTG and anti-EMA tests may be reduced in people who maintain a gluten-free diet, an increasingly common scenario.[47] If a patient wishes to maintain a gluten-free diet, HLA-DQ2/DQ8 haplotype testing can be used to exclude CD as 99% of patients with CD will test positive for HLA-DQ2/DQ8.[48]

Among the various etiologies of IBS, de novo and persistent GI symptoms occurring after an enteric infection have been well described and termed postinfectious (PI-IBS).[49] The exact mechanisms responsible for the development of PI-IBS remain unknown, but investigators have shown that infectious gastroenteritis in animals and humans is associated with the development of circulating antibodies to cytolethal distending toxin B (CdtB) and vinculin.[50] Vinculin is an actin-binding protein, and it is hypothesized that anti-CdtB and anti-vinculin disrupt vinculin-mediated processes in the enteric nervous system to induce alterations in motility, contractility, epithelial barrier formation, and cell adhesion.[50,51] In a multicenter 2375-person validation study, Pimentel and colleagues[52] found that anti-vinculin and anti-CdtB were significantly higher in IBS-D subjects compared with healthy subjects, patients with IBD, or patients with CD. Based on their observations, a serum panel testing for anti-CdtB and anti-vinculin levels identified antibody thresholds that distinguished between IBS and IBD with a likelihood ratio of 5.2 for anti-CdtB and 2.0 for anti-vinculin. Similar likelihood ratios also were observed in a study of 30 patients in Mexico for distinguishing IBS from organic disease.[53] In the pivotal trial by Pimentel and colleagues,[52] however, the specificity for the diagnosis of IBS with each antibody was in the 80% to 90% range, with sensitivity less than 50%. A community-based study in Australia evaluated the ability of anti-CdtB and anti-vinculin to differentiate between patients with IBS-D, functional dyspepsia (FD), and organic disease and observed higher levels of anti-CdtB in patients with FD and IBS/FD overlap versus healthy controls, but there were no differences in anti-vinculin levels.[54] Based on accumulated evidence, the role of anti-CdtB and anti-vinculin testing in patients with IBS symptoms remains unclear and additional data are needed to determine if these tests can confidently distinguish between patients with IBS and other organic conditions.

## Stool Testing

Fecal calprotectin and fecal lactoferrin are stool neutrophil–derived markers released into the gut lumen in the presence of intestinal and colonic inflammation. In a systematic review and meta-analysis, Menees and colleagues[44] showed that CRP levels of less than or equal to 0.5 mg/dL or fecal calprotectin levels of less than or equal to 40 μg/g essentially excluded IBD in patients with IBS symptoms. These tests do appear to be helpful in excluding IBD in patients with suspected IBS but should not be used to rule-in IBS. Fecal lactoferrin has been shown to have a lower sensitivity and higher specificity than fecal calprotectin for distinguishing between IBD and IBS; however, it is not as widely available and not as widely studied in this clinical scenario. The recent ACG clinical guideline on the management of IBS recommends obtaining a CRP serologic test in combination with a fecal calprotectin test as a screen for IBD in patients presenting with symptoms of IBS.[55] It bears emphasizing that this recommendation does not apply to patients with alarm signs/symptoms, such as hematochezia or fistulas. It is common for patients with IBD to have a previous diagnosis of IBS, but alarm signs or symptoms should prompt appropriate endoscopic and/or radiologic evaluation.

Stool analysis for bacteria, ova, and parasites are widely available and frequently ordered by clinicians as part of the evaluation of patients with IBS symptoms, especially those with a diarrheal component. The updated ACG IBS guideline recommends against routine testing for bacterial or viral pathogens in patients with chronic IBS symptoms.[55] One reason for this recommendation is that GI infection with these organisms rarely causes chronic diarrhea. Additionally, antibiotic therapy has been identified as a possible risk factor for PI-IBS.[56] Tolliver and colleagues[33] performed stool ova and parasite examinations in 170 patients with suspected IBS and found none had evidence of enteric infection. Similar studies by Hamm and colleagues[57] found 1.7% (19 out of 1154) of patients with suspected IBS had an intestinal pathogen found on standard stool ova and parasite examination, with approximately half of those being colonized with *Blastocystis hominis*, a relatively common organism of unclear clinical significance.

Special consideration should be given to *Giardia lamblia*. This protozoan is found worldwide and in every region of the United States.[58] *G lamblia* is the most common parasite in adults with chronic diarrhea.[59] The infection typically lasts 2 weeks to 6 weeks in immunocompetent adults but can become chronic and can recur after treatment. Although *G lamblia* can be found in 5% to 7% of stool cultures in the United States, many individuals infected with *G lamblia* are asymptomatic, and the protozoan has been observed more frequently in the stool samples of asymptomatic individuals than among individuals with acute diarrheal illness.[60,61] Therefore, the pretest probability of *G lamblia* should be considered before ordering routine stool analysis. The 2019 American Gastroenterological Association (AGA) guidelines on chronic diarrhea and IBS-D recommend routine stool testing for *G lamblia*[62] whereas the recent ACG IBS guideline recommends stool evaluation for *G lamblia* only if there is a high pretest probability and definite risk factors for *G lamblia* exposure.[55]

### Testing for Bile Acid Malabsorption

Bile acid malabsorption (BAM) is thought to be a common cause of diarrhea in adults and may mirror IBS symptoms, with some studies estimating the prevalence of BAM in patients with IBS-D to be between 25% and 33% based on SeHCAT testing.[62–64] A recent 300-person observational study found a 38% prevalence of BAM in patients fulfilling Rome IV criteria for IBS-D.[65] The diagnosis of BAM can be challenging. The most definitive test is SeHCAT testing, a nuclear medicine procedure involving administration of selenium-labeled homocholyltaurine, a bile acid that is resistant to bacterial degradation or passive absorption by the small intestine. Whole-body retention is measured by means of gamma-camera scanning on days 1 and 7 to provide an indirect assessment of absorption and fecal excretion of bile acids. SeHCAT testing has a reported sensitivity of 89% and specificity of 100% for BAM as well as a dose-response relationship that has been demonstrated between the malabsorption severity and treatment success with bile acid sequestrants.[66,67] SeHCAT testing is not available in the United States, however, and its use in other countries is restricted due to the required infrastructure and time necessary to perform this testing.

Three other biomarkers currently are available to evaluate for BAM: (1) 48-hour stool collection with total bile acid measurement and the serum tests, (2) fasting serum FGF19, and (3) fasting serum $7\alpha$-hydroxy-4-cholesten-3-one (7-C4). Decreased serum FGF19 levels are associated with increased bile wasting and increased hepatic bile acid synthesis and a fasting FGF19 less than 145 pg/mL predicts a SeHCAT less than 10% with a negative predictive value of 82% and a positive predictive value of 61%.[68] As an alternative test, the bile acid precursor 7-C4 can be measured in the blood by high-performance liquid chromatography. Brydon and colleagues[69] evaluated SeHCAT and serum 7-C4 in 164 patients with chronic diarrhea and calculated that a 7-C4 level greater than 35 ng/mL has a positive predictive value of 74% and negative predictive value of 98% for SeHCAT 7-day retention of less than 10%. The current AGA guidelines on chronic diarrhea and IBS-D recommend testing for BAM (or empiric therapy if testing is not available)[62] and the recent ACG IBS guidelines do not address testing for BAM in patients with IBS.[55] Given the lack of broadly generalizable studies evaluating the yield of these diagnostic tests for BAM, they do not represent a standard of care at this time.

Some experts argue that a clinical response to an empiric trial of bile-acid sequestrants, such as cholestyramine, colestipol, and colesevelam is sufficient to diagnose BAM.[70] Although this may be considered by some to be a pragmatic approach, this course of action does not definitively establish BAM as a cause of IBS symptoms. In addition, many bile acid sequestrants are poorly tolerated and can interfere with the absorption and bioavailability of other medicines. Whether a diagnostic or an empiric trial is pursued, international consensus is clear that BAM should be considered in patients with IBS-D symptoms.[71,72]

### Breath Testing

Breath testing remains an important investigative tool for multiple GI symptoms and there are numerous testable substrates (glucose, fructose, lactose, lactulose, sucrose, inulin, sorbitol, and isomaltase) that can be used, depending on the symptoms being investigated and the suspected condition.[73] Currently the diagnoses for which breath testing is commonly employed in the setting of IBS symptoms are microbiota alterations, such as small intestinal bacterial overgrowth (SIBO), small intestinal methanogen overgrowth (SIMO), and carbohydrate maldigestion.

Small intestine bacterial overgrowth and SIMO have been implicated in the pathogenesis of IBS in multiple studies.[74–76] Although SIBO has been linked most commonly to IBS subtypes with a diarrheal component, SIMO has been linked to IBS-C. Methanogens are prokaryotic organisms belonging to the domain Archaea that produce methane as a metabolic byproduct in hypoxic conditions. Archaea are distinguished from true bacteria due to the non-peptidoglycan structure of their cell walls and their lack of nuclei and are thought to be among the most ancient life forms on Earth. There is wide heterogeneity among studies evaluating the prevalence of SIBO and SIMO in patients with IBS symptoms that can be explained in part due to the variation in clinical criteria used to diagnose IBS, differences in patient populations, and diversity of breath test substrates, techniques, and criteria used to diagnose these conditions. In a meta-analysis of 12 studies containing 1921 subjects meeting criteria for IBS, the pooled prevalence of a positive lactulose breath test was 54% (95% CI, 32%–76%), positive glucose breath test 31% (95% CI, 14%–50%), and positive jejunal aspirate and culture 4% (95% CI, 2%–9%). IBS patients were 3.3 times more likely to have an abnormal breath test than controls.[73] In another pooled meta-analysis, breath testing more often was abnormal among IBS subjects than healthy controls (OR 4.46; 95% CI, 1.69–11.80) and was able to distinguish the diagnosis of IBS with a sensitivity of 43.6% and specificity of 83.6%.[76] The gold standard for the diagnosis of SIBO remains a quantitative culture of small bowel aspirate of greater than $10^3$ colony-forming units/mL, but the practicality, cost, potential for oropharyngeal cross-contamination, and inability to culture the entire small bowel have led experts to favor breath tests using glucose or lactulose over small bowel aspirate to diagnose SIBO.[77,78]

Incomplete digestion of carbohydrates, such as lactose, fructose, sorbitol, and sucrose, can exacerbate and contribute to IBS symptoms. In a large population study of 2390 patients, Goebel-Stengel and colleagues[79] investigated the prevalence of symptomatic lactose and fructose maldigestion in patients with IBS-like symptoms based on Rome II criteria and found that 35% had lactose maldigestion, 64% had fructose maldigestion, and 25% had combined carbohydrate malabsorption. Corlew-Roath and Di Palma[80] found a similar incidence in carbohydrate maldigestion in patients with and without IBS. In a prospective European study, Beyerlein and colleagues[81] found that the risk and severity of symptoms were increased in IBS patients with positive hydrogen breath testing for lactose maldigestion. Yang and colleagues[82] were able to show that this risk also was related to the ingested dose of lactose. Current US IBS guidelines do not comment on routine breath testing in patients with IBS symptoms. Given the relative lack of breath testing capability outside of larger or academic gastroenterology practices, the wide availability of appropriate and standardized recommendations for lactose-restricted diets, and easy access to dairy-free substitutes or over-the-counter enzyme replacement therapy, breath testing to identify lactose maldigestion as part of the diagnosis of IBS cannot be recommended routinely.

A relatively recent concept in the differential diagnosis of adults with IBS symptoms is the possibility of sucrase-isomaltase deficiency (SID). This brush border enzyme is necessary to cleave the disaccharide sucrose into glucose and fructose, which then can be absorbed in the small intestine. SID can manifest as meal-related symptoms that mimic those of IBS. The current gold standard for diagnosing SID is quantitative disaccharidase testing from duodenal biopsies, requiring special handling and a reference laboratory. Sucrase maldigestion also can be diagnosed via $^{13}$C-sucrose breath testing.[83] The exact prevalence of SID in patients with IBS symptoms is unknown, although a recent small prospective pilot study using disaccharidase assays suggested that the prevalence of SID in patients with IBS-D and IBS-M symptoms was 35%.[84] Additional data from larger, prospective studies are required before routine testing to exclude SID in patients with IBS symptoms can be advocated.

### Lower Gastrointestinal Endoscopy

Colonoscopy frequently is used in the evaluation and management of patients with IBS. A national database analysis identified that 25% of all colonoscopes performed in the United States were for IBS-related symptoms and that 10% of all colonoscopies performed in patients under the age of 50 were for IBS symptoms.[85] The yield of colonoscopy as part of the diagnostic process in patients with typical IBS symptoms and absent alarm signs/symptoms is minimal and does not justify the risk or burden on patients or payers when considered in totality. In a prospective, multicenter, case-control study of 466 patients, Chey and colleagues[86] performed colonoscopy with rectosigmoid biopsies in patients with nonconstipated IBS symptoms and no alarm features. Colonoscopy did not alter the diagnosis of IBS in more than 98% (457/466). A notable exception from this study, which subsequently influenced clinical guidelines, was the prevalence of microscopic colitis in patients with IBS symptoms, which was 1.5% overall (7/466) and 2.3% (4/171) in patients greater than or equal to 45 years of age.

These findings were consistent with a randomized controlled trial by Begtrup and colleagues,[87] showing that a positive diagnostic strategy, based on the use of the Rome III criteria, CBC, and CRP, was noninferior to an exclusionary diagnostic strategy involving blood and stool tests and sigmoidoscopy with biopsies. Follow-up at 5 years demonstrated that that the positive diagnostic strategy delivered a durable IBS diagnosis in a majority of patients and was associated with significantly lower direct health care costs compared with the exclusionary strategy, including lower GI endoscopy and biopsy.[88] Similarly, Tolliver and colleagues[33] evaluated the yield of sigmoidoscopy, barium enema, and/or colonoscopy in 196 patients with IBS symptoms and found 2 patients (1.0%) with organic disease that could have caused their symptoms.

Similar to the diagnostic prevalence of IBS in patients eventually diagnosed with IBD, several studies have found that 28% to 33% of patients with microscopic colitis previously have been diagnosed with IBS.[89–91] There is controversy regarding the need for colonoscopy and right-sided colon biopsies to confidently exclude microscopic colitis.[92,93] A recent retrospective study by Bjørnbak and colleagues[94] concluded that biopsies from the left colon are sufficient to exclude microscopic colitis and reported that less than 2.5% of cases of microscopic colitis would have been missed if right colon biopsies were not obtained. In a meta-analysis of 10 studies,

Kamp and colleagues[95] found that the pooled prevalence of IBS in patients with microscopic colitis was 33.4%.

The accumulated evidence from these studies lends support for the recommendations of the ACG IBS task force to reserve colonoscopy in the evaluation of patients with IBS symptoms to those older than 45 years (primarily for the purpose of CRC screening) and those with alarm signs/symptoms suggestive of organic colorectal disease.[35] When colonoscopy is performed in patients with suspected IBS-D, it has been suggested that clinicians obtain random mucosal biopsies to rule out microscopic colitis, but the evidence supporting this suggestion is weak, and additional data are needed. Otherwise, routine lower GI endoscopy or radiographic imaging is not recommended to exclude organic disease in patients younger than 45 years of age with typical IBS symptoms and no alarm signs/symptoms.

## SUMMARY

Based on accumulated evidence, the development and subsequent refinement of symptom-based criteria have facilitated the appropriate initial diagnostic approach for the majority of patients with IBS symptoms. Despite the fact that the, diagnosis of IBS in clinical practice often occurs only after extensive diagnostic testing to exclude organic disease. One reason for this is the legitimate concern surrounding the possibility of a missed diagnosis as well as the emerging availability of additional tests and theories regarding the cause of IBS symptoms. The yield and role, however, for many of these emerging tests in the diagnostic process of IBS has yet to be established. Current best evidence supports a positive diagnosis of IBS based on fulfillment of clinical criteria and the absence of alarm signs/symptoms from the history, physical examination, and judicious use of diagnostic testing (**Fig. 1**). This approach is recommended in the recent ACG IBS management guidelines for improved cost-effectiveness and was anchored with a strong recommendation based on high-quality evidence. Such an approach is supported further by the stability of the diagnosis of IBS in multiple longitudinal follow-up studies, demonstrating that subsequent diagnosis of organic disease judged

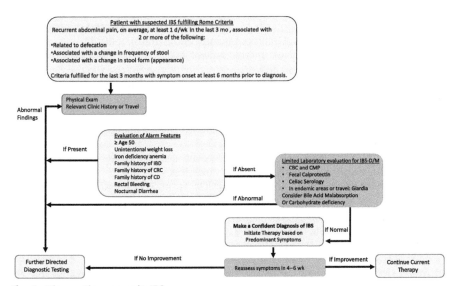

**Fig. 1.** Diagnostic process in IBS.

to be responsible for IBS symptoms is rare. The presence of alarm signs/symptoms should prompt an appropriate diagnostic evaluation directed by those signs/symptoms. Current recommendations support obtaining tests for CD and serum/stool markers of inflammation in patients with IBS symptoms, including diarrhea, and performing lower GI endoscopy with consideration of mucosal sampling in select patient populations. Additional evaluations, including radiography, breath testing, blood tests, and stool samples, have not shown sufficient diagnostic yield to be recommended in a blanket fashion for the evaluation of patients with IBS symptoms and should be individualized when there is an increased pretest probability of specific organic disease.

## CLINICS CARE POINTS

- Symptom-based criteria for diagnosing and characterizing IBS subtypes are sufficient for making the diagnosis of IBS in patients without alarm signs or symptoms.
- Minimal laboratory or endoscopic testing is needed to establish a diagnosis of IBS.
- Alarm signs and symptoms identified in patients with IBS symptoms should prompt additional diagnostic evaluation.

## DISCLOSURE

R.S. Goldstein has no disclosures. B.D. Cash has served a consultant and speaker for QOL Medical.

## REFERENCES

1. Creed F, Ratcliffe J, Fernandez L, et al. Health-related quality of life and health care costs in severe, refractory irritable bowel syndrome. Ann Intern Med 2001; 134(9 Pt 2):860–8.
2. Lovell RM, Ford AC. Global prevalence of and risk factors for irritable bowel syndrome: a meta-analysis. Clin Gastroenterol Hepatol 2012;10(7):712–21.
3. Canavan C, West J, Card T. Review article: the economic impact of the irritable bowel syndrome. Aliment Pharmacol Ther 2014;40(9):1023–34.
4. Sandler RS, Everhart JE, Donowitz M, et al. The burden of selected digestive diseases in the United States. Gastroenterology 2002;122(5):1500–11.
5. Sandler RS. Epidemiology of irritable bowel syndrome in the United States. Gastroenterology 1990;99(2):409–15.
6. Spiegel B, Harris L, Lucak S, et al. Developing valid and reliable health utilities in irritable bowel syndrome: results from the IBS PROOF Cohort. Am J Gastroenterol 2009;104(8):1984–91.
7. Manning AP, Thompson WG, Heaton KW, et al. Towards positive diagnosis of the irritable bowel. Br Med J 1978;2(6138):653–4.
8. Thompson WG, Dotewall G, Drossman DA, et al. Irritable bowel syndrome: guidelines for the diagnosis. Gastroenterol Int 1989;2:92–5.
9. Thompson WG, Longstreth GF, Drossman DA, et al. Functional bowel disorders and functional abdominal pain. Gut 1999;45(Suppl 2):1143–7.
10. Longstreth GF, Thompson WG, Chey WD, et al. Functional bowel disorders. Gastroenterology 2006;130(5):1480–91.
11. Drossman DA. Functional gastrointestinal disorders: history, pathophysiology, clinical features and Rome IV. Gastroenterology 2016;150:1262–79.
12. Jeong H, Lee HR, Yoo BC, et al. Manning criteria in irritable bowel syndrome: its diagnostic significance. Korean J Intern Med 1993;8(1):34–9.

13. Doğan UB, Unal S. Kruis scoring system and Manning's criteria in diagnosis of irritable bowel syndrome: is it better to use combined? Acta Gastroenterol Belg 1996;59(4):225–8.
14. Ford AC, Bercik P, Morgan DG, et al. Validation of the Rome III criteria for the diagnosis of irritable bowel syndrome in secondary care. Gastroenterology 2013;145(6):1262–70.
15. Mearin F, Lacy BE, Chang L, et al. Bowel disorders. Gastroenterology 2016;150: 1393–407.
16. Spiegel BM, Bolus R, Agarwal N, et al. Measuring symptoms in the irritable bowel syndrome: development of a framework for clinical trials. Aliment Pharmacol Ther 2010;32(10):1275–91.
17. Palsson OS, Whitehead WE, van Tilburg MA, et al. Rome IV diagnostic question-naires and tables for investigators and clinicians. Gastroenterology 2016;150: 1481–91.
18. Palsson OS, Whitehead W, Tornblom H, et al. Prevalence of Rome IV functional bowel disorders among adults in the Unites States, Canada, and the United Kingdom. Gastroenterology 2020;158:1262–73.
19. Garrigues V, Mearin F, Badía X, et al. Change over time of bowel habit in irritable bowel syndrome: a prospective, observational, 1-year follow-up study (RITMO study). Aliment Pharmacol Ther 2007;25(3):323–32.
20. Drossman DA, Morris CB, Hu Y, et al. A prospective assessment of bowel habit in irritable bowel syndrome in women: defining an alternator. Gastroenterology 2005;128(3):580–9.
21. Wong RK, Palsson OS, Turner MJ, et al. Inability of the Rome III criteria to distin-guish functional constipation from constipation-subtype irritable bowel syndrome. Am J Gastroenterol 2010;105(10):2228–34.
22. Owens DM, Nelson DK, Talley NJ. The irritable bowel syndrome: long-term prog-nosis and the physician-patient interaction. Ann Intern Med 1995;122(2):107–12.
23. Brandt LJ, Chey WD, Foxx-Orenstein AE, et al. An evidence-based position state-ment on the management of irritable bowel syndrome. Am J Gastroenterol 2009; 104(Suppl 1):S1–35.
24. Lewis SJ, Heaton KW. Stool form scale as a useful guide to intestinal transit time. Scand J Gastroenterol 1997;32:920–4.
25. Patel P, Bercik P, Morgan DG, et al. Prevalence of organic disease at colonos-copy in patients with symptoms compatible with irritable bowel syndrome: cross-sectional survey. Scand J Gastroenterol 2015;50(7):816–23.
26. Ford AC, Talley NJ, Veldhuyzen van Zanten SJ, et al. Will the history and physical examination help establish that irritable bowel syndrome is causing this patient's lower gastrointestinal tract symptoms? JAMA 2008;300(15):1793–805.
27. Sood R, Camilleri M, Gracie DJ, et al. enhancing diagnostic performance of symptom-based criteria for irritable bowel syndrome by additional history and limited diagnostic evaluation. Am J Gastroenterol 2016;111(10):1446–54.
28. Hammer J, Eslick GD, Howell SC, et al. Diagnostic yield of alarm features in irri-table bowel syndrome and functional dyspepsia. Gut 2004;53(5):666–72.
29. Ford AC, Lacy BE, Talley NJ. Irritable bowel syndrome. N Engl J Med 2017; 376(26):2566–78.
30. Kamboj AK, Hoversten P, Oxentenko AS. Chronic abdominal wall pain: a common yet overlooked etiology of chronic abdominal pain. Mayo Clin Proc 2019;94: 139–44.

31. Noelting J, Eaton JE, Choung RS, et al. The incidence rate and characteristics of clinically diagnosed defecatory disorders in the community. Neurogastroenterol Motil 2016;28(11):1690–7.
32. Brandler J, Camilleri M. Pretest and post-test probabilities of diagnoses of rectal evacuation disorders based on symptoms, rectal exam, and basic tests: a systematic review. Clin Gastroenterol Hepatol 2020;18(11):2479–90.
33. Tolliver BA, Herrera JL, DiPalma JA. Evaluation of patients who meet clinical criteria for irritable bowel syndrome. Am J Gastroenterol 1994;89(2):176–8.
34. Cash BD, Lee D, Riddle M, et al. Yield of diagnostic testing in patients with suspected irritable bowel syndrome (IBS): a prospective, US multicenter trial. Am J Gastroenterol 2008;103(Suppl 1):S462.
35. Tovoli F, Masi C, Guidetti E, et al. Clinical and diagnostic aspects of gluten related disorders. World J Clin Cases 2015;3(3):275–84.
36. Choung RS, Larson SA, Khaleghi S, et al. Prevalence and morbidity of undiagnosed celiac disease from a community-based study. Gastroenterology 2017; 152(4):830–9.
37. Rubio-Tapia A, Ludvigsson JF, Brantner TL, et al. The prevalence of celiac disease in the United States. Am J Gastroenterol 2012;107(10):1538–45.
38. Dubé C, Rostom A, Sy R, et al. The prevalence of celiac disease in average-risk and at-risk Western European populations: a systematic review. Gastroenterology 2005;128(4 Suppl 1):S57–67.
39. Sanders DS, Carter MJ, Hurlstone DP, et al. Association of adult coeliac disease with irritable bowel syndrome: a case-control study in patients fulfilling ROME II criteria referred to secondary care. Lancet 2001;358(9292):1504–8.
40. Almazar AE, Talley NJ, Larson JJ, et al. Celiac disease is uncommon in irritable bowel syndrome in the USA. Eur J Gastroenterol Hepatol 2018;30(2):149–54.
41. Cash BD, Rubenstein JH, Young PE, et al. The prevalence of celiac disease among patients with non-constipated irritable bowel syndrome is similar to controls. Gastroenterology 2011;141(4):1187–93.
42. Irvine AJ, Chey WD, Ford AC. Screening for celiac disease in irritable bowel syndrome: an updated systematic review and meta-analysis. Am J Gastroenterol 2017;112(1):65–76.
43. Ford AC, Chey WD, Talley NJ, et al. Yield of diagnostic tests for celiac disease in individuals with symptoms suggestive of irritable bowel syndrome: systematic review and meta-analysis. Arch Intern Med 2009;169(7):651–8.
44. Menees SB, Powell C, Kurlander J, et al. A meta-analysis of the utility of C-reactive protein, erythrocyte sedimentation rate, fecal calprotectin, and fecal lactoferrin to exclude inflammatory bowel disease in adults with IBS. Am J Gastroenterol 2015;110(3):444–54.
45. Rubio-Tapia A, Hill ID, Kelly CP, et al. ACG clinical guidelines: diagnosis and management of celiac disease. Am J Gastroenterol 2013;108(5):656–77.
46. Ludvigsson JF, Bai JC, Biagi F, et al. Diagnosis and management of adult coeliac disease: guidelines from the British Society of Gastroenterology. Gut 2014;63(8): 1210–28.
47. Niland B, Cash BD. Health benefits and adverse effects of a gluten-free diet in non-celiac disease patients. Gastroenterol Hepatol (N Y) 2018;14(2):82–91.
48. Lewis D, Haridy J, Newnham ED. Testing for coeliac disease. Aust Prescr 2017; 40(3):105–8.
49. Spiller R, Lam C. An update on post-infectious irritable bowel syndrome: role of genetics, immune activation, serotonin and altered microbiome. J Neurogastroenterol Motil 2012;18(3):258–68.

50. Pimentel M, Chatterjee S, Chang C, et al. A new rat model links two contemporary theories in irritable bowel syndrome. Dig Dis Sci 2008;53(4):982–9.
51. Pimentel M, Morales W, Pokkunuri V, et al. Autoimmunity links vinculin to the pathophysiology of chronic functional bowel changes following *Campylobacter jejuni* infection in a rat model. Dig Dis Sci 2015;60(5):1195–205.
52. Pimentel M, Morales W, Rezaie A, et al. Development and validation of a biomarker for diarrhea-predominant irritable bowel syndrome in human subjects. PLoS One 2015;10(5):e0126438.
53. Schmulson M, Balbuena R, Corona de Law C. Clinical experience with the use of anti-CdtB and anti-vinculin antibodies in patients with diarrhea in Mexico. Rev Gastroenterol Mex 2016;81(4):236–9.
54. Talley NJ, Holtmann G, Walker MM, et al. Circulating anti-cytolethal distending toxin b and anti-vinculin antibodies as biomarkers in community and healthcare populations with functional dyspepsia and irritable bowel syndrome. Clin Transl Gastroenterol 2019;10(7):e00064.
55. Lacy BE, Pimentel M, Brenner DM, et al. ACG clinical guideline: management of irritable bowel syndrome. Am J Gastroenterol 2021;116(1):17–44.
56. Klem F, Wadhwa A, Prokop LJ, et al. Prevalence, risk factors, and outcomes of irritable bowel syndrome after infectious enteritis: a systematic review and meta-analysis. Gastroenterology 2017;152(5):1042–54.
57. Hamm LR, Sorrells SC, Harding JP, et al. Additional investigations fail to alter the diagnosis of irritable bowel syndrome in subjects fulfilling the Rome criteria. Am J Gastroenterol 1999;94(5):1279–82.
58. Feng Y, Xiao L. Zoonotic potential and molecular epidemiology of Giardia species and giardiasis. Clin Microbiol Rev 2011;24(1):110–40.
59. Huang DB, White AC. An updated review on Cryptosporidium and Giardia. Gastroenterol Clin North Am 2006;35(2):291–314.
60. Ortega YR, Adam RD. Giardia: overview and update. Clin Infect Dis 1997;25(3): 545–50.
61. Muhsen K, Levine MM. A systematic review and meta-analysis of the association between Giardia lamblia and endemic pediatric diarrhea in developing countries. Clin Infect Dis 2012;55(Suppl 4):S271–93.
62. Smalley W, Falck-Ytter C, Carrasco-Labra A, et al. AGA clinical practice guidelines on the laboratory evaluation of functional diarrhea and diarrhea-predominant irritable bowel syndrome in adults (IBS-D). Gastroenterology 2019;157(3):851–4.
63. Slattery SA, Niaz O, Aziz Q, et al. Systematic review with meta-analysis: the prevalence of bile acid malabsorption in the irritable bowel syndrome with diarrhoea. Aliment Pharmacol Ther 2015;42(1):3–11.
64. Aziz I, Mumtaz S, Bholah H, et al. High prevalence of idiopathic bile acid diarrhea among patients with diarrhea-predominant irritable bowel syndrome based on Rome III Criteria. Clin Gastroenterol Hepatol 2015;13(9):1650–5.
65. Shiha MG, Ashgar Z, Fraser EM, et al. High prevalence of primary bile acid diarrhoea in patients with functional diarrhoea and irritable bowel syndrome-diarrhoea, based on Rome III and Rome IV criteria. EClinicalMedicine 2020;25: 100465.
66. Sciarretta G, Vicini G, Fagioli G, et al. Use of 23-selena-25-homocholyltaurine to detect bile acid malabsorption in patients with ileal dysfunction or diarrhea. Gastroenterology 1986;91(1):1–9.
67. Wedlake L, A'Hern R, Russell D, et al. Systematic review: the prevalence of idiopathic bile acid malabsorption as diagnosed by SeHCAT scanning in patients

with diarrhoea-predominant irritable bowel syndrome. Aliment Pharmacol Ther 2009;30(7):707–17.

68. Pattni SS, Brydon WG, Dew T, et al. Fibroblast growth factor 19 in patients with bile acid diarrhoea: a prospective comparison of FGF19 serum assay and SeH-CAT retention. Aliment Pharmacol Ther 2013;38(8):967–76.

69. Brydon WG, Nyhlin H, Eastwood MA, et al. Serum 7 alpha-hydroxy-4-cholesten-3-one and selenohomocholyltaurine (SeHCAT) whole body retention in the assessment of bile acid induced diarrhoea. Eur J Gastroenterol Hepatol 1996;8(2):117–23.

70. Carrasco-Labra A, Lytvyn L, Falck-Ytter Y, et al. AGA technical review on the evaluation of functional diarrhea and diarrhea-predominant irritable bowel syndrome in adults (IBS-D). Gastroenterology 2019;157(3):859–80.

71. Sadowski DC, Camilleri M, Chey WD, et al. Canadian Association of Gastroenterology clinical practice guideline on the management of bile acid diarrhea. Clin Gastroenterol Hepatol 2020;18(1):24–41.

72. Arasaradnam RP, Brown S, Forbes A, et al. Guidelines for the investigation of chronic diarrhoea in adults: British Society of Gastroenterology, 3rd edition. Gut 2018;67(8):1380–99.

73. Gasbarrini A, Corazza GR, Gasbarrini G, et al. Methodology and indications of H2-breath testing in gastrointestinal diseases: the Rome Consensus Conference. Aliment Pharmacol Ther 2009;29(Suppl 1):1–49.

74. Ghoshal UC, Shukla R, Ghoshal U, et al. The gut microbiota and irritable bowel syndrome: friend or foe? Int J Inflam 2012;2012:151085.

75. Ford AC, Spiegel BM, Talley NJ, et al. Small intestinal bacterial overgrowth in irritable bowel syndrome: systematic review and meta-analysis. Clin Gastroenterol Hepatol 2009;7(12):1279–86.

76. Shah ED, Basseri RJ, Chong K, et al. Abnormal breath testing in IBS: a meta-analysis. Dig Dis Sci 2010;55(9):2441–9.

77. Ghoshal UC. How to interpret hydrogen breath tests. J Neurogastroenterol Motil 2011;17(3):312–7.

78. Rezaie A, Buresi M, Lembo A, et al. Hydrogen and methane-based breath testing in gastrointestinal disorders: the North American consensus. Am J Gastroenterol 2017;112(5):775–84.

79. Goebel-Stengel M, Stengel A, Schmidtmann M, et al. Unclear abdominal discomfort: pivotal role of carbohydrate malabsorption. J Neurogastroenterol Motil 2014;20(2):228–35.

80. Corlew-Roath M, Di Palma JA. Clinical impact of identifying lactose maldigestion or fructose malabsorption in irritable bowel syndrome or other conditions. South Med J 2009;102(10):1010–2.

81. Beyerlein L, Pohl D, Delco F, et al. Correlation between symptoms developed after the oral ingestion of 50 g lactose and results of hydrogen breath testing for lactose intolerance. Aliment Pharmacol Ther 2008;27(8):659–65.

82. Yang J, Deng Y, Chu H, et al. Prevalence and presentation of lactose intolerance and effects on dairy product intake in healthy subjects and patients with irritable bowel syndrome. Clin Gastroenterol Hepatol 2013;11(3):262–8.e1.

83. Robayo-Torres CC, Opekun AR, Quezada-Calvillo R, et al. 13C-breath tests for sucrose digestion in congenital sucrase isomaltase-deficient and sacrosidase-supplemented patients. J Pediatr Gastroenterol Nutr 2009;48(4):412–8.

84. Kim SB, Calmet FH, Garrido J, et al. Sucrase-isomaltase deficiency as a potential masquerader in irritable bowel syndrome. Dig Dis Sci 2020;65(2):534–40.

85. Lieberman DA, Holub J, Eisen G, et al. Utilization of colonoscopy in the United States: results from a national consortium. Gastrointest Endosc 2005;62(6): 875–83.
86. Chey WD, Nojkov B, Rubenstein JH, et al. The yield of colonoscopy in patients with non-constipated irritable bowel syndrome: results from a prospective, controlled US trial. Am J Gastroenterol 2010;105(4):859–65.
87. Begtrup LM, Engsbro AL, Kjeldsen J, et al. A positive diagnostic strategy is non-inferior to a strategy of exclusion for patients with irritable bowel syndrome. Clin Gastroenterol Hepatol 2013;11(8):956–62.
88. Engsbro AL, Begtrup LM, Haastrup P, et al. A positive diagnostic strategy is safe and saves endoscopies in patients with irritable bowel syndrome: A five-year follow-up of a randomized controlled trial. Neurogastroenterol Motil 2020;33(3): e14004.
89. Limsui D, Pardi DS, Camilleri M, et al. Symptomatic overlap between irritable bowel syndrome and microscopic colitis. Inflamm Bowel Dis 2007;13(2):175–81.
90. Kao KT, Pedraza BA, McClune AC, et al. Microscopic colitis: a large retrospective analysis from a health maintenance organization experience. World J Gastroenterol 2009;15(25):3122–7.
91. Madisch A, Bethke B, Stolte M, et al. Is there an association of microscopic colitis and irritable bowel syndrome–a subgroup analysis of placebo-controlled trials World. J Gastroenterol 2005;11(41):6409.
92. Tanaka M, Mazzoleni G, Riddell RH. Distribution of collagenous colitis: utility of flexible sigmoidoscopy. Gut 1992;33(1):65–70.
93. Carpenter HA, Tremaine WJ, Batts KP, et al. Sequential histologic evaluations in collagenous colitis. Correlations with disease behavior and sampling strategy. Dig Dis Sci 1992;37(12):1903–9.
94. Bjørnbak C, Engel PJ, Nielsen PL, et al. Microscopic colitis: clinical findings, topography and persistence of histopathological subgroups. Aliment Pharmacol Ther 2011;34(10):1225–34.
95. Kamp EJ, Kane JS, Ford AC. Irritable bowel syndrome and microscopic colitis: a systematic review and meta-analysis. Clin Gastroenterol Hepatol 2016;14(5): 659-e55.

# Diet Interventions for Irritable Bowel Syndrome

## Separating the Wheat from the Chafe

Emily Haller, MS, RDN[a],*, Kate Scarlata, MPH, RDN[b]

## KEYWORDS

- Irritable bowel syndrome • Diet therapy • Nutrition • Gluten • Carbohydrates
- Histamine • Low FODMAP diet • Sucrase-isomaltase deficiency

## KEY POINTS

- As a heterogeneous condition, irritable bowel syndrome (IBS)-based diet therapy requires individualization.
- Consider IBS masqueraders or overlapping conditions that may prompt food intolerance in patients with IBS who are unresponsive to traditional therapies.
- The mechanisms responsible for food-related symptom induction in patients with IBS is multifactorial and, as yet, incompletely defined.

## INTRODUCTION

Individuals living with irritable bowel syndrome (IBS) have frequently identified food as a trigger to their digestive distress. In one survey study of nearly 200 patients with IBS, 84% perceived that eating any food would induce gastrointestinal (GI) symptoms. Carbohydrates were the most common food group identified as problematic in 70% of those surveyed, including dairy products (49%), beans/lentils (36%), apple (28%), flour (24%), and plum (23%), all potential fermentable, oligo-,di-mono-saccharide and polyol (FODMAP) carbohydrate sources. Interestingly, 58% of this cohort identified foods rich in histamine, such as wine/beer (31%), salami (22%), and cheese (20%), as prompting symptoms.[1]

Food can impact a variety of physiologic factors that are relevant to the pathogenesis of IBS, such as motility, visceral sensation, brain–gut interactions, microbiome, gut permeability, immune activation, and neuro-endocrine function.[2] To comprehend the intricacy of the relationship between food and gut symptoms in patients with IBS, it

[a] Division of Gastroenterology and Hepatology, Michigan Medicine, 3912 Taubman Center, 1500 East Medical Center Drive SPC, 5362, Ann Arbor, MI 48109-5362, USA; [b] For a Digestive Peace of Mind, LLC Medway, MA 02053, USA
* Corresponding author.
*E-mail address:* emilyhal@umich.edu
Twitter: @emilyhaller_rdn (E.H.); @KateScarlata_RD (K.S.)

Gastroenterol Clin N Am 50 (2021) 565–579
https://doi.org/10.1016/j.gtc.2021.03.005
0889-8553/21/© 2021 Elsevier Inc. All rights reserved.

is imperative to understand that food, in and of itself, is complex. Different components in a food can vary depending on a number of factors, including the ripeness and processing of food. These variables can impact the role of food intolerance. To further elucidate this concept, mechanically processing or separating fibers from grains will alter the particle size of the fiber. Larger particle size in insoluble fibers has been shown to enhance colonic mechanical irritation and laxation.[3] Ripeness can alter the nature of the carbohydrates in food; for example, unripe bananas are rich in resistant starch, whereas some varieties when ripened have greater amounts of fructans, a source of rapidly fermentable oligosaccharides, known to prompt GI distress in patients with IBS.[4,5]

Given that IBS is a heterogeneous condition and that the symptomology present in patients with IBS is common in other GI disorders, one needs to consider other potential overlapping or alternative diagnoses that may incite food intolerance, such as the connection between celiac disease and gluten or bile acid diarrhea and a high-fat diet. Gluten, a protein found in wheat, barley, and rye has been clearly identified as the trigger of immune activation and inflammation in celiac disease, but gluten's role in patients with IBS is less clear. Celiac disease occurs in approximately 1% of the population, but those who present with IBS-like symptoms appear to have an increased risk. A systematic review and meta-analysis showed a higher pooled prevalence of biopsy-proven celiac disease across all subtypes of IBS.[6] Moreover, more than 1/3 of Rome IV IBS-diarrhea or functional diarrhea have been shown to be experiencing primary bile acid diarrhea.[7] Once considered solely a pediatric condition, sucrase-isomaltase deficiency (SID) may be an IBS-D mimicker in adults. Adults presenting with genetic mutations related to congenital SID can present with IBS-D symptomology and have a greater likelihood of not responding to a low FODMAP diet (LFD).[8]

## THE COMPLEXITY OF WHEAT INTOLERANCE IN IRRITABLE BOWEL SYNDROME

Wheat, a type of grass plant, is second only to rice as the key food crop consumed by humans. The physiologic effects of wheat bran can be split into nutritional effects, mechanical effects (on the GI tract) and antioxidant effects via phytonutrients in wheat.[9]

Whole wheat provides a rich source of carbohydrates, including insoluble fiber (wheat bran) and soluble fibers such as rapidly fermentable fructans. The various components in wheat have the potential to elicit different food intolerance symptom responses in those with IBS.[10]

Wheat-based fructans have been identified as part of the short-chain, rapidly fermentable carbohydrate family, coined FODMAPs. FODMAPs are found in many everyday foods and can prompt GI symptoms via their osmotic or fermentation effects in the gut.[11] Gluten, amylose trypsin inhibitors (ATIs), and other proteins present in grains, including wheat, barley, and rye, also may incite GI symptoms. ATIs found in higher levels in wheat and other gluten-containing cereals activate an innate immune response in mice and increase intestinal inflammation.[12] The potential role of ATIs in humans with IBS remains to be explored.

The use of novel confocal laser endomicroscopy (CLE), an endoscopic imaging tool that enables a high-resolution assessment of GI mucosal histology at a cellular and subcellular level, allowing identification of changes such as increased intraepithelial immune cells, epithelial leaks/gaps, and widened intervillous spaces that can be observed in real time, has revealed interesting data in patients with IBS. CLE research has uncovered that an atypical allergy to wheat and to a lesser degree with yeast, may be present in some individuals with IBS. Fritscher-Ravens and colleagues[13] used CLE to assess food sensitivity in patients with IBS and found a significant proportion reacted to wheat and then felt better on a wheat-free diet. Seventy-six (70%) of 109 patients with IBS reacted to 1 of 5 tested food antigen mixtures (CLE+) delivered to the duodenal mucosa: wheat (61%), yeast (20%), milk (9.2%), soy (6.6%), or egg white (4%). CLE+ patients experienced immediate changes in tight junction proteins including increases in expression of claudin-2, decreases in occludin, as well as increased eosinophil degranulation. The researchers postulate these CLE+ patients with IBS have a form of non–immunoglobulin (Ig)E-mediated atypical food allergy that involves enhanced eosinophil and intraepithelial lymphocyte activation. When food antigens that elicited a positive CLE response were excluded from the diet, patients demonstrated a 70% average improvement in Francis IBS severity score after 3 months and a 76% improvement at 6 months. Impressively, 68% of CLE+ patients showed at least an 80% improvement in symptoms, whereas only 4% did not respond at all.[13] This innovative research using CLE highlights that some patients with IBS may be experiencing epithelial dysfunction due to atypical food allergy. Two recent publications of CLE in patients with IBS suggest the potential use of this technology to identify atypical food allergy and guide specific food elimination diets.[13,14]

When all of these data are taken into consideration, it is clear that wheat is complex and contains several compounds that could produce a symptomatic response in patients with IBS, see **Table 1**.

## GLUTEN INTOLERANCE IN IRRITABLE BOWEL SYNDROME

Both the popularity of following a gluten-free diet (GFD) and the market for gluten-free products have increased at astounding rates. Kim and colleagues[17] analyzed data from the National Health and Nutrition Examination Surveys (NHANES) 2009 to 2014 and found the prevalence of celiac disease remained steady while the self-reported adherence to a GFD among individuals without celiac disease increased over the same period. Based on their findings, approximately 2.7 million people adhere to a GFD without a celiac disease diagnosis. Self-reported wheat sensitivity is associated with functional gastrointestinal disorders, including IBS.[18] It appears that many individuals are gravitating toward a GFD because they believe it is healthier for them or that it could lessen their GI symptoms. It should be noted there is no evidence that a GFD is healthier than a gluten-containing diet. In fact, many gluten-free products, such as crackers, breads, and snack foods, are devoid of the enrichment of key nutrients, such as iron, thiamin, riboflavin, and folic acid found in their enriched wheat-based counterparts.[19]

The data supporting a GFD for those with IBS are lacking, yet there may be benefit in an unclear proportion of patients. A 2018 systematic review and meta-analysis of randomized controlled trials (RCTs) assessing the impact of a GFD or LFD in improving IBS symptoms found insufficient evidence to recommend a GFD to reduce IBS symptoms.[20] There were only 2 RCTs looking at a GFD that met the inclusion criteria for this meta-analysis. Participants in both trials who had their diets spiked with gluten had increased IBS symptoms compared with those who remained on a GFD. Each study had separately reported a statistically significant result, but the significance was lost when results were pooled due to the marked heterogeneity between individual trial results.[20] A recent prospective study demonstrated patients with IBS who tested positive for deamidated antigliadin antibodies (AGA+), IgG and IgA, experienced greater GI symptom improvement (75%) on a GFD than those who were without the antibodies (AGA−) (38%). After adhering to a GFD for 4 weeks, GI symptoms improved overall in AGA+ patients with IBS, specifically constipation ($P$ = .01), diarrhea

**Table 1**
**The complexity of wheat and GI symptom induction in IBS**

| Component of Wheat | Definition | Pathomechanism for GI Symptom Induction in IBS |
|---|---|---|
| Gluten | A family of proteins found in wheat, as well as other grains including rye and barley. Gluten is composed of gliadins and glutenins in wheat, secalins in rye and hordeins in barley. | Alters bowel barrier function and/or leads to increased stool frequency, particularly in HLA-DQ2/8–positive patients.[15–17] |
| Fructan | A polymer of fructose molecules found in wheat, as well as other grains including rye and barely. | Microbial fermentation of fructans gives rise to gas in the colon, contributing to luminal distention. Although the gas production is normal, those with IBS may experience an exaggerated symptom response of discomfort, pain, bloating due to visceral hypersensitivity.[11] |
| Amylase trypsin inhibitors | Proteins found in wheat as well as other grains including rye and barely. | Increases intestinal inflammation via activating toll-like receptor 4 (TLR4) on myeloid cells in the intestine of mice.[15] Studies lacking in humans. |
| Wheat-germ agglutinin | A protein found in wheat. | May initiate an inflammatory immune reaction in the gut.[16] |
| Wheat bran | An insoluble fiber found in wheat. | Large particle wheat bran mechanically stimulates/irritates the gut mucosa which increases fecal mass and colonic transit rate. Fermentable fiber. Shown to be ineffective at normalizing bowel habits in patients with IBS as well as increase bloating, gas, and pain.[3] |
| Wheat protein | Four classes of proteins found in wheat (albumin, globulin, gliadin, glutenin). | IGE allergy or atypical allergy noted via CLE in patients with IBS.[13,14] |

*Abbreviations:* CLE, confocal laser endomicroscopy; GI, gastrointestinal; IBS, irritable bowel syndrome; IGE, Immunoglobulin E.

($P$ = .001), and abdominal pain ($P$<.001), whereas AGA− patients with IBS experienced improvements only in abdominal pain ($P$ = .01). There were limitations to this trial, however, as it was a small study and participants were not blinded to the GFD intervention.[21] Larger studies are needed to validate the usefulness of AGA as a potential marker to identify a subgroup of patients with IBS who may benefit from a GFD.

## IS IT GLUTEN OR FRUCTAN INTOLERANCE?

When one goes on a GFD, eliminating wheat, rye, and barely, gluten is not the only food component that is removed from the diet. Fructans, also present in these grains, are reduced on a GFD and thus may be responsible for symptom improvement. A double-blind, placebo-controlled (DBPC) study in participants with self-reported gluten sensitivity found fructans were more likely to induce symptoms than gluten. IBS symptom scores, both overall and for bloating, were higher with fructans compared with gluten. Surprisingly, only 13 of 59 participants had their highest symptom score after the gluten challenge, whereas 27 participants had their lowest symptom score after the gluten challenge.[22] These data support that fructans are a more likely culprit than gluten. Research by Biesiekierski and colleagues[23] further substantiates that the presence of fructans in wheat drives IBS symptoms and not gluten. In a placebo-controlled, crossover rechallenge study, patients who habitually consumed a GFD diet experienced symptom relief with FODMAP reduction and did not have specific or dose-dependent reactions with gluten challenges. In this same cohort of patients, elevated biomarkers of intestinal injury were found in patients on a self-selected GFD and improved once they reduced their FODMAP intake. In addition, the reintroduction of gluten at various dosages did not negatively influence markers of intestinal epithelial injury and barrier function.[24]

## THE POWER OF THE PLACEBO AND NOCEBO EFFECT

The placebo and nocebo effect cannot be overlooked, especially in a patient population such as IBS that has demonstrated high rates of the placebo effect, ranging from 16.0% to 71.4%, with a pooled placebo response of 40.2%.[25] On social media and in alternative medicine clinics, gluten is often promoted as inflammatory or toxic; this perception could play a role in the nocebo response often found in clinical trials involving patients with IBS who believe they are gluten sensitive. An eye-opening systematic review by Molina-Infante and Carroccio[26] found 80% of patients with suspected non-celiac gluten sensitivity cannot be diagnosed formally after a DBPC crossover gluten challenge and revealed that 40% of patients undergoing a DBPC challenge showed a nocebo response.

## LEVERAGING BIOMARKERS TO PREDICT RESPONSE TO DIET IN IRRITABLE BOWEL SYNDROME

Using biomarkers to help predict those who might benefit from the LFD is highly desirable, as this would reduce the overuse of a complex elimination diet while selecting patients who are the most likely to respond to this diet intervention.

A potentially promising area for the development of biomarkers is the gut microbiome and/or metabolome. An exciting exploratory study found fecal volatile organic compounds (VOC) profiling was able to predict response to an LFD and a probiotic intervention.

Rossi and colleagues[27] found 15 VOC profile features that classified response to an LFD with a mean accuracy of 97% (95% confidence interval [CI] 96%–99%). This study highlighted a noninvasive, cost-effective tool may be a promising method to help predict response to diet interventions in those with IBS. In addition, several studies have identified characteristics of the microbiome or metabolome that predict a greater likelihood of response to the LFD. Children who responded to the LFD were at baseline enriched in *Bacteroides,* Ruminococcaceae, *Faecalibacterium prausnitzii*, taxa with known saccharolytic metabolic capacity.[28] Adult patients with IBS demonstrated distinct differences in bacterial DNA profiles between responders and nonresponders to the LFD.[29] Bennet and colleagues[30] demonstrated fecal bacterial profiles from stools collected before starting the LFD were able to discriminate responders from nonresponders.

Food sensitivity testing using IgG antibodies to various foods in patients with IBS lacks proper validation in methodologically rigorous RCTs.[31,32] Despite their lack of validation, food sensitivity tests are quite popular, often recommended by functional practitioners, and can be costly to patients with limited coverage via health insurance. Several major medical organizations including the American Academy of Allergy, Asthma & Immunology, the Canadian Society of Allergy and Clinical Immunology, and the European Academy of Allergy and Clinical Immunology recommend against using IgG testing to diagnose food allergies or food intolerances/sensitivities due to the lack of evidence to support their use.[33] Furthermore, food-specific serum IgG levels have been proposed to reflect exposure to food components versus an intolerance or hypersensitivity.[34] Patients often present to clinic with questions regarding food sensitivity testing or with results from a test they have previously taken. It is important to have a thorough discussion with patients regarding the lack of evidence behind their use and the risks of "false positives," which ultimately lead to unnecessary food avoidance and escalation of food fears. Studies on IgG-based food sensitivity testing are ongoing and will hopefully shed light on whether these tests offer any benefit to patients with IBS.

An RCT of 58 patients with IBS found that a 4-week exclusion diet guided by leukocyte activation testing (LAT) led to significant global improvement and decreased symptom severity compared with a matched comparison diet. It should be noted that several of the foods (apple, onion, pear, and chickpea) removed based on LAT are high in FODMAPs, which may have contributed to the symptom reduction experienced by those in the intervention arm. Although the results are compelling, a larger trial is needed to assess the usefulness of LAT in guiding elimination diets for those with IBS.[35]

The Lifestyle Eating and Performance Mediator Release Test (LEAP MRT) is another commercially available food sensitivity test that lacks validation. There is currently no published, peer-reviewed research to support the anecdotal claims that MRT can identify potential food sensitivities in those with IBS.

## LOW FERMENTABLE, OLIGO-,DI-MONO-SACCHARIDE AND POLYOL DIET AND IRRITABLE BOWEL SYNDROME

For years, patients with IBS have identified food as a trigger for their GI symptoms, but the medical community had little to offer in terms of diet interventions. The LFD emerged in the literature in 2005, and through ongoing research has validated a connection between diet and IBS symptom induction. Pioneered by Monash University researchers, FODMAPs were first *speculated* as a potential link to diet-induced changes in small bowel ecology and injurious effects on the colonic epithelium with increases in intestinal permeability, potentially predisposing one to IBD.[36] The LFD is done in 3 phases and ideally, should be administered by a trained GI dietitian, see **Fig. 1**. Gibson and colleagues[37] continue to hypothesize that hyperfermentation

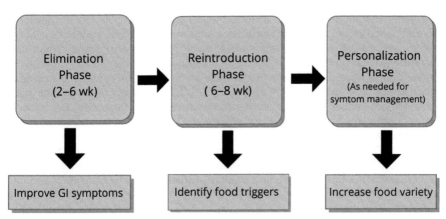

**Fig. 1.** The low FODMAP diet approach.

related to FODMAPs may be problematic in GI patients, prompting potential inflammatory and intestinal permeability effects as observed in animal studies. FODMAPs are prevalent in the diet in everyday foods, including milk, wheat, onion, garlic, apples, and watermelon, to name a few, and even in popular manufacturing process, such as the addition of fiber additives to our food supply in the form of chicory root extract. Because of their small size, FODMAP carbohydrates are rapidly fermented and osmotically active, prompting luminal distention and gut symptoms in patients with IBS who often have underlying abnormalities in motility and visceral sensation.[11,38,39] The full mechanism for how FODMAPs induce IBS symptoms has yet to be elucidated. Metabolomic research reveals that a high FODMAP diet consumed by patients with IBS increases urinary histamine and an increase in bacterial endotoxin, lipopolysaccharides.[40,41] The dynamics between diet and the gut microbiome, in addition to luminal distention in individuals with IBS appears to play a key role.

Dionne and colleagues,[20] in a systematic review of the LFD, identified 7 RCTs comparing a LFD to a number of different types of control interventions in 397 participants. The LFD was noted to have a reduced relative risk for global symptoms compared with control interventions (Relative risk = 0.69; 95% CI 0.54–0.88). Unfortunately, there was a high degree of heterogenicity in the study designs, limiting the quality of the data.[20] Another systematic review and meta-analysis by Schumann and colleagues[42] found 9 RCTs with a total of 596 subjects. This meta-analysis found significant group differences for LFD compared with other diets with regard to gastrointestinal symptoms (standardized mean difference [SMD] −0.62; 95% CI −0.93 to −0.31; $P = .0001$), abdominal pain (SMD −0.50; 95% CI −0.77 to −0.22; $P = .008$), and health-related quality of life (SMD 0.36; 95% CI 0.10–0.62; $P = .007$).

There is great interest in the LFD in the IBS community. A plethora of food manufacturers are emerging with low FODMAP offerings. In part, the diet has validated the patient's experience that food does impact their GI symptoms. The LFD has metaphorically opened up a Pandora's box for the use of nutritional interventions in patients with IBS.

## THE LOW FERMENTABLE, OLIGO-,DI-MONO-SACCHARIDE AND POLYOL DIET AND NUTRIENT ADEQUACY

Removing a number of fruits, vegetables, wheat, and the omnipresent garlic and onion from one's diet can be a challenge on the low FODMAP elimination diet; however, this dietary intervention does include all food groups and can be nutritionally balanced. The elimination phase of the LFD includes a wide variety of fruits, vegetables, whole grains, nuts, seeds, legumes, lactose-free dairy, and animal proteins. When well planned, the LFD can meet a person's nutrient, both macronutrient and micronutrient, needs. Studies have demonstrated individuals on an LFD have decreased intakes of carbohydrate,[43–46] calcium, [45,46] and energy.[43,44,46] Although other studies have found nutrient intakes to remain similar between an LFD intervention, the habitual diet, or control arm.[47–50] Once adjusting for energy intake, Eswaran and colleagues[46] found the only statistically significant decrease in micronutrient intake observed during a 4-week LFD was for riboflavin. Many patients at baseline were observed to have intakes below the recommended daily intake (DRIs) for several nutrients, including vitamin D, vitamin E, vitamin C, and calcium. A dietitian-led elimination phase can actually enhance micronutrient intake from baseline, as was demonstrated by the increased intake of vitamins A, C, E, K, niacin, B-6, Cu, and Mg on a 4-week LFD, with significant increases in niacin ($P<.05$) and vitamin B-6 ($P<.01$).[46] Moreover, when the LFD was compared with a sham diet, no difference was observed between the 2 groups' total energy, macronutrients, or fiber intake.[47] In this trial, both groups were noted to be consuming approximately 13 g of fiber per day, which is below daily recommended fiber intakes of 25 to 38 g.[51] A recent pilot study demonstrated a dietitian-led LFD in adults older than 65 years did not significantly reduce a participant's nutrient intake from their baseline, but at baseline, most participants consumed less than DRIs of several macronutrients and micronutrients.[49] Long-term nutrient intake in those educated on an LFD appears also to be adequate. Patients who were educated on an LFD and continued some form of restriction, termed 'FODMAP adapted,' were found to be consuming a nutritionally adequate diet up to 18 months after initial education.[50] In addition to improving GI symptoms, any nutrition therapy or diet intervention should be tailored to address and prevent nutrient intake shortfalls.

## ROLE OF HISTAMINE INTOLERANCE

Histamine intolerance occurs when there is an imbalance of accumulated histamine and a reduced capacity for histamine degradation.[52] Within the GI tract, exogenous histamine can be impacted by a reduction in diamine oxidase (DAO), the enzyme required to degrade dietary histamine, consumption of a diet rich in histamine content, and the gut microbial metabolism of histidine, which produces histamine. Small bowel inflammation or reduced surface area may reduce DAO production, as it is produced on the apical enterocytes of the upper intestinal villi.[53] Symptoms of histamine intolerance can present with both common IBS symptoms as well as extraintestinal symptoms, including abdominal pain, diarrhea, flushing, urticaria, headaches, vertigo, hypotension, bronchoconstriction, nausea and vomiting.[52] As mentioned previously, one survey study revealed almost 60% of patients with IBS identify histamine-containing foods as a trigger to their digestive distress.[1] The histamine content of foods can vary depending on the microbial composition in the food as well as how the food product is stored and prepared.[54]

Presently, the diagnosis of histamine intolerance is based on the following criteria[55]:

- Presentation of 2 or more histamine-intolerance symptoms
- Improvement with a low-histamine diet
- Improvement with antihistamine medications

Some general recommendations to reduce dietary histamine include reducing high histamine foods, freezing leftover protein-rich foods to retard histamine production, and consuming fresh, minimally processed foods over ultraprocessed foods. See **Table 2** for histamine-rich foods.

The role of a low-histamine diet has not been properly evaluated in patients with IBS but provides another potential area of research in the intersection of diet and IBS.

| Table 2<br>Foods rich in histamine | |
| --- | --- |
| **Food Type** | **High Histamine Foods** |
| Fruit | Avocado, citrus, strawberries, kiwifruit, papayas, pineapples, dried fruit |
| Vegetable | Tomatoes, spinach, eggplant |
| Animal protein | Mackerel, tuna, sardines, anchovies, herring, eggs, aged beef, cured meats, leftover meat or fish |
| Dairy | Aged cheeses, Kefir, yogurt |
| Alcohol | All |
| Other | Nuts, chocolate, vinegar, fermented foods such as kimchi, sauerkraut |

*Data from* Refs.[55–57]

## THE SIXTH FERMENTABLE, OLIGO-,DI-MONO-SACCHARIDE AND POLYOL? SUCROSE INTOLERANCE

The LFD does not exclude sucrose, as this disaccharide is typically well digested and absorbed. When there is an absence or reduction in sucrase and isomaltase, however, malabsorption of dietary carbohydrates such as sucrose and starches may prompt GI distress similar to malabsorbed FODMAP carbohydrates due to resultant fermentative and osmotic effects. SID can be either congenital (CSID) or acquired (for example, in association with mucosal injury). SID may be a factor in patients who do not benefit from traditional IBS therapy, such as the LFD. Research revealed patients who carried hypomorphic (pathogenic) sucrase-isomaltase (*SI*) gene variants were significantly less likely to experience adequate symptom relief from the LFD compared with non-carriers (43.5% vs 60.9%; *P* = .031; odds ratio [OR] 4.66).[8]

Although a condition more on the radar for the pediatric gastroenterologists, there may be benefit for assessing for SID in adult patients with IBS who do not benefit from traditional therapy. Symptomology in adults includes frequent, postprandial diarrhea, along with gas and bloating.[58] Patients with CSID tend to have lifelong symptoms. On the other hand, acquired SID may result transiently due to villous atrophy or small intestinal inflammation, such as in untreated celiac disease, Crohn's disease, malnutrition, or in some cases of small intestinal bacterial overgrowth.[59]

Recent studies reveal that heterozygous carriers of *SI* variants experience GI symptoms. One recent study found that CSID genetic mutations were more common in patients with IBS (n = 1031) than asymptomatic controls (*P* = .074; OR 1.84).[60] In a 6-year retrospective study involving disaccharidase assay in nearly 28,000 mucosal biopsy samples in symptomatic children, researchers found that 9.3% of the cohort was deficient in sucrase and maltase.[61] A small study (n=31) in adults with presumed diarrhea-predominant IBS and mixed presentation IBS found SID present in 35% of patients. Among patients with SID, 63.6% had diarrhea, 45.4% had abdominal pain, and 36.4% had bloating.[58] SID (genetic or acquired) should be a consideration, particularly in IBS-D or IBS-M patients who do not respond to an LFD and demonstrate intolerance to foods rich in sucrose, see **Table 3**.

**Table 3**
**Sample of foods rich in sucrose**

| Food Type | High-Sucrose Foods[62] |
|---|---|
| Fruit | Apples, apricots, cantaloupe, dates, mango, nectarines, oranges, peaches, tangerines |
| Vegetable | Beets, carrots, corn, green peas, sweet potatoes/yams |
| Sweeteners and ingredients | Sucrose (table sugar), many other types of sugar: brown, cane, beet, coconut, date, and powdered, maple syrup, jam and jelly |
| Dairy | Products (yogurt, milk, milk shakes) sweetened with the preceding ingredients or containing high-sucrose fruits |
| Baked and processed foods | Breakfast cereals, baked goods, candy granola bars, pastries, pudding |

*Not a complete list.

## THE POTENTIAL FOR DISORDERED EATING AND EATING DISORDERS IN IRRITABLE BOWEL SYNDROME

When eating leads to debilitating GI symptoms, there may be a normal adaptive response to avoid food triggers. Determining when eating behavior becomes disordered in a patient with GI symptoms can be challenging. Eating and feeding disorder tools have not been validated in IBS, so one must be cautious when assigning a diagnosis of an eating behavior in this population. A higher prevalence of disordered eating (DE) has been found in patients with GI disorders compared with healthy controls. A systematic review demonstrated 23.43% of general gastroenterology patients engaged in DE behaviors.[63] The 2 most common eating disorders (EDs), anorexia nervosa and bulimia nervosa, can result in digestive distress, and studies reveal 41% to 52% of patients with an ED history have IBS.[64] In addition, in an IBS patient cohort, greater adherence to an LFD was shown to be associated with ED behavior.[65] Recently, research has started to examine Avoidant/Restrictive Food Intake Disorder (ARFID), an ED first included in the *Diagnostic and Statistical Manual of Mental Disorders, 5th Edition*, in the adult gastroenterology population. In general, little research has examined the assessment, treatment, and impact of ARFID in adults. Although the prevalence of ARFID in the adult GI population is not well known, 2 studies found 12.6% to 21.0% of patients met ARFID criteria.[66,67] In addition, a prospective screening study using the 9-item ARFID screen (NIAS) identified a 19.6% positive ARFID screen risk in adult patients with GI disorders.[68] These studies highlight this may be an underrecognized disorder among this population.

When considering the use of diet therapy for a person with IBS, it is essential for clinicians to understand a patient's current dietary habits and history, which includes assessing/screening for maladaptive eating habits and past or present history of an ED. An elimination diet is not appropriate for a patient who has already implemented significant restrictions and/or may be struggling with DE or an active ED. As with all IBS patient care, an integrated care approach is optimal, and for a patient with DE or an ED a mental health provider and dietitian who specializes in ED should be part of their treatment team.

## SUMMARY

Diet interventions for patients with IBS are not a "one-size-fits-all" proposition. Depending on the degree of symptomology, initial therapy may simply include adjusting meal timing, limiting overly processed foods and additives, and adding balance of macronutrients to the diet. In patients with low to moderate symptomology and/or very poor background diet, these slight changes may be all that is warranted. Patients with IBS who were frequently under eating during the day and consuming most of their nutrition in the evening through a larger main meal experienced symptom improvement on a balanced Mediterranean diet. The balanced Mediterranean diet focused mostly on increasing dietary fiber and improving food habits by recommending regular meals and snacks throughout the day. Not surprisingly, this diet approach was preferred by patients over the LFD and GFD.[69] If the patient has failed "cleaning up" the diet, one may consider an LFD intervention as long as there are no contraindications of doing so, such as an active ED or extreme food fears. Details for potential contraindications of the LFD have been reviewed elsewhere.[70] In addition to full diet protocols, such as the LFD for symptom management, one may also consider adding certain foods to offer therapeutic benefit, such as 2 green kiwifruit per day, to aid symptoms of constipation.[71,72] The use of prebiotics combined with diet changes such as the Mediterranean diet are being explored and may provide benefit.[73] Patients with IBS who are interested in diet therapy will benefit from receiving a referral to an experienced GI dietitian. GI dietitians perform a full nutrition assessment, provide detailed instructions, including grocery shopping, menu planning, and label reading, while individualizing the diet intervention to the patient's lifestyle and personal clinical needs.

## CLINICS CARE POINTS

- The low FODMAP diet is the 3 phase nutritional approach with the most evidence supporting its efficacy for symptom control in IBS.
- Patients with IBS are at increased risk for maladaptive eating and should be screened for disordered eating and/or eating disorders, particularly prior to prescribing restrictive diet therapies.
- IBS masqueraders such as sucrase isomaltase deficiency, bile acid diarrhea and celiac disease may prompt the necessity of diet therapies other than the low FODMAP diet.
- A GI dietitian referral is recommended for IBS patients to help guide individualized nutritional advice based on lifestyle, symptoms, socio-economics and complete medical history.

## DISCLOSURE

Consultant: GI OnDemand (E. Haller). Paid Board Member/Advisory Panel, FODY food company, GI OnDemand Consultant: A2 milk company, Beckon, Gastro Girl. Stock/Shareholder: Fody foods, Epicured, GI OnDemand (K. Scarlata).

## REFERENCES

1. Böhn L, Störsrud S, Törnblom H, et al. Self-reported food-related gastrointestinal symptoms in IBS are common and associated with more severe symptoms and reduced quality of life. Am J Gastroenterol 2013;108:634–41.
2. Chey WD. Food: the main course to wellness and illness in patients with irritable bowel syndrome [review]. Am J Gastroenterol 2016;111(3):366–71.
3. McRorie JW Jr. Evidence-based approach to fiber supplements and clinically meaningful health benefits, part 2: what to look for and how to recommend an effective fiber therapy. Nutr Today 2015;50(2):90–7.

4. Falcomer AL, Riquette RFR, de Lima BR, et al. Health benefits of green banana consumption: a systematic review. Nutrients 2019;11(6):1222.

5. Shalini R, Antony U. Fructan distribution in banana cultivars and effect of ripening and processing on Nendran banana. J Food Sci Technol 2015;52(12):8244–51.

6. Irvine AJ, Chey WD, Ford AC. Screening for celiac disease in irritable bowel syndrome: an updated systematic review and meta-analysis. Am J Gastroenterol 2017;112(1):65–76.

7. Shiha MG, Ashgar Z, Fraser EM, et al. High prevalence of primary bile acid diarrhoea in patients with functional diarrhea and irritable bowel syndrome based on Rome III and Rome IV criteria. EClinicalMedicine 2020;25:100465.

8. Zheng T, Eswaran S, Photenhauer AL, et al. Reduced efficacy of low FODMAPs diet in patients with IBS-D carrying sucrase-isomaltase (SI) hypomorphic variants. Gut 2020;69(2):397–8.

9. Stevenson L, Phillips F, O'Sullivan K, et al. Wheat bran: its composition and benefits to health, a European perspective. Int J Food Sci Nutr 2012;63(8):1001–13.

10. Shewry PR, Hey SJ. The contribution of wheat to human diet and health. Food Energy Secur 2015;4(3):178–202.

11. Major G, Pritchard S, Murray K, et al. Colon hypersensitivity to distension, rather than excessive gas production, produces carbohydrate-related symptoms in individuals with irritable bowel syndrome. Gastroenterology 2017;152(1):124–33.e2.

12. Zevallos V, Raker V, Tenzer S, et al. Nutritional wheat amylase-trypsin inhibitors promote intestinal inflammation via activation of myeloid cells. Gastroenterology 2017;152(5):1100–13.e12.

13. Fritscher-Ravens A, Pflaum T, Mösinger M, et al. Many patients with irritable bowel syndrome have atypical food allergies not associated with immunoglobulin E. Gastroenterology 2019;157(1):109–18.e5.

14. Fritscher-Ravens A, Schuppan D, Ellrichmann M, et al. Confocal endomicroscopy shows food-associated changes in the intestinal mucosa of patients with irritable bowel syndrome. Gastroenterology 2014;147(5):1012–20.e4.

15. Schuppan D, Pickert G, Ashfaq-Khan M, et al. Non-celiac wheat sensitivity: differential diagnosis, triggers and implications. Best Pract Res Clin Gastroenterol 2015;29(3):469–76.

16. de Punder K, Pruimboom L. The dietary intake of wheat and other cereal grains and their role in inflammation. Nutrients 2013;5(3):771–87.

17. Kim H, Patel K, Orosz E, et al. Time trends in the prevalence of celiac disease and gluten-free diet in the US Population. JAMA Intern Med 2016;176(11):1716.

18. Potter M, Walker M, Jones M, et al. Wheat intolerance and chronic gastrointestinal symptoms in an Australian population-based study: association between wheat sensitivity, celiac disease and functional gastrointestinal disorders. Am J Gastroenterol 2018;113(7):1036–44.

19. Melini V, Melini F. Gluten-free diet: gaps and needs for a healthier diet. Nutrients 2019;11(1):170.

20. Dionne J, Ford AC, Yuan Y, et al. A systematic review and meta-analysis evaluating the efficacy of a gluten-free diet and a low FODMAPs diet in treating symptoms of irritable bowel syndrome. Am J Gastroenterol 2018;113(9):1290–300.

21. Pinto-Sanchez MI, Nardelli A, Borojevic R, et al. Gluten-Free Diet Reduces Symptoms, Particularly Diarrhea, in Patients With Irritable Bowel Syndrome and Anti-gliadin IgG. Clin Gastroenterol Hepatol. 2020;S1542-3565(20)31149-6.

22. Skodje G, Sarna V, Minelle I, et al. Fructan, rather than gluten, induces symptoms in patients with self-reported non-celiac gluten sensitivity. Gastroenterology 2018; 154(3):529–39.e2.

23. Biesiekierski J, Peters S, Newnham E, et al. No effects of gluten in patients with self-reported non-celiac gluten sensitivity after dietary reduction of fermentable, poorly absorbed, short-chain carbohydrates. Gastroenterology 2013;145(2): 320–8.e3.

24. Ajamian M, Rosella G, Newnham E, et al. Effect of gluten ingestion and FODMAP restriction on intestinal epithelial integrity in patients with irritable bowel syndrome and self-reported non-coeliac gluten sensitivity. Mol Nutr Food Res. 2021;65(5):e1901275.

25. Patel SM, Stason WB, Legedza A, et al. The placebo effect in irritable bowel syndrome trials: a meta-analysis. Neurogastroenterol Motil 2005;17(3):332–40.

26. Molina-Infante J, Carroccio A. Suspected nonceliac gluten sensitivity confirmed in few patients after gluten challenge in double-blind, placebo-controlled trials. Clin Gastroenterol Hepatol 2017;15:339–48.

27. Rossi M, Aggio R, Staudacher HM, et al. Volatile organic compounds in feces associate with response to dietary intervention in patients with irritable bowel syndrome. Clin Gastroenterol Hepatol 2018;16(3):385–91.e1.

28. Chumpitazi BP, Cope JL, Hollister EB, et al. Randomised clinical trial: gut microbiome biomarkers are associated with clinical response to a low FODMAP diet in children with the irritable bowel syndrome. Aliment Pharmacol Ther 2015;42(4): 418–27.

29. Valeur J, Småstuen MC, Knudsen T, et al. Exploring gut microbiota composition as an indicator of clinical response to dietary FODMAP restriction in patients with irritable bowel syndrome. Dig Dis Sci 2018;63(2):429–36.

30. Bennet SMP, Böhn L, Störsrud S, et al. Multivariate modelling of faecal bacterial profiles of patients with IBS predicts responsiveness to a diet low in FODMAPs. Gut 2018;67(5):872–81.

31. Croft N. IgG food antibodies and irritating the bowel. Gastroenterology 2005; 128(4):1135–6.

32. Atkinson W. Food elimination based on IgG antibodies in irritable bowel syndrome: a randomised controlled trial. Gut 2004;53(10):1459–64.

33. AAAAI. The American Academy of Allergy, Asthma & Immunology. | The myth of IgG food panel testing. 2020. Available at: https://www.aaaai.org/conditions-and-treatments/library/allergy-library/IgG-food-test. Accessed November 22, 2020.

34. Stapel S, Asero R, Ballmer-Weber B, et al. Testing for IgG4 against foods is not recommended as a diagnostic tool: EAACI Task Force Report*. Allergy 2008; 63(7):793–6.

35. Ali A, Weiss TR, McKee D, et al. Efficacy of individualised diets in patients with irritable bowel syndrome: a randomised controlled trial. BMJ Open Gastroenterol 2017;4(1):e000164.

36. Gibson P, Shepherd S. Personal view: food for thought - western lifestyle and susceptibility to Crohn's disease. The FODMAP hypothesis. Aliment Pharmacol Ther 2005;21(12):1399–409.

37. Gibson P, Halmos E, Muir J. Review article: FODMAPS, prebiotics and gut health-the FODMAP hypothesis revisited. Aliment Pharmacol Ther 2020;52(2):233–46.

38. Barrett JS, Gearry RB, Muir JG, et al. Dietary poorly absorbed, short-chain carbohydrates increase delivery of water and fermentable substrates to the proximal colon. Aliment Pharmacol Ther 2010;31(8):874–82.

39. Ong DK, Mitchell SB, Barrett JS, et al. Manipulation of dietary short chain carbohydrates alters the pattern of gas production and genesis of symptoms in irritable bowel syndrome. J Gastroenterol Hepatol 2010;25(8):1366–73.

40. McIntosh K, Reed DE, Schneider T, et al. FODMAPs alter symptoms and the metabolome of patients with IBS: a randomised controlled trial. Gut 2017;66(7): 1241–51 [published correction appears in Gut. 2019;68(7):1342].

41. Zhou SY, Gillilland M 3rd, Wu X, et al. FODMAP diet modulates visceral nociception by lipopolysaccharide-mediated intestinal inflammation and barrier dysfunction. J Clin Invest 2018;128(1):267–80.

42. Schumann D, Klose P, Lauche R, et al. Low fermentable, oligo-, di-, monosaccharides and polyol diet in the treatment of irritable bowel syndrome: a systematic review and meta-analysis. Nutrition 2018;45:24–31.

43. Eswaran SL, Chey WD, Han-Markey T, et al. A randomized controlled trial comparing the low FODMAP diet vs. modified NICE guidelines in US adults with IBS-D. Am J Gastroenterol 2016;111:1824–32.

44. Böhn L, Störsrud S, Liljebo T, et al. Diet low in FODMAPs reduces symptoms of irritable bowel syndrome as well as traditional dietary advice: a randomized controlled trial. Gastroenterology 2015;149(6):1399–407.e2.

45. Staudacher HM, Lomer MC, Anderson JL, et al. Fermentable carbohydrate restriction reduces luminal bifidobacteria and gastrointestinal symptoms in patients with irritable bowel syndrome. J Nutr 2012;142(8):1510–8.

46. Eswaran S, Dolan RD, Ball SC, et al. The impact of a 4-week low-FODMAP and mNICE diet on nutrient intake in a sample of US adults with irritable bowel syndrome with diarrhea. J Acad Nutr Diet 2020;120(4):641–9.

47. Staudacher HM, Lomer MCE, Farquharson FM, et al. A diet low in FODMAPs reduces symptoms in patients with irritable bowel syndrome and a probiotic restores bifidobacterium species: a randomized controlled trial. Gastroenterology 2017;153(4):936–47.

48. Staudacher HM, Ralph FSE, Irving PM, et al. Nutrient intake, diet quality, and diet diversity in irritable bowel syndrome and the impact of the low FODMAP diet. J Acad Nutr Diet 2020;120(4):535–47 [published correction appears in J Acad Nutr Diet 2020;120(12):2098].

49. O'Brien L, Skidmore P, Wall C, et al. A low FODMAP diet is nutritionally adequate and therapeutically efficacious in community dwelling older adults with chronic diarrhoea. Nutrients 2020;12(10):3002.

50. O'Keeffe M, Jansen C, Martin L, et al. Long-term impact of the low-FODMAP diet on gastrointestinal symptoms, dietary intake, patient acceptability, and healthcare utilization in irritable bowel syndrome. Neurogastroenterol Motil 2018;30(1). doi: 10.1111/nmo.13154.

51. Institute of Medicine. Dietary reference intakes for energy, carbohydrate, fiber, fat, fatty acids, cholesterol, protein, and amino acids. Washington, DC: The National Academies Press; 2005. https://doi.org/10.17226/10490.

52. Maintz L, Novak J. Histamine and histamine intolerance. Am J Clin Nutr 2007; 85(5):1185–96.

53. Rosell-Camps A, Zobetto S, Perez-Esteban G, et al. Histamine Intolerance as a cause of chronic digestive complaints in pediatric patients. Rev Esp Enferm Dig 2013;105(4):201–7.

54. Doeun D, Davaatseren M, Chung MS. Biogenic amines in foods. Food Sci Biotechnol 2017;26(6):1463–74.

55. Tuck Caroline J, Biesiekierski JR, Schmid-Grendelmeier, et al. Food intolerances. Nutrients 2019;11:1684.

56. Spencer M, Chey WD, Eswaran S. Dietary renaissance in IBS: has food replaced medications as a primary treatment strategy? Curr Treat Options Gastroenterol 2014;12:424–40.
57. Sánchez-Pérez S, Comas-Basté O, Rabell-González J, et al. Biogenic amines in plant-origin foods: are they frequently underestimated in low-histamine diets? Foods 2018;7(12):205.
58. Kim SB, Calmet FH, Garrido J, et al. Sucrase-isomaltase deficiency as a potential masquerader in irritable bowel syndrome. Dig Dis Sci 2020;65(2):534–40.
59. Chey WD, Cash B, Lembo A, et al. Congenital sucrase-isomaltase deficiency: what, when, and how? Gastroenterol Hepatol 2020;16(10):1-11.
60. Henström M, Diekmann L, Bonfiglio F, et al. Functional variants in the sucrase-isomaltase gene associate with increased risk of irritable bowel syndrome. Gut 2018;67(2):263–70.
61. Nichols BL Jr, Adams B, Roach CM, et al. Frequency of sucrase deficiency in mucosal biopsies. J Pediatr Gastroenterol Nutr 2012;55(Suppl 2):S28–30.
62. Sucraid® and Diet Therapy for Adults. 2019. Available at: https://www.sucraidassist.com/pdf/adult-diet-guide.pdf. Accessed December 12, 2020.
63. Satherley R, Howard R, Higgs S. Disordered eating practices in gastrointestinal disorders. Appetite 2015;84:240–50.
64. Sato Y, Fukudo S. Gastrointestinal symptoms and disorders in patients with eating disorders. Clin J Gastroenterol 2015;8(5):255–63.
65. Mari A, Hosadurg D, Martin L, et al. Adherence with a low-FODMAP diet in irritable bowel syndrome: are eating disorders the missing link? Eur J Gastroenterol Hepatol 2019;31(2):178–82.
66. Harer K, Jagielski C, Riehl M, Chey W. 272 – Avoidant/restrictive food intake disorder among adult gastroenterology behavioral health patients: Demographic and clinical characteristics. Gastroenterology. 2019;156(6):S-53.
67. Zia JK, Riddle M, DeCou CR, et al. Prevalence of eating disorders, especially DSM-5's avoidant restrictive food intake disorder, in patients with functional gastrointestinal disorders: a cross-sectional online survey. Gastroenterology 2017;152(5 Suppl 1):S715–6.
68. Harer K, Baker J, Reister N, et al. Avoidant/restrictive food intake disorder in the adult gastroenterology population: an under-recognized diagnosis? Am J Gastroenterol 2018;113(Supplement):S247–8.
69. Paduano D, Cingolani A, Tanda E, et al. Effect of three diets (low-FODMAP, gluten-free and balanced) on irritable bowel syndrome symptoms and health-related quality of life. Nutrients 2019;11(7):1566.
70. Halmos EP, Gibson PR. Controversies and reality of the FODMAP diet for patients with irritable bowel syndrome. J Gastroenterol Hepatol 2019;34(7):1134–42.
71. Chang CC, Lin YT, Lu YT, et al. Kiwifruit improves bowel function in patients with irritable bowel syndrome with constipation. Asia Pac J Clin Nutr 2010;19(4):451–7.
72. Chey S, Chey W, Jackson K, et al. S0454  Randomized, comparative effectiveness trial of green kiwifruit, psyllium, or prunes in U.S. patients with chronic constipation. Am J Gastroenterol 2020;115(1):S229.
73. Huaman JW, Mego M, Manichanh C, et al. Effects of prebiotics vs a diet low in FODMAPs in patients with functional gut disorders. Gastroenterology 2018;155(4):1004–7.

# Behavioral Strategies for Irritable Bowel Syndrome
## Brain-Gut or Gut-Brain?

Christina H. Jagielski, PhD, MPH[a],*, Megan E. Riehl, PsyD[b]

KEYWORDS

- Gut-brain axis • Gut-brain psychotherapies • Cognitive behavioral therapy
- Gut-directed hypnosis • Irritable bowel syndrome

KEY POINTS

- Irritable bowel syndrome (IBS) is a common disorder of gut-brain interaction.
- IBS is associated with significant physical, emotional, and occupational burden.
- IBS is associated with several factors that influence gut-brain communication, including early life stress, sleep disruption, maladaptive coping strategies, symptom hypervigilance, and visceral hypersensitivity.
- Gut-brain psychotherapies, such as gastrointestinal-specific cognitive behavioral therapy, gut-directed hypnosis, and mindfulness-based strategies are effective at treating gut-brain dysregulation, including IBS.

## INTRODUCTION

Irritable bowel syndrome (IBS) is a disorder of gut-brain interaction (DGBI), formerly known as a functional gastrointestinal disorder. The transition to conceptualizing IBS as a DGBI highlights the manner in which symptoms are driven by brain and gut interactions and significantly affected by biopsychosocial factors.[1] Gut-directed psychotherapies are recommended in the context of multidisciplinary care for patients with global symptoms of IBS (**Table 1**).[2–4] Rome IV diagnostic criteria include the presence of recurrent bouts of abdominal pain, as well as altered bowel habits.[5] IBS is one of several DGBIs that do not have an identifiable structural or biochemical abnormality to account for their symptoms. Therefore, diagnosis is based on symptom patterns. Rome IV criteria are considered the most widely accepted standard for IBS diagnosis. In addition to IBS, other DGBIs include functional constipation, functional diarrhea, functional abdominal bloating/distention, opioid-inducted constipation, and unspecified bowel disorder. A 2020 study revealed a prevalence of 27.8% of patients across

[a] Internal Medicine-Gastroenterology, Michigan Medicine, 380 Parkland Plaza, Ann Arbor, MI 48103, USA; [b] Internal Medicine-Gastroenterology, Michigan Medicine, 3912 Taubman Center, SPC 5362, Suite 3436, 1500 East Medical Center Drive, Ann Arbor, MI 48109-5362, USA
* Corresponding author.
*E-mail address:* cjagiels@med.umich.edu

Gastroenterol Clin N Am 50 (2021) 581–593
https://doi.org/10.1016/j.gtc.2021.03.006
0889-8553/21/© 2021 Elsevier Inc. All rights reserved.

gastro.theclinics.com

**Table 1**
**Integrating behavioral health services into the care of patients with irritable bowel syndrome**

| Have Resources Available | Encourage Discussions in Clinic | Multidisciplinary and Holistic Care | Locating Mental Health Providers and Resources |
|---|---|---|---|
| Create a referral list of qualified GI–mental health providers in your area<br>Characteristics of the mental health provider include expertise in clinical health psychology, behavioral medicine, CBT treatment approaches, chronic health conditions, stress, anxiety, and mood disorders | Highlight to patients that emotional health is as important as physical health<br>Ask patients about the impact of their IBS on mood, stress, anxiety, and pandemic concerns to ensure early intervention<br>Provide patients with information about the brain-gut axis and the brain-gut psychotherapies most effective in addressing this pathway | Ensure that you will remain a part of your patient's care when you recommend a GI–mental health provider<br>Recommend referral to GI–mental health provider early in treatment to aid patient in the management of IBS | Rome Foundation therapist finder: www.romegipsych.org/<br>Psychology Today therapist finder: www.therapists.psychologytoday.com/<br>Directory of Cognitive Behavioral Therapists: www.abct.org/<br>Society of Behavioral Medicine: www.sbm.org/<br>Gut-directed hypnotherapy providers: www.ibshypnosis.com/<br>GI-specific educational resources: www.giondemand.com/ |

*Abbreviations:* CBT, cognitive behavioral therapy; GI, gastrointestinal.

the United States, Canada, and the United Kingdom who met criteria for a functional bowel disorder.[6]

IBS is a complex, multifactorial condition that is often viewed through the lens of the biopsychosocial model. The model as a means of conceptualizing IBS was first described by Dr Douglas Drossman[7] in 1998 and shows the interactions between genetic factors and environmental factors such as early life stress; parental beliefs and behaviors; culture; the role of psychological factors, including psychiatric comorbidity, health-related anxiety, and somatization; symptom hypervigilance; central nervous system (CNS) structure and function; structural brain abnormalities; functional network connection; emotion and cognitive modulation of visceral afferent signals and classic fear conditions; and the interaction with gut physiology, including gut permeability, motility, sensation, the gut microbiome, inflammation, and immune dysfunction (**Fig. 1**).[8]

The brain-gut axis (BGA) is a bidirectional pathway between the brain and gastrointestinal (GI) tract. More specifically, this bidirectional pathway occurs between the CNS and enteric nervous system (ENS) through numerous pathways. The ENS is a self-regulatory system that can function independently of CNS input.[9] The BGA involves communication between the autonomic nervous system, endocrine system (via the hypothalamic pituitary adrenal [HPA] axis), and immune system, as well as the gut microbiome. It plays a critical role in regulation of digestive processes, modulation of the immune system, and coordination of physical and emotional states.[10]

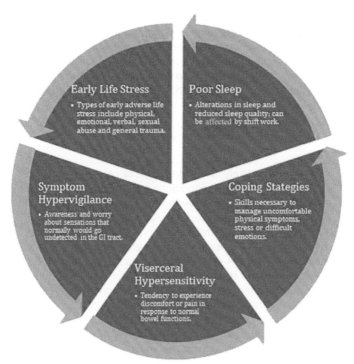

**Fig. 1.** Factors that contribute to a diagnosis of irritable bowel syndrome.

ENS nerves in patients with IBS send amplified pain signals to the brain in response to normal GI functioning, which may explain why normal amounts of gas in the intestines or muscle contractions of the colon can be perceived as highly painful for someone with IBS, but typically do not bother patients without IBS.[11] Although the initial onset of symptoms may be explained by dysregulation of brain-gut functioning, chronicity of symptoms is most likely related to neuroplastic and structural changes in the nervous system and the GI tract.[10] Because of this strong connection in brain-gut interaction, alterations in the BGA are suspected as a significant factor in the onset or exacerbation of DGBI.

## BURDEN OF IRRITABLE BOWEL SYNDROME

People living with IBS report significant physical, emotional, and occupational burden. IBS is associated with higher levels of depression and anxiety compared with healthy controls.[12,13] A meta-analysis found the presence of anxiety or depression at baseline doubled the risk of IBS symptom onset.[14] IBS is also associated with increased risk of suicidality, largely because of the impact of GI symptoms.[15] Patients with IBS with anxiety and depression reported higher GI and non-GI symptom burden, as well as higher GI-specific anxiety and poorer GI-specific quality of life, compared with patients without anxiety or depression.[16] IBS is also associated with other aspects of mental health, including higher somatization scores compared with healthy controls.[17] Obsessive-compulsive disorder is associated with higher prevalence of IBS and GI symptom severity.[18]

Patients with IBS reported significantly lower health-related quality of life.[19,20] IBS is associated with greater absenteeism and presenteeism, as well as decreased work productivity,[20,21] and increased health care use and disability.[22] Resiliency, characterized by the ability to cope during periods of stress, is an important factor in how people are affected by disease and respond to available treatment.[23] Patients with IBS showed lower resilience compared with healthy controls. Lower resilience was associated with increased IBS symptom severity and poorer GI-specific quality of life.[23] Having other bodily symptoms in addition to IBS criteria was associated with increased functional impairment, psychological distress, and health care seeking, and poorer quality of life.[24]

## FACTORS THAT CONTRIBUTE TO IRRITABLE BOWEL SYNDROME
### Early Life Stress

Patients with IBS are more likely to report physical or sexual abuse in childhood compared with patients with other GI conditions or controls.[25–29] A study by Bradford and colleagues[25] highlighted the often overlooked impact of emotional abuse on IBS. Emotional abuse was the strongest predictor for the development of IBS compared with other types of early adverse life stress, such as physical and sexual abuse and general trauma. Early adverse life events (EALs) were also associated with lower levels of resilience in patients with IBS.[23] A meta-analysis revealed posttraumatic stress disorder was a significant risk factor for developing IBS.[30] Exposure to EALs is associated with numerous physiologic changes, including an impact on the HPA axis.[31–33] Patients with a history of abuse are more likely to have comorbid psychiatric conditions such as panic, depression, sleep disturbances, and somatic complaints.[34] Further, childhood trauma has been linked to significant increase in levels of the inflammatory markers C-reactive protein, interleukin-6, and tumor necrosis factor alpha.[35]

### Sleep

In a study of patients in a tertiary GI clinic, 72% of patients with IBS reported poor sleep and 51% had clinical insomnia.[36] Alterations in sleep and sleep quality have been shown to affect IBS symptoms. Sleep awakenings were significantly associated with increased abdominal pain and GI distress. Both sleep awakenings and poor sleep quality were associated with non-GI pain such as headache and back pain, as well as somatoform complaints.[37] In addition, depression, anxiety, and GI-specific anxiety all correlated with waking episodes.[37] Knutsson and Bøggild[38] also found a negative impact of shift work on GI symptoms. People who engage in shift work, which can dramatically affect people's sleep, can also experience other health problems. In a study of nurses, those with rotating shift work had significantly higher prevalence of abdominal pain compared with those with daytime or nighttime shifts.[39]

### Coping Strategies and Coping Responses

Research has shown differences in particular coping strategies for patients with IBS. Catastrophizing is a cognitive coping method that involves exaggerated negative thoughts about experiences and/or a tendency to minimize the ability to cope with these experiences. Catastrophizing is commonly expressed by patients with IBS and is associated with worse IBS symptom severity[17] and poorer health-related quality of life.[40] A study by Lackner and colleagues[41] revealed that catastrophizing partially mediated the relationship between depression and abdominal pain severity in patients with IBS and the connection between both anxiety and depression and pediatric abdominal pain.[42]

Patients with IBS were more likely to use problem-focused coping strategies (active coping, planning, and use of instrumental support), as well as avoidant coping strategies (behavioral disengagement, self-blame, self-distraction, denial, and substance use [drugs and alcohol]) compared with healthy controls.[19] The use of active coping may play a role in the tendency of patients with IBS toward hypervigilance and higher use of health care advice and treatment.

### Symptom Hypervigilance/Attentional Bias

Patients with IBS report increased attention to physical symptoms and more difficulty tuning out unpleasant sensations. This tendency can lead these patients to notice and become worried about sensations that normally would go undetected. Patients with IBS report higher rates of hypervigilance compared with those with organic GI disorders.[43]

### Visceral Hypersensitivity

Many patients with IBS report a tendency to experience discomfort or pain in response to normal bowel functions, known as visceral hypersensitivity. It is suspected that, in patients with IBS, ENS nerves send stronger pain signals to the brain in response to normal activity in the GI tract, including typically undetectable muscle contractions moving through the GI tract or normal gas patterns, which are then experienced as discomfort. This condition has primarily been shown through balloon distension research showing that patients with IBS have lower pain tolerance to distension compared with healthy controls[44,45] and can lead to abnormal pain processing in the CNS.[46,47] Explaining this concept to patients with IBS can aid in their understanding of how the brain and gut interact and why gut-brain psychological interventions can be of benefit (**Box 1**).

### BEHAVIORAL TREATMENTS FOR IRRITABLE BOWEL SYNDROME

Research into the role of behavioral psychotherapies for IBS began in the 1980s. These treatments differ from traditional psychotherapies in several ways, including being brief, GI symptom focused, and skills based. In addition, patients with severe

---

**Box 1**
**The art of discussing the irritable bowel syndrome diagnosis**

Communicating a diagnosis of IBS to a patient and introducing the recommendation for gut-brain psychotherapies
  Patient: "Doctor, it is very frustrating that these tests tell me nothing is wrong. The pain I endure every day and the amount of time I am in the bathroom indicate something is very wrong. I'm afraid I am going to lose my job because my symptoms are so bad in the morning, which is causing me significant stress and more anxiety. There has to be some other test you can run. This is not all in my head."
  Physician: "I understand these symptoms are very debilitating. We are sure that you have IBS and no further testing is required. I'd like to discuss this complicated diagnosis and the available treatment options that will get you feeling better. The symptoms you experience are definitely not made up or in your head. They are affected by the interaction between your brain and your gut, though. In patients with IBS, the nerves that run throughout your digestive tract communicate too much with your brain, which can cause symptoms in your gut, a concept known as visceral hypersensitivity. Stress can also exacerbate the symptoms you experience. Sometimes patients will respond to our available medical treatments or to making changes to their diet, but often a combination of several interventions is needed. Given that your symptoms cause significant stress and anxiety related to getting to work, you will likely benefit greatly from a consultation with our colleague, a GI-specific mental health professional, who provides psychological interventions that specifically address the brain-gut connection and your IBS symptoms."

psychiatric comorbidities are typically not good candidates for GI-specific behavioral treatments, because these patients are more likely to benefit from pharmacologic support or work with a general mental health provider to treat the psychiatric condition.[48] The most commonly used behavioral treatments for IBS include GI-specific cognitive behavioral therapy (CBT), gut-directed hypnotherapy, and mindfulness-based strategies.

### Cognitive Behavioral Therapy

CBT is a "short-term, skills-based therapy approach that focuses on modifying behaviors and altering dysfunctional thinking patterns to influence mood and physiological symptoms."[11] This therapy was originally developed for the treatment of anxiety and depression in the 1950s and 1960s and has been studied across numerous health conditions, including gastrointestinal conditions. CBT has been used to target maladaptive cognitive processes, including catastrophizing, visceral anxiety, hypervigilance/attentional bias to benign gut sensations, and cognitive inflexibility, as well as avoidance behaviors and regulation of autonomic arousal through relaxation training.[11]

CBT for IBS can be delivered in as few as 4 sessions over the course of 10 weeks.[49] CBT can be delivered in a group setting[50] or via telehealth,[51] and in a self-guided format with minimal therapist contact.[52] Some patients prefer face-to-face provision of CBT, especially those with lower motivation to make behavioral change or to conduct the self-monitoring exercises that are an important part of CBT.[53] GI-CBT has also shown benefit for noncardiac chest pain.[54–56]

Exposure therapy for IBS was developed using panic-based CBT models, because of similarities of patients with IBS to patients with panic. Specifically, patients with IBS have a high likelihood of visceral hypersensitivity and symptom hypervigilance, which is similar to the acute focus on somatic sensations seen in people with panic attacks.[57] Hypervigilance toward bodily sensations can produce anxiety, which can then provoke increased autonomic arousal, which may increase the feared sensations, leading to an unhelpful cycle of fear and sensations that leads to a panic attack. A similar pattern can be seen in patients with IBS, where hypervigilance toward the presence of unpleasant sensations can lead to increased autonomic arousal, which can intensify GI sensations, further reinforcing patient fear of GI symptoms.[57] As such, a form of interoceptive exposure therapy was developed for patients with IBS. There is some evidence that interoceptive exposure was superior to attention control and in some ways superior to stress management alone.[57] In a Swedish study, exposure therapy for IBS was studied using a single-case experimental design of 13 patients. Seventy percent of patients had significant improvement in GI symptoms, pain catastrophizing, and GI quality of life. There was a modest effect on avoidance behaviors.[58]

## GUT-DIRECTED HYPNOSIS

Gut-directed hypnosis (GDH) is a therapeutic technique that cultivates a state of enhanced receptiveness to GI-specific suggestions in order to support therapeutic changes, and control and normalize GI functioning. Treatment typically involves 7 to 12 weekly sessions. There are 2 standard protocols for gastrointestinal conditions. The Manchester Protocol was developed by Whorwell and colleagues[59] in 1984, and the North Carolina Protocol was developed by Olafur Palsson and William Whitehead in 1994.[60] Targets of GDH include regulating smooth muscle activity, reducing the impact of stress on GI symptoms, reducing abdominal pain perception and attention to symptoms, and increased sense of control over symptoms.[48]

More than 15 randomized controlled trials have been conducted on the use of hypnosis for IBS.[61] GDH was associated with reduction in anger, frustration, embarrassment, and shame, as well as reduced bowel performance anxiety and improved self-efficacy.[62] Reductions in anxiety, depression, and quality of life were also shown.[63]

In a study comparing patients with IBS with controls with normal rectal sensation to balloon distension, GDH failed to reduce pain sensation for the entire sample, but did lead to significant reductions in those patients with the highest levels of baseline rectal sensitivity. Patients with normal sensation before GDH did not experience a change in sensation, leading the investigators to speculate that GDH seems to normalize visceral hypersensitivity.[64] For patients with pediatric abdominal pain, GDH led to an impressive 85% symptom improvement after 1 year[65] and 68% at 5-year follow-up.[66]

However, the results for GDH have not been consistent, with some studies finding no effect on visceral sensation.[67,68] This inconsistency may be explained by methodology, because the experimental stimuli are often administered in locations (ie, balloon inflation in the rectum or sigmoid colon) that may or may not align with the anatomic source of clinical symptoms.[69] GDH had a normalizing effect on central processing of visceral signals in patients with IBS using functional MRI.[70] GDH has also been shown to be as effective as the low-FODMAP (fermentable oligosaccharides, disaccharides, monosaccharides, and polyols) diet for patients with IBS.[71] Given that many patients with IBS restrict their diets in an attempt to avoid symptoms, GDH should be considered if there is concern for disordered or overly restrictive eating.[72]

### Mindfulness and Acceptance-based Treatments

The use of mindfulness and acceptance-based treatments can be particularly helpful for patients coping with unpleasant physical sensations. Mindfulness can be described as a willingness to remain in contact with the present moment, which may involve acceptance of unpleasant sensations or emotions. Participants are encouraged to notice and observe details about their symptoms without passing judgment or reacting to triggers. In these treatments, reduction of symptoms is not the primary target. The goal is to be able to notice and accept discomfort. In a study of 90 patients with IBS randomized to mindfulness-based stress reduction (MBSR) or waitlist control, both groups showed symptom improvement over time; however, the MBSR group showed a clinically meaningful decrease in symptom severity (characterized as going from constantly to occasionally present). At 6-month follow-up, the MBSR group maintained their clinically meaningful improvement in symptoms compared with the waitlist group.[73] A meta-analysis revealed that, across 6 studies, mindfulness-based therapies yielded significant improvements for patients with DGBI. Pooled effects were statistically significant for IBS severity and GI-specific quality of life.[74] In addition, a study of 75 patients with IBS found that mindfulness training provided benefits by promoting nonreactivity to visceral anxiety and catastrophic thinking about the significance of abdominal sensations.[75]

Acceptance and commitment therapy (ACT) is a newer treatment that incorporates mindfulness and acceptance-based strategies, as well as commitment to values-based action. ACT takes a particular approach to the notion of suffering, emphasizing that suffering stems not specifically from experiences such as physical symptoms or psychological distress, but how the person reacts to these experiences.[76] The treatment incorporates several core principles, including maintaining contact with the present moment (mindfulness), identifying one's core values, commitment to values-based action, acceptance, and mindfulness. ACT includes a focus on the patient's tendency toward experiential avoidance (unwillingness to acknowledge or experience unpleasant sensations or emotions), which often leads individuals to disengage from their values in an effort to prevent feelings of discomfort (eg, not going on a desired family trip out of fear that GI symptoms will affect the ability to enjoy the trip).

Although there is limited research on the efficacy of ACT in IBS, smaller studies have shown that ACT reduced symptom severity and GI-specific anxiety and improved quality of life for patients with refractory IBS.[77] These improvements occurred through the reduction in avoidance behaviors and increased psychological flexibility around IBS symptoms. Although there is less research support for ACT, it may be a valuable tool, particularly for patients who show experiential avoidance.[77]

## AGE OF VIRTUAL CARE

With the onset of the pandemic, many clinical practices shifted to virtual care. Literature supports efficacy for the delivery of gut-brain psychotherapies via telehealth, and therefore patients with IBS can receive their valuable care in a time when risk of increased mental health concerns is prevalent.[61] Patients with IBS can benefit from receiving their care in the comfort of their homes, especially if symptomatic. Symptomatic patients may be less inclined to cancel their appointments if they are not required to commute.

Although the pandemic has caused various psychosocial stressors, some patients have recognized improvements in their symptoms caused by working from home, ease of bathroom access, decreased anxiety about social interactions, or reduced extracurricular commitments. Working with a GI-specific mental health professional to ease back into personal and professional commitments outside the home will likely be incorporated into future treatment.

## DISCUSSION

Increasing knowledge of the bidirectional pathway that is the gut-brain axis has yielded exciting opportunities for effective treatments for IBS. Gut-brain psychotherapies can assist with downregulation of unpleasant GI sensations, decreasing avoidance behaviors associated with fears of having GI symptoms and improving coping and resilience to stress related to having a chronic health condition.[48]

As discussed, patients with IBS are more likely to engage in problem-focused and avoidant strategies. Although problem-focused strategies have been found to be helpful for controllable stressors, it is the use of emotion-focused coping strategies (such as use of emotional support, acceptance, humor, positive reframing, constructive self-talk, and religion or spirituality) that is helpful for coping with uncontrollable stressors,[78] including the unpredictability of IBS. Working with a GI-specific mental health provider can assist patients with identifying and effectively implementing appropriate strategies for the varying situations and stressors associated with IBS. Treatment can help to reduce the physical and emotional stress associated with ineffective coping. Patients also develop more confidence in their ability to manage their symptoms, meaning that they have strategies to use even if symptoms occur in unpredictable circumstances.

As previously discussed, IBS is often multifactorial; therefore, involving behavioral providers to the treatment team not only improves patient care by providing more comprehensive treatment but may also reduce physician burnout.[79] As to whether behavioral strategies affect gut-to-brain or brain-to-gut function, the answer is both. Strategies such as relaxation training and hypnosis can improve gut-to-brain functioning, whereas techniques such as CBT can improve brain-to-gut communication.[79] The American Gastroenterological Association (AGA)[4] and the American College of Gastroenterology (ACG)[2] recommend psychological interventions for patients with global symptoms of IBS or patients with refractory symptoms, or patients for whom psychological factors exacerbate symptoms.[2,48] The Rome Foundation has developed an internal psychogastroenterology section including a list of providers trained in providing the behavioral treatments discussed in this article. Gastroenterologists are encouraged to partner with a GI-specific mental health provider and to view these providers as part of the treatment team. The collection of best practices by Keefer and colleagues[80] is an essential read and was developed to assist in the incorporation of psychogastroenterology practices for clinicians in gastroenterology.

## CLINICS CARE POINTS

- IBS is a complex condition that is best viewed through the biopsychosocial model to understand the role of genetics, early life stress and other psychological factors, the gut microbiome, health behaviors such as sleep quality, and physiologic factors such as visceral hypersensitivity and gut permeability.

- Evidence-based treatments such as GI-specific CBT, GDH, and mindfulness-based therapies can be used in combination with medical treatments and nutritional therapies, such as the low-FODMAP diet, to improve gut-brain communication and teach patients effective use of behavioral strategies to reduce the negative impact of stress on GI symptoms.

- Gut-brain psychological interventions can be effectively delivered in person or via telehealth modalities, which can allow increased access to these valuable treatment options.

- Gastroenterologists are encouraged to partner with GI-specific mental health providers in order to develop an effective pathway for referral and bidirectional communication between medical and psychological providers to improve patient quality of care.

## DISCLOSURE

Dr C.H. Jagielski has no commercial or financial conflicts of interest, nor any funding sources to disclose. M.E. Riehl, Gastro Girl, coparent owner of GI OnDEMAND, consultant fee; Health Union, LLC, consultant fees.

## REFERENCES

1. Drossman DA, Hasler WL. Rome IV-functional GI disorders: disorders of gut-brain interaction. Gastroenterology 2016;150(6):1257–61.
2. Lacy BE, Pimentel M, Brenner DM, et al. ACG Clinical Guideline: Management of irritable bowel syndrome. Am J Gastroenterol 2021;116(1):17–44.
3. Ford AC, Moayyedi P, Chey WD, et al. American College of Gastroenterology Monograph on management of irritable bowel syndrome. Am J Gastroenterol 2018;113(Suppl 2):1–18.
4. Drossman DA, Camilleri M, Mayer EA, et al. AGA technical review on irritable bowel syndrome. Gastroenterology 2002;123(6):2108–31.
5. Lacy BE, Mearin F, Chang L, et al. Bowel disorders. Gastroenterology 2016; 150(6):1393–407.
6. Palsson OS, Whitehead W, Törnblom H, et al. Prevalence of Rome IV functional bowel disorders among adults in the United States, Canada, and the United Kingdom. Gastroenterology 2020;158(5):1262–73.
7. Drossman DA. Presidential address: Gastrointestinal illness and the biopsychosocial model. Psychosom Med 1998;60(3):258–67.
8. Van Oudenhove L, Levy RL, Crowell MD, et al. Biopsychosocial aspects of functional gastrointestinal disorders: How central and environmental processes

contribute to the development and expression of functional gastrointestinal disorders. Gastroenterology 2016;150(6):1355–67.

9. Hansen MB. The enteric nervous system I: organisation and classification. Phar-. macol Toxicol 2003;92(3):105–13.

10. Mayer EA, Tillisch K. The brain-gut axis in abdominal pain syndromes. Annu Rev Med 2011;62:381–96.

11. Kinsinger SW. Cognitive-behavioral therapy for patients with irritable bowel syndrome: current insights. Psychol Res Behav Manag 2017;10:231–7.

12. Lee C, Doo E, Choi JM, et al. The increased level of depression and anxiety in irritable bowel syndrome patients compared with healthy controls: Systematic review and meta-analysis. J Neurogastroenterol Motil 2017;23(3):349–62.

13. Zamani M, Alizadeh-Tabari S, Zamani V. Systematic review with meta-analysis: the prevalence of anxiety and depression in patients with irritable bowel syndrome. Aliment Pharmacol Ther 2019;50(2):132–43.

14. Sibelli A, Chalder T, Everitt H, et al. A systematic review with meta-analysis of the role of anxiety and depression in irritable bowel syndrome onset. Psychol Med 2016;46(15):3065–80.

15. Miller V, Hopkins L, Whorwell PJ. Suicidal ideation in patients with irritable bowel syndrome. Clin Gastroenterol Hepatol 2004;2(12):1064–8.

16. Midenfjord I, Polster A, Sjövall H, et al. Anxiety and depression in irritable bowel syndrome: Exploring the interaction with other symptoms and pathophysiology using multivariate analyses. Neurogastroenterol Motil 2019;31(8):e13619.

17. van Tilburg MA, Palsson OS, Whitehead WE. Which psychological factors exacerbate irritable bowel syndrome? Development of a comprehensive model. J Psychosom Res 2013;74(6):486–92.

18. Turna J, Grosman Kaplan K, Patterson B, et al. Higher prevalence of irritable bowel syndrome and greater gastrointestinal symptoms in obsessive-compulsive disorder. J Psychiatr Res 2019;118:1–6.

19. Stanculete MF, Matu S, Pojoga C, et al. Coping strategies and irrational beliefs as mediators of the health-related quality of life impairments in irritable bowel syndrome. J Gastrointestin Liver Dis 2015;24(2):159–64.

20. Buono JL, Carson RT, Flores NM. Health-related quality of life, work productivity, and indirect costs among patients with irritable bowel syndrome with diarrhea. Health Qual Life Outcomes 2017;15(1):35.

21. Frändemark Å, Törnblom H, Jakobsson S, et al. Work productivity and activity impairment in irritable bowel syndrome (IBS): A multifaceted problem. Am J Gastroenterol 2018;113(10):1540–9.

22. Poulsen CH, Eplov LF, Hjorthøj C, et al. Irritable bowel symptoms, use of healthcare, costs, sickness and disability pension benefits: A long-term population-based study. Scand J Public Health 2019;47(8):867–75.

23. Park SH, Naliboff BD, Shih W, et al. Resilience is decreased in irritable bowel syndrome and associated with symptoms and cortisol response. Neurogastroenterol Motil 2018;30(1):e13155.

24. Vandvik PO, Wilhelmsen I, Ihlebaek C, et al. Comorbidity of irritable bowel syndrome in general practice: a striking feature with clinical implications. Aliment Pharmacol Ther 2004;20(10):1195–203.

25. Bradford K, Shih W, Videlock EJ, et al. Association between early adverse life events and irritable bowel syndrome. Clin Gastroenterol Hepatol 2012;10(4):385–90.

26. Drossman DA, Leserman J, Nachman G, et al. Sexual and physical abuse in women with functional or organic gastrointestinal disorders. Ann Intern Med 1990;113(11):828–33.

27. Halland M, Almazar A, Lee R, et al. A case-control study of childhood trauma in the development of irritable bowel syndrome. Neurogastroenterol Motil 2014; 26(7):990–8.

28. Heitkemper MM, Cain KC, Burr RL, et al. Is childhood abuse or neglect associated with symptom reports and physiological measures in women with irritable bowel syndrome? Biol Res Nurs 2011;13(4):399–408.

29. Ju T, Naliboff BD, Shih W, et al. Risk and protective factors related to early adverse life events in irritable bowel syndrome. J Clin Gastroenterol 2020; 54(1):63–9.

30. Ng QX, Soh AYS, Loke W, et al. Systematic review with meta-analysis: The association between post-traumatic stress disorder and irritable bowel syndrome. J Gastroenterol Hepatol 2019;34(1):68–73.

31. Keeshin BR, Cronholm PF, Strawn JR. Physiologic changes associated with violence and abuse exposure: an examination of related medical conditions. Trauma Violence Abuse 2012;13(1):41–56.

32. Labus JS, Dinov ID, Jiang Z, et al. Irritable bowel syndrome in female patients is associated with alterations in structural brain networks. Pain 2014;155(1):137–49.

33. Videlock EJ, Adeyemo M, Licudine A, et al. Childhood trauma is associated with hypothalamic-pituitary-adrenal axis responsiveness in irritable bowel syndrome. Gastroenterology 2009;137(6):1954–62.

34. Drossman DA, Li Z, Leserman J, et al. Health status by gastrointestinal diagnosis and abuse history. Gastroenterology 1996;110(4):999–1007.

35. Baumeister D, Akhtar R, Ciufolini S, et al. Childhood trauma and adulthood inflammation: a meta-analysis of peripheral C-reactive protein, interleukin-6 and tumour necrosis factor-$\alpha$. Mol Psychiatry 2016;21(5):642–9.

36. Ballou S, Alhassan E, Hon E, et al. Sleep disturbances are commonly reported among patients presenting to a gastroenterology clinic. Dig Dis Sci 2018; 63(11):2983–91.

37. Patel A, Hasak S, Cassell B, et al. Effects of disturbed sleep on gastrointestinal and somatic pain symptoms in irritable bowel syndrome. Aliment Pharmacol Ther 2016;44(3):246–58.

38. Knutsson A, Bøggild H. Gastrointestinal disorders among shift workers. Scand J Work Environ Health 2010;36(2):85–95.

39. Nojkov B, Rubenstein J, Chey WD, et al. The impact of rotating shift work on the prevalence of irritable bowel syndrome in nurses. Am J Gastroenterol 2010; 105(4):842–7.

40. Sherwin LB, Leary E, Henderson WA. The association of catastrophizing with quality-of-life outcomes in patients with irritable bowel syndrome. Qual Life Res 2017;26(8):2161–70.

41. Lackner JM, Quigley BM, Blanchard EB. Depression and Abdominal Pain in IBS Patients: The Mediating Role of Catastrophizing. Psychosom Med 2004;66(3): 435–41.

42. Hollier JM, van Tilburg MA, Liu Y, et al. Multiple psychological factors predict abdominal pain severity in children with irritable bowel syndrome. Neurogastroenterol Motil 2019;31(2):e13509.

43. Posserud I, Svedlund J, Wallin J, et al. Hypervigilance in irritable bowel syndrome compared with organic gastrointestinal disease. J Psychosom Res 2009;66(5): 399–405.

44. Ritchie J. Pain from distension of the pelvic colon by inflating a balloon in the irritable colon syndrome. Gut 1973;14(2):125–32.
45. Mertz H, Naliboff B, Munakata J, et al. Altered rectal perception is a biological marker of patients with irritable bowel syndrome. Gastroenterology 1995; 109(1):40–52.
46. Mertz H, Morgan V, Tanner G, et al. Regional cerebral activation in irritable bowel syndrome and control subjects with painful and nonpainful rectal distension. Gastroenterology 2000;118(5):842–8.
47. Tillisch K, Mayer EA, Labus JS. Quantitative meta-analysis identifies brain regions activated during rectal distension in irritable bowel syndrome. Gastroenterology 2011;140(1):91–100.
48. Palsson OS, Whitehead WE. Psychological treatments in functional gastrointestinal disorders: a primer for the gastroenterologist. Clin Gastroenterol Hepatol 2013;11(3):208–16.
49. Lackner JM, Gudleski GD, Keefer L, et al. Rapid response to cognitive behavior therapy predicts treatment outcome in patients with irritable bowel syndrome. Clin Gastroenterol Hepatol 2010;8(5):426–32.
50. van Dulmen AM, Fennis JF, Bleijenberg G. Cognitive-behavioral group therapy for irritable bowel syndrome: effects and long-term follow-up. Psychosom Med 1996; 58(5):508–14.
51. Hunt MG, Moshier S, Milonova M. Brief cognitive-behavioral internet therapy for irritable bowel syndrome. Behav Res Ther 2009;47(9):797–802.
52. Moss-Morris R, McAlpine L, Didsbury LP, et al. A randomized controlled trial of a cognitive behavioural therapy-based self-management intervention for irritable bowel syndrome in primary care. Psychol Med 2010;40(1):85–94.
53. Tonkin-Crine S, Bishop F, Ellis M, et al. Exploring patients' views of a cognitive behavioral therapy-based website for the self-management of irritable bowel syndrome symptoms. J Med Internet Res 2013;15(9):e190.
54. Klimes I, Mayou RA, Pearce MJ, et al. Psychological treatment for atypical non-cardiac chest pain: a controlled evaluation. Psychol Med 1990;20(3):605–11.
55. Mayou RA, Bryant BM, Sanders D, et al. A controlled trial of cognitive behavioural therapy for non-cardiac chest pain. Psychol Med 1997;27(5):1021–31.
56. Van Peski-Oosterbaan AS, Spinhoven P, Van der Does AJ, et al. Cognitive change following cognitive behavioural therapy for non-cardiac chest pain. Psychother Psychosom 1999;68(4):214–20.
57. Craske MG, Wolitzky-Taylor KB, Labus J, et al. A cognitive-behavioral treatment for irritable bowel syndrome using interoceptive exposure to visceral sensations. Behav Res Ther 2011;49(6–7):413–21.
58. Boersma K, Ljótsson B, Edebol-Carlman H, et al. Exposure-based cognitive behavioral therapy for irritable bowel syndrome. A single-case experimental design across 13 subjects. Cogn Behav Ther 2016;45(6):415–30.
59. Whorwell PJ, Prior A, Faragher EB. Controlled trial of hypnotherapy in the treatment of severe refractory irritable-bowel syndrome. Lancet 1984;2(8414):1232–4.
60. Palsson OS. Standardized hypnosis treatment for irritable bowel syndrome: The North Carolina protocol. Int J Clin Exp Hypn 2006;54(1):51–64.
61. Black CJ, Thakur ER, Houghton LA, et al. Efficacy of psychological therapies for irritable bowel syndrome: systematic review and network meta-analysis. Gut 2020;69(8):1441–51.
62. Gonsalkorale WM, Toner BB, Whorwell PJ. Cognitive change in patients undergoing hypnotherapy for irritable bowel syndrome. J Psychosom Res 2004;56(3): 271–8.

63. Gonsalkorale WM, Houghton LA, Whorwell PJ. Hypnotherapy in irritable bowel syndrome: a large-scale audit of a clinical service with examination of factors influencing responsiveness. Am J Gastroenterol 2002;97(4):954–61.
64. Lea R, Houghton LA, Calvert EL, et al. Gut-focused hypnotherapy normalizes disordered rectal sensitivity in patients with irritable bowel syndrome. Aliment Pharmacol Ther 2003;17(5):635–42.
65. Vlieger AM, Menko-Frankenhuis C, Wolfkamp SC, et al. Hypnotherapy for children with functional abdominal pain or irritable bowel syndrome: a randomized controlled trial. Gastroenterology 2007;133(5):1430–6.
66. Vlieger AM, Rutten JM, Govers AM, et al. Long-term follow-up of gut-directed hypnotherapy vs. standard care in children with functional abdominal pain or irritable bowel syndrome. Am J Gastroenterol 2012;107(4):627–31.
67. Vlieger AM, van den Berg MM, Menko-Frankenhuis C, et al. No change in rectal sensitivity after gut-directed hypnotherapy in children with functional abdominal pain or irritable bowel syndrome. Am J Gastroenterol 2010;105(1):213–8.
68. Palsson OS, Turner MJ, Johnson DA, et al. Hypnosis treatment for severe irritable bowel syndrome: investigation of mechanism and effects on symptoms. Dig Dis Sci 2002;47(11):2605–14.
69. Palsson OS. Hypnosis treatment of gastrointestinal disorders: A comprehensive review of the empirical evidence. Am J Clin Hypn 2015;58(2):134–58.
70. Lowén MB, Mayer E A, Sjöberg M, et al. Effect of hypnotherapy and educational intervention on brain response to visceral stimulus in the irritable bowel syndrome. Aliment Pharmacol Ther 2013;37(12):1184–97.
71. Peters SL, Yao CK, Philpott H, et al. Randomised clinical trial: the efficacy of gut-directed hypnotherapy is similar to that of the low FODMAP diet for the treatment of irritable bowel syndrome. Aliment Pharmacol Ther 2016;44(5):447–59.
72. Kamal A, Pimentel M. Influence of dietary restriction on irritable bowel syndrome. Am J Gastroenterol 2019;114(2):212–20.
73. Zernicke KA, Campbell TS, Blustein PK, et al. Mindfulness-based stress reduction for the treatment of irritable bowel syndrome symptoms: a randomized wait-list controlled trial. Int J Behav Med 2013;20(3):385–96.
74. Aucoin MA, Lalonde-Parsi MJ, Cooley K. Mindfulness-based therapies in the treatment of functional gastrointestinal disorders: a meta-analysis. Evid Based Complement Alternat Med 2014;2014:140724.
75. Garland EL, Gaylord SA, Palsson OS, et al. Therapeutic mechanisms of a mindfulness-based treatment for IBS: effects on visceral sensitivity, catastrophizing, and affective processing of pain sensations. J Behav Med 2012;35(6):591–602.
76. Hayes SC, Strosahl KD, Wilson KG. Acceptance and commitment therapy: the process and practice of mindful change. New York: Guilford Press; 2011.
77. Ferreira NB, Gillanders D, Morris PG, et al. Pilot study of acceptance and commitment therapy for irritable bowel syndrome: a preliminary analysis of treatment outcomes and processes of change. Clin Psychol 2018;22(2):241–50.
78. Park CL, Armeli S, Tennen H. Appraisal-coping goodness of fit: a daily internet study. Pers Soc Psychol Bull 2004;30(5):558–69.
79. Chey WD, Keefer L, Whelan K, et al. Behavioral and diet therapies in integrated care for patients with irritable bowel syndrome. Gastroenterology 2021;160(1):47–62.
80. Keefer L, Palsson OS, Pandolfino JE. Best Practice Update: Incorporating psychogastroenterology into management of digestive disorders. Gastroenterology 2018;154:1249–57.

# Irritable Bowel Syndrome and Eating Disorders

## A Burgeoning Concern in Gastrointestinal Clinics

Andrea McGowan, MPH[a], Kimberly N. Harer, MD, ScM[b],*

### KEYWORDS

- Irritable bowel syndrome • Eating disorder • Disordered eating • ARFID • Orthorexia

### KEY POINTS

- Most patients with IBS report worsening of their symptoms with eating, and up to 90% of patients with IBS exclude certain foods in the hopes of avoiding or improving their GI symptoms.
- Dietary restriction in the setting of GI symptoms are a normal, adaptive response or a pathologic, maladaptive process.
- Eating disorders and GI disorders, such as IBS, often occur simultaneously and are not mutually exclusive diagnoses. Eating disorders can present before GI symptom onset, concomitantly with GI symptoms, or as a result of chronic GI symptoms. Simultaneous management of both conditions is imperative.
- Treatment of patients with IBS and an eating disorder involves a multidisciplinary approach, which includes gastroenterologists, psychologists, psychiatrists, and dietitians.

### INTRODUCTION

There is increasing interest and growing evidence of the bidirectional relationship between irritable bowel syndrome (IBS) and eating disorders. Eating disorders are illnesses associated with dietary intake, eating behaviors, and metabolism; therefore, it is intuitive that eating disorders might be further associated with gastrointestinal (GI) symptoms and IBS. Up to 90% of patients with IBS exclude certain foods to improve their GI symptoms,[1] and evidence has shown patients with diet-controlled illnesses are at higher risk of disordered eating and eating disorders than the general population.[2]

[a] University of Michigan School of Public Health, c/o Kimberly Harer, 1500 East Medical Center Drive, 3912 TC SPC 5362, Ann Arbor, MI 48109, USA; [b] University of Michigan, Division of Gastroenterology, Department of Internal Medicine, 1500 East Medical Center Drive, 3912 TC SPC 5362, Ann Arbor, MI 48109, USA
* Corresponding author.
*E-mail address:* kharer@med.umich.edu

Gastroenterol Clin N Am 50 (2021) 595–610
https://doi.org/10.1016/j.gtc.2021.03.007
0889-8553/21/© 2021 Elsevier Inc. All rights reserved.

Although the bidirectional relationship is known, the temporal relationship between eating disorders and GI conditions is complex and poorly understood. Eating disorders among GI patients can occur independently of GI symptoms, concomitantly with GI symptoms, or secondary to chronic GI symptoms. The latter category is of particular interest to gastroenterologists treating patients with IBS because a high index of suspicion is required to identify pathologic dietary habits in the setting of chronic GI symptoms. Often, the dietary adjustments implemented by patients with IBS are appropriate adaptations. However, these normal adaptive dietary modifications can spiral out of control and result in maladaptive behaviors. These maladaptive behaviors, which are classified as eating disorders, and their association with IBS serve as the focus of this review.

Aims:
- Discuss the difference between eating disorders and disordered eating
- Outline the diagnostic criteria for the most common eating disorders
- Compare the prevalence of IBS symptoms among patients with eating disorders versus the prevalence of eating disorders among patients with IBS symptoms
- Highlight the role gastroenterologists play in the multidisciplinary approach to treatment in patients with concomitant IBS and eating disorders

## EATING DISORDER VERSUS DISORDERED EATING

Eating disorders are defined by stringent criteria via the Diagnostic and Statistical Manual of Mental Disorders (DSM); however, many patients have disordered eating behaviors that do not fit perfectly into these criteria.[3] Disordered eating is typically defined as eating behavior including, but not limited to, bingeing, purging, or restricting without meeting the criteria for a specific eating disorder.[4,5] These "nonnormative" eating behaviors are not as pathologic or persistent as a full syndrome eating disorder and exist across individuals of all weights and body mass indexes (BMI).[4,5] Research suggests that disordered eating is significantly more prevalent than full syndrome eating disorders.[3,5] In a cross-sectional study of women ages 25 to 45 years old (n = 4023), nearly one-third of participants reported purging to control weight and nearly three-quarters of participants reported preoccupations with body weight and shape.[5] A systematic review of cross-sectional and cohort studies on eating behavior suggested that disordered eating among nonclinical populations is twice as prevalent as full syndrome eating disorders.[3] This same review, pooling more than 26,000 participants, suggested that participants with disordered eating or partial syndrome eating disorders reported such behaviors as dieting, restricting, diuretics/laxatives, and purging less frequently than full syndrome eating disorders.[3]

## GASTROINTESTINAL DISORDERS AS A RISK FACTOR FOR EATING DISORDERS

GI patients seem to be at higher risk for eating disorders than the normal population.[6,7] Among GI patients, there is growing evidence patients with IBS are at risk of developing disordered eating behaviors and eating disorders. Most of the current evidence evaluating the relationship between IBS and eating disorders focuses on restrictive eating disorders, such as anorexia nervosa or avoidant/restrictive food intake disorder (ARFID). This is likely secondary to the high prevalence of food-induced GI symptoms and the tendency of patients to avoid GI symptom triggers.

All eating disorders are harmful and pathologic; however, not all disordered eating behaviors among GI patients are harmful or pathologic. Disordered eating behaviors is either a normal adaptive response to GI symptoms or a pathologic maladaptive response (Fig. 1). This differentiation is paramount when understanding dietary

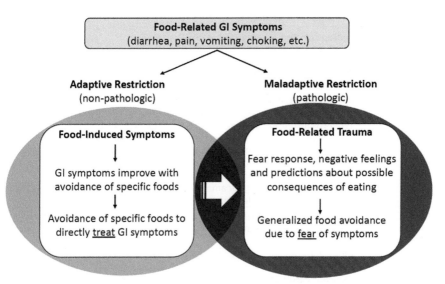

**Fig. 1.** Adaptive dietary restriction versus maladaptive restriction.

habits among patients with IBS or GI symptoms. For example, a patient may implement a low FODMAP diet for 4 to 6 weeks to treat IBS symptoms, followed by a reintroduction phase to identify specific food triggers. The patient may then choose to avoid their identified food triggers. This is a normal dietary restriction response to dietary-induced GI symptoms. An example of maladaptive eating behavior is a patient with IBS who restricted their diet to 10 "safe foods" within the low FODMAP diet, refused to reintroduce foods, and required supplement beverages to help maintain a normal weight. Note that many experts view disordered eating as a spectrum, and research suggests that disordered eating behavior can progress to a pathologic eating disorder.[3] Thus, it is imperative for gastroenterologists to recognize disordered eating habits and monitor for evidence that the restriction could be spiraling out of control.

## OVERVIEW OF EATING DISORDER DIAGNOSTIC CRITERIA

Feeding and eating disorders (**Table 1**) are described as pathologic disturbances of eating behavior and comprise an entire chapter in the DSM-5.[8] The DSM-5 includes several modifications from the previous publication in 1994.[9] These changes include the addition of binge eating disorder as a separate diagnosis and the transformation of "Feeding and Eating Disorders of Infancy or Early Childhood" to three disorders: (1) ARFID, (2) pica, and (3) rumination disorder.[10] It is critical for gastroenterologists to be aware of the diagnostic criteria to recognize these conditions in their patients.

## WHAT IS KNOWN ABOUT THE OVERLAP OF IRRITABLE BOWEL SYNDROME AND EATING DISORDERS?

There is a paucity of evidence evaluating the prevalence of eating disorders among GI patients. Most research to date has focused on the prevalence of GI symptoms among patients with eating disorders. The heterogeneity of IBS symptoms and the inconsistent criteria used to diagnose IBS across studies further complicates the arduous task

**Table 1**
**Feeding and eating disorders and primary clinical manifestations**

| Eating Disorder | Primary Clinical Manifestation |
|---|---|
| Anorexia nervosa | Characterized by restriction of energy intake resulting in low body weight. Individuals present with a pathologic fear of gaining weight and body dysmorphia.<br>Two recognized subtypes: restricting type characterized by an absence of bingeing or purging behavior, and binge-eating/purging type characterized by binge/purging behavior in the last 3 mo.<br>Disease onset is more common in adolescence and young adulthood, especially surrounding the onset of puberty.[8]<br>Clinical prevalence is higher among females than males, although those that identify as male are less represented in studies.[11] |
| Bulimia nervosa | Characterized by reoccurring episodes of binge eating (consumption of atypically large amounts of food in a discrete period of time and a feeling of lack of control).<br>Binge episodes are followed by compensatory behaviors (ie, vomiting, laxative and diuretic use, fasting, or excessive exercise).<br>Behavior occurs at least once per week for 3 mo and may be motivated by shape or weight preoccupation.[8]<br>More common in females than males and occurs in older adolescents and young adults.[8] |
| Binge eating disorder | Characterized by episodes of bingeing associated with 3 or more of the following behaviors: eating more rapidly than normal, eating until uncomfortably full, eating alone out of embarrassment, eating large amounts while not hungry, or feeling shame following a binge.<br>Behavior occurs at least once a week for 3 mo and is not followed by subsequent compensatory behavior like vomiting, laxative and diuretic use, fasting, or excessive exercise.[8]<br>Prevalence seems to be similar across different racial and ethnic groups.[8] |
| ARFID | Characterized by an eating or feeding disturbance associated with at least one of the following: weight loss, nutritional deficiency, dependence on supplementary nutrition, or interference with psychosocial behavior.<br>Disturbance is seen as a lack of interest in food, sensory aversions, or concerns about consequences of eating (ie, GI symptoms).<br>The eating disturbance is not motivated by a lack of food availability, weight/shape concerns, or another mental disorder.<br>This diagnosis presents at any age, but existing literature focuses on presentation in children.[8] |
| Orthorexia nervosa | Not formally recognized in the DSM-5, but it is important to address in GI patients[12] and can be mistaken for ARFID because of the dietary restriction.<br>Manifestations include obsession over purity of diet, planning and preparing healthful food, and superiority of one's dietary choices compared with others.[13]<br>Additional criterion includes extreme stress surrounding food choices without weight loss being the main intention,[14] paired with one of the following: medical consequences from dietary choices (weight loss, malnutrition, deficiency), hindered day-to-day functioning because of dietary choices (social, academic, vocational, intrapersonal), or a body image and/or worth that is dependent on dietary choices.[14]<br>Screening for orthorexia relies on ORTO-15 scores, a validated questionnaire developed in 2005 from a sample of 525.[15] |

*(continued on next page)*

| Table 1 (continued) | |
|---|---|
| **Eating Disorder** | **Primary Clinical Manifestation** |
| Pica | Characterized by persistent eating of nonfood/nonnutritive substances (ie, ice, soap, paint, pebbles, charcoal, hair, soil) over a period of at least 1 mo. Behavior is not representative of a cultural or social practice and is inappropriate for the individual's developmental stage. Prevalence is understudied, but onset in childhood is most typical. Diagnosis is illuminated from bloodwork and bowel obstructions.[8] |
| Rumination disorder | Characterized by repeated regurgitation of food over a period of 1 mo or more. Regurgitated food can be spit out, rechewed, or reswallowed. The regurgitation is not a result of a GI condition. Prevalence data remain inconclusive, and onset can occur between infancy and adulthood.[8] |
| Other specified feeding or eating disorder | Characterized by symptoms of feeding and eating disorders that do not meet all of the criteria for a specific eating disorder diagnosis. Examples include atypical anorexia nervosa (all criteria present except the individual's weight is normal or high), bulimia nervosa (infrequent or limited duration of symptoms), binge eating disorder (infrequent or limited duration of symptoms), purging disorder, and night eating syndrome. |

of understanding the relationship between eating disorders and IBS. The available data regarding IBS and eating disorders are discussed, and the more global association between GI symptoms and eating disorders.

## Irritable Bowel Syndrome and Eating Disorders/Disordered Eating

### Disordered eating among patients with irritable bowel syndrome

A systematic review including nine studies demonstrated the prevalence of disordered eating is higher among gastroenterology patients than healthy control subjects, with a prevalence up to 44%.[7] In a case-control study measuring food frequency and lifestyle habits among a sample of patients with IBS and healthy control subjects (n = 78 and n = 79), patients with IBS had 3.96 higher odds of engaging in irregular eating habits (eg, skipping meals, going long periods without eating, not having regular meals) compared with healthy control subjects.[16] Similarly, in a sample of 2639 students, the female participants with IBS had significantly higher patterns of irregular meal times and skipped meals compared with female participants without IBS.[17] Male students did not have significant differences within the groups.[17] These irregular behaviors do not indicate a full syndrome eating disorder, but could become more pathologic on the eating disorder spectrum. In a study of adolescents, no statistically significant differences were found in disordered eating symptoms in an attempt to influence shape or weight as measured by the Eating Disorders Examination Questionnaire comparing patients with IBS (n = 48) and healthy control subjects (n = 51).[18] However, adolescents with IBS tried to control symptoms by avoiding the offending food (97.9% IBS vs 15.7% healthy control subjects; $P<.001$), not eating any food even when hungry (41.7% IBS vs 9.8% healthy control subjects; $P<.001$), or vomiting after eating (12.5% IBS vs 2% healthy control subjects; $P<.05$).

Although disordered eating behavior might be motivated by GI symptom control, rather than weight and shape control, it is still of concern because of the potential for symptoms to progress into more pathologic disordered eating.[18] Additionally, the Eating Attitude Test (EAT) was administered to inflammatory bowel disease (IBD), IBS, and eating disorder patients and a control group. When not including the eating disorder patients, patients with IBS had statistically significantly higher EAT scores compared with patients with IBD,[19] suggesting that patients with IBS might be more likely to experience disordered eating than patients with IBD.

There is also growing awareness of the association between weight-related teasing and disordered eating behaviors. Adolescents with a diagnosed bowel disorder (eg, celiac disease, IBD, IBS) are more likely to report weight-related teasing in their childhood.[20] Although weight-related teasing does not necessitate disordered eating behavior, longitudinal studies have shown that this teasing can predict disordered eating behaviors later in life.[21] It is possible that elevated teasing could precede manifestation of disordered eating in patients with IBS.

### Eating disorders among patients with irritable bowel syndrome

Shifting focus from disordered eating to eating disorders, it is widely believed that individuals with GI disorders may be more at risk for an eating disorder.[7] This relationship has been exemplified in adolescents with celiac disease[22] and in individuals with other diet-related health conditions.[6] Furthermore, a large longitudinal twin study indicated that a history of constipation and diarrhea correlated with a significantly higher Eating Disorders Inventory-2 (EDI) score.[23] A study of 100 patients with IBS diagnosed via Rome-IV criteria and 100 healthy adults demonstrated that patients with IBS are at higher risk of having disordered eating than healthy adults (odds ratio, 5.3; 95% confidence interval, 4.3–9.3; $P<.001$), as identified by the EAT questionnaire.[24] In that study, there was no statistically significant difference in EAT scores between the various subtype of IBS.[24] Although causality is uncertain, temporality has been self-reported in at least one small study. In a prospective cohort study of 48 eating disorder patients (most with anorexia nervosa), 17% had a previous IBS diagnosis before admission for treatment of an eating disorder.[25]

In a sample of patients with IBS (n = 60), IBS symptom severity was correlated with perfectionism and ineffectiveness subscales on the EDI,[26] two character traits that are frequently implicated in individuals with an eating disorder.[27] Additionally, there was an association between patients with IBS who reported significant vomiting and nausea on the EDI bulimia subscale and a "desire for lower body weight."[26]

### Irritable bowel syndrome among patients with eating disorders

**Anorexia nervosa.** Given the paucity of evidence regarding the prevalence of eating disorders among patients with IBS, the data regarding IBS among patients with eating disorders is often used to explore the association between these two conditions. IBS is common among patients with eating disorders, but the cause of this association is unclear. GI dysmotility and intestinal dysbiosis have been hypothesized causes of IBS symptoms secondary to malnutrition, restricted diversity of foods consumed, and altered metabolic or hormonal processes. In a cross-sectional study of 234 predominately female individuals with a previous or current eating disorder diagnosis, 64% fulfilled the Manning criteria for IBS.[28] Of the 144 individuals who met IBS criteria, 87% reported developing their eating disorder, before IBS onset,[28] providing some insight into temporality in this study. In a cohort of 100 patients with eating disorders, 41% met the Rome III criteria for IBS on admission to treatment.[29] In a demographically similar cohort of 160 patients with an eating disorder, 45% met the Rome II criteria for IBS on admission for treatment.[29] In a sample of 184 women in an eating disorder unit with anorexia nervosa, 42.9% met Rome II criteria for IBS.[30]

Regarding the relationship between IBS symptom severity and eating disorders, 30 outpatients with anorexia nervosa were included in a cross-sectional study that indicated IBS symptom severity is correlated with Eating Disorder Examination Questionnaire scores.[31] This study further suggested that eating disorder pathology and somatization scores accounted for half of the variance in GI symptoms.[31] Although it is a small study with potential bias from self-reporting, GI symptoms and somatization should be addressed by clinicians to remove barriers to eating disorder recovery. Temporality of IBS remains unclear in this study.

**Bulimia nervosa.** A study evaluated the prevalence of IBS in 64 participants with bulimia nervosa or eating disorder not otherwise specified (EDNOS)/bulimia nervosa, and found 68.8% (n = 44) met Manning criteria for IBS.[32] Patients with IBS in this sample reported higher frequency of self-induced vomiting in comparison with those who did not meet IBS criteria.[32] Additionally, in a sample of 33 women admitted to an eating disorder unit for bulimia nervosa, 54.5% met Rome II IBS criteria.[30] Thus, the prevalence of IBS seems to be at least as high in those with bulimia nervosa as in individuals with anorexia nervosa or mixed eating disorder diagnoses.[28,30,32] However, there are comparatively fewer studies that address bulimia nervosa in comparison with anorexia nervosa.

**Binge eating disorder.** In a cross-sectional study using data from a Swedish twin study, 16.9% (n = 55) of total individuals with binge eating (n = 362) met criteria for IBS compared with 7.4% (n = 548) of total individuals without binge eating behavior (n = 7955).[33] This statistically significant result suggested elevated IBS prevalence among those with binge eating behavior.[33] More data need to be collected on this eating disorder diagnosis, especially among males.

**Avoidant/restrictive food intake disorder.** ARFID is an eating disorder characterized by avoidance or restriction of foods associated with clinically significant weight loss, nutritional deficiency, dependence on tube feeds/oral supplements, or significant psychosocial interference. As discussed in the overview of eating disorders, ARFID describes an inability to meet energy and nutrient requirements that is not attributed to food insecurity, eating disorder behavior, or shape or weight concerns.[8] Unlike orthorexia, the dietary restriction in ARFID is primarily driven by a fear of negative consequences or desire to avoid GI symptoms instead of a compulsion with eating "healthy" foods. The diet-responsive nature of IBS symptoms places patients with IBS at particular risk for ARFID. Although some dietary restriction is normal and healthy, in some patients the success of dietary exclusions can promote extreme and pathologic restriction. Because of this feedback cycle and the increasing popularity of restrictive diet interventions for patients with IBS, ARFID is a topic of growing interest and importance among gastroenterologists.[12,34]

There is currently a substantial knowledge gap in understanding how ARFID complicates the clinical presentation of patients with IBS; however, there is growing awareness of the connection between these disorders. In a retrospective chart review of adolescents with ARFID admitted as underweight (n = 27), GI symptoms were identified as the reason for restriction in 81.5%.[35] This finding highlights why gastroenterologists should closely monitor eating behavior and look for red flag symptoms in patients with IBS. Although ARFID is more studied in children and adolescents, attention has started to shift to adults with GI diagnoses. There is increasing awareness of ARFID among adult GI patients, with a prevalence of approximately 20%.[36,37] Oftentimes, these patients present with extremely restrictive diets and develop fear of certain foods because of the potential GI consequences.[38]

**Eating disorder not otherwise specified.** There are little data on the prevalence of IBS in patients with EDNOS. In a sample of 67 women in an eating disorder unit diagnosed with EDNOS, 44.8% met Rome II criteria for IBS.[30]

## GLOBAL GASTROINTESTINAL SYMPTOMS AND EATING DISORDERS

Given the lack of robust data evaluating eating disorders specifically in the IBS population and that a diagnosis of IBS includes common GI symptoms (ie, abdominal pain, constipation, diarrhea), it is worthwhile to look at studies that evaluated eating disorders in the general GI population as a whole. In a prospective cohort of eating disorder patients, GI symptoms were common. Ninety-six percent of participants reported post-prandial fullness and 90% of participants reported abdominal distention.[25] Similarly, in a sample of 160 individuals in an eating disorder unit, 93% reported a functional GI disorder.[39] Specifically, IBS and functional constipation was associated with quality of life in eating disorder patients based on Eating Disorder Quality of life scores,[39] suggesting that IBS and functional constipation have a greater impact on quality of life among this patient population. Data on GI symptoms are more robust for anorexia nervosa than bulimia nervosa, binge eating disorder, and atypical presentations of eating disorders as described in the sections that follow.

Anorexia nervosa is associated with a host of GI symptoms including Barrett esophagus, delayed gastric emptying, delayed intestinal transit and motility, celiac disease, and constipation.[40,41] In a study sample of 348 adolescent patients with anorexia nervosa including predominately females, 27.6% reported constipation with no observed association to BMI.[42] GI symptoms could enhance eating-associated discomfort, further delaying eating disorder recovery.[43,44]

GI symptoms may perpetuate the perseverance of anorexia nervosa[44] and current evidence has shown most GI symptoms in individuals with anorexia nervosa are reported following eating disorder development.[45] Specifically, in a cohort of 23 individuals with anorexia nervosa followed throughout a 22-week recovery period, they all reported that their weight loss intentions occurred before onset of their GI symptoms.[45] When working with anorexia nervosa patients, it is challenging to determine if GI symptoms are reported as a consequence of abnormal GI function, a result of the refeeding/recovery process, or reported as secondary to the underlying eating disorder in an effort to avoid oral intake.[46] It is generally thought that most GI symptoms in patients with anorexia nervosa improve on completion of the refeeding and recovery periods.[41]

A systematic review found that bulimia nervosa is associated with constipation, one of the cardinal symptoms of IBS, and bloating, heartburn, and delayed gastric emptying.[40] Binge eating disorder is associated with heartburn, nausea, abdominal pain, altered perception of satiety, acid regurgitation, and bloating.[40] In a population-based survey of 250 individuals with binge eating disorder, diarrhea (16%) was more common than constipation (6%).[47] Additionally, fecal urgency was reported among 16% of individuals with binge eating disorder compared with 5.1% (n = 178) of the sample without binge eating disorder (n = 3481).[47]

## ASSOCIATION BETWEEN IRRITABLE BOWEL SYNDROME TREATMENT AND EATING DISORDERS

As nutrition-based IBS treatments like the low FODMAP diet rise in use with increasing evidence,[12,48] research has started to explore how adherence to a restrictive diet for GI symptom management might be associated with the development of an eating disorder or disordered eating. In 2003, nearly 30% of patients with IBS identified in a retrospective chart review received nonpharmacologic treatment recommendations including diet and lifestyle[49] and in 2015 more than half of gastroenterologists reported recommending dietary strategies to most of their patients.[34] In a prospective cohort study of IBS patients (n=233), adherence of the FODMAP diet was significantly greater in individuals that demonstrated eating disorder behavior according to the SCOFF eating disorder screen[50]. Commentary on these findings suggest that these patients weren't necessarily demonstrating eating disorder behavior, but rather had increased drive to modify their diets due to IBS-related symptoms[51]. With this in mind, it is suggested to be cautious when recommending elimination diets as treatment for IBS patients if previous eating disorder history is reported[12]. Specifically, it might not be a coincidence that females with IBS are more likely to manipulate their diet than males with IBS in response to symptoms[52] and females have higher prevalence of eating disorder and IBS.[2,11]

Similarly, in a matched case-control study analyzing individuals with diet-related chronic health conditions (including IBS, IBD, cystic fibrosis, celiac disease, and type 1 diabetes), patients were more likely than control subjects to exercise excessively and abuse medication to manipulate their weight, but were less likely to feel pressure from the media to meet body image standards.[6] Although this is not specific to IBS, the results are still indicative of added food preoccupation that can occur in diet-related health conditions, predisposing individuals to further disordered eating behavior that is not motivated by body image ideals perpetuated by media.

## WHAT IS THE ROLE OF THE GASTROENTEROLOGIST?
### Recognition of Eating Disorders

There is an underappreciation and poor recognition of eating disorders among GI patients. The first duty of gastroenterologists is to be aware eating disorders complicate the clinical picture of GI patients and understand the red flag symptoms of eating disorders (**Table 2**). Red flag symptoms include consuming a very restricted diet, identifying a short list of "safe foods," implementing strong or fixed rules around food, unwillingness to introduce new foods into the diet, obsessive exercising, isolating from friends and family, not eating in front of others, skipping meals, weight loss or large weight fluctuations, or reliance on tube feeds/supplement beverages to maintain weight.

Common misunderstandings that can inhibit recognition of eating disorders in GI patients include the ideas that eating disorders are uncommon among patients with IBS, eating disorders occur in only children and adolescents, patients with eating disorders are underweight/have a low BMI, and all eating disorders are driven by body dysmorphia.[53]

### Judicious Prescription of Restrictive Diets

A study demonstrated that 23% of patients with IBS who were prescribed a low-FODMAP diet were classified to be at risk for eating disorder behavior. Although there is ongoing discussion regarding if the restriction noted in that study was due to eating disorder behavior versus a desire to control IBS symptoms[50], the study clearly showed these patients were at risk of severe dietary restriction. Given the increasing popularity of restrictive diets to treat IBS symptoms (ie, low FODMAP diet), it is imperative gastroenterologists understand these restrictive diets are not appropriate for all patients. Restrictive diets are contraindicated for patients who already have a restricted diet, are underweight, are actively losing weight unintentionally, or have a history of a restrictive eating disorder. Prescribing restrictive diets for patients who already struggle with their relationship with food has the potential to further increase food-related anxiety.

**Table 2**
**Red flag behaviors of harmful dietary restriction or an eating disorder**

| Behavior | Examples and Comments |
| --- | --- |
| Dietary changes | |
| Consumption of a very restricted diet | Restricted caloric intake<br>Consumes high volume of very-low-calorie foods<br>Excludes entire food groups, and often multiple food groups |
| Identification of a short list of "safe foods" and declines to introduce new foods into the diet; "safe foods" and "unsafe foods" do NOT follow expected restrictions to treat GI symptoms | Identifies 10 safe foods within the already restrictive low FODMAP diet, and declines to perform the reintroduction phase<br>Will drink ice tea, but not water or juice |
| Requires supplemental nutrition to maintain weight or nutrition | Requires tube feeds, total parenteral nutrition, or supplement beverages, with the need inconsistent or discordant with severity of GI diagnosis |
| Implements strong or fixed rules around food | Abnormal or ritualistic eating habits, such as eating foods in a certain order, excessive chewing, or rearranging food on a plate<br>Fixed rules about which "healthy foods" are acceptable |
| Behavioral changes | |
| Does not eat in front of others or in social settings | Because of desire to hide restricted diet, embarrassment, fear of developing GI side effects in social settings, and so forth |
| Skips meals or consistently makes excuses to avoid mealtimes | Because of desire to avoid eating, hide restricted diet, fear of developing GI side effects in social settings, and so forth |
| Obsessive exercising | Evidence of weight control and body dysmorphia |
| Depressed mood or irritability | Isolates from friends and family<br>Stops doing previously enjoyed activities<br>Thoughts of suicide |
| High anxiety about gaining weight | Driven by body dysmorphia<br>Not seen in ARFID |
| Frequently talks about dieting | Preoccupation with food, calories, diet, "healthy" foods, and so forth |
| Hoarding and rapid disappearance of food | Evidence of bingeing |
| Frequently leaving to use the restroom immediately after meals | Evidence of vomiting/purging |

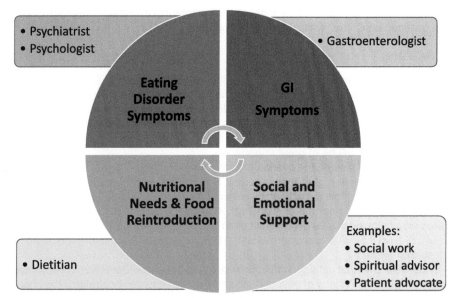

• Psychiatrist
• Psychologist

• Gastroenterologist

Eating Disorder Symptoms

GI Symptoms

Nutritional Needs & Food Reintroduction

Social and Emotional Support

• Dietitian

Examples:
• Social work
• Spiritual advisor
• Patient advocate

**Fig. 2.** Multidisciplinary treatment approach to patients with concomitant gastrointestinal symptoms and an eating disorder.

### Role in the Multidisciplinary Treatment Team

Most patients with eating disorders concomitantly suffer from IBS symptoms. Gastro-enterologists play a key role in the multidisciplinary team of providers treating this cohort of patients. The multidisciplinary, collaborative, integrated care approach is key given the complexity and multidimensional nature of these patients' management. In general, gastroenterologists do not spearhead the treatment of patients with an eating disorder unless they have specific expertise and training in the area. The key individuals on the multidisciplinary integrated care team include a gastroenterologist, psychiatrist, psychologist, and dietitian (**Fig. 2**).

The role of the gastroenterologist is to manage GI symptoms and monitor for evidence of maladaptive dietary behaviors. GI symptoms may occur as a result of the eating disorder/malnutrition (ie, constipation, gastroparesis) or may be caused by an underlying disorder independent of the eating disorder. Regardless of the cause, the presence of uncontrolled GI symptoms may act as negative reinforcement or a trigger for eating disorder behaviors. This is of particular concern in patients with restrictive eating disorders, such as anorexia nervosa, ARFID, or orthorexia. It is also imperative for gastroenterologists to periodically monitor patients' dietary habits, particularly before prescribing dietary restrictions or referring the patient to a dietitian for a highly restrictive diet (ie, low FODMAP diet). Psychiatry and psychology should spearhead treatment of the eating disorder. It is imperative to treat the behavioral aspect in tandem with management of the GI symptoms. Dietitians are a crucial part of the team and guide the food reintroduction aspect of care, particularly for patients with restrictive eating behaviors.

Eating disorder behavior is detrimental to resolution of GI symptoms and GI symptoms are detrimental to resolution of an eating disorder.[46,54] The multidisciplinary model requires each provider to work in tandem to tackle their respective tasks, because GI symptoms and eating disorder behaviors exacerbate one another. Clinical awareness and understanding of theses associations is vital when treating patients with overlapping GI and eating disorder symptoms.

## LIMITATIONS

Although the prevalence of IBS is high among current and past eating disorder patients, temporality and differences among the various eating disorders needs further study. Additionally, different studies use different instruments to assess IBS and eating disorders. To accelerate the understanding of eating disorders in patients with IBS, standardization and validation of eating disorder tools for use in patients with GI symptoms will be of great importance.

Many studies evaluating the overlap of eating disorders and GI symptoms excluded participants who were higher than a certain BMI.[31] This weight exclusion could bias published research. This is particularly relevant for disorders, such as ARFID, where most patients have a normal or high BMI. A study of GI patients with ARFID who were being followed in a GI behavioral health clinic demonstrated 10% had an underweight BMI (<18.5), 68% had a normal BMI (18.5–24.9), and 22% had an overweight or obese BMI (>25).[55]

Evidence shows that patients with other restrictive eating disorders can have a normal or overweight BMI. A study of patients with anorexia nervosa demonstrated 37% of patients had an overweight or obese BMI. Furthermore, patients with anorexia nervosa with an overweight or obese BMI went twice as long before being diagnosed.

Finally, females are overrepresented in these studies. A common misconception is that eating disorders only occur in women. However, approximately 25% of adult patients with eating disorders are men.[56] Among pediatric patients with ARFID, about half are male.[57] Studies that ensure adequate male gender representation are needed.

## SUMMARY

There is growing awareness and appreciation for the overlap between IBS and eating disorders. However, understanding this relationship has proven to be challenging, and the question of temporality remains entangled.

Eating disorders and IBS potentially manifest with similar symptoms, and eating disorders can be secretive in nature. Therefore, patients might mask eating disorders with IBS symptoms, further muddying the ability to identify maladaptive or pathologic behaviors.

It is a challenge to disentangle each patient's lived experience and the underlying cause for the maladaptive eating behaviors. Further research is sorely needed to help gastroenterologists differentiate between normal, adaptive restriction and pathologic, maladaptive restriction. Given how common dietary modification and restriction is implemented among patients with IBS, it is imperative for gastroenterologists to ask about dietary habits. This is particularly important given the rise in popularity of restriction diets to treat IBS symptoms. Although gastroenterologists do not directly treat eating disorders, they are in a key position to identify and help monitor maladaptive eating behaviors and play a key role in the multidisciplinary, collaborative treatment team for patients with IBS with concomitant eating disorders.

## CLINICS CARE POINTS

- Most patients with IBS report worsening of their symptoms with eating, and up to 90% of patients with IBS exclude certain foods in the hopes of avoiding or improving their GI symptoms.

- Gastroenterologists need to be aware of the potential negative consequences of prescribing restrictive diets in patients with IBS with maladaptive eating patterns and eating disorders.
- Gastroenterologists need to be aware of the red flag symptoms of an eating disorder.
- Treatment of patients with IBS and an eating disorder involves a collaborative, multidisciplinary approach, which includes gastroenterologists, psychologists, psychiatrists, and dieticians.
- Greater than 35% of patients with eating disorders have a normal BMI and approximately 25% of eating disorder patients are men.

## DISCLOSURE

Authors state they do not have any relevant disclosures.

## REFERENCES

1. Hayes P, Corish C, O'Mahony E, et al. A dietary survey of patients with irritable bowel syndrome. J Hum Nutr Diet 2014;27:36–47.
2. Quick VM, Byrd-Bredbenner C, Neumark-Sztainer D. Chronic illness and disordered eating: a discussion of the literature. Adv Nutr 2013;4:277–86.
3. Shisslak CM, Crago M, Estes LS. The spectrum of eating disturbances. Int J Eat Disord 1995;18:209–19.
4. Grilo C. Eating and weight disorders. New York: Taylor & Francis Group; 2006.
5. Reba-Harrelson L, Von Holle A, Hamer RM, et al. Patterns and prevalence of disordered eating and weight control behaviors in women ages 25-45. Eat Weight Disord EWD 2009;14:e190–8.
6. Quick VM, McWilliams R, Byrd-Bredbenner C. Case–control study of disturbed eating behaviors and related psychographic characteristics in young adults with and without diet-related chronic health conditions. Eat Behav 2012;13:207–13.
7. Satherley R, Howard R, Higgs S. Disordered eating practices in gastrointestinal disorders. Appetite 2015;84:240–50.
8. American Psychiatric Association. Diagnostic and statistical manual of mental disorders. 5th edition. Washington, DC: American Psychiatric Association; 2013.
9. American Psychiatric Association, editor. Diagnostic and statistical manual of mental disorders: DSM-IV; includes ICD-9-CM codes effective 1. Oct. 96. 4. ed., 7. Washington, DC: American Psychiatric Publishing; 1998.
10. Call C, Walsh BT, Attia E. From DSM-IV to DSM-5: changes to eating disorder diagnoses. Curr Opin Psychiatry 2013;26:532–6.
11. Lindvall Dahlgren C, Wisting L, Rø Ø. Feeding and eating disorders in the DSM-5 era: a systematic review of prevalence rates in non-clinical male and female samples. J Eat Disord 2017;5:56.
12. Chey WD. Elimination diets for irritable bowel syndrome: approaching the end of the beginning. Am J Gastroenterol 2019;114:201–3.
13. Donini LM, Marsili D, Graziani MP, et al. Orthorexia nervosa: a preliminary study with a proposal for diagnosis and an attempt to measure the dimension of the phenomenon. Eat Weight Disord - Stud Anorex Bulim Obes 2004;9:151–7.
14. Dunn TM, Bratman S. On orthorexia nervosa: a review of the literature and proposed diagnostic criteria. Eat Behav 2016;21:11–7.
15. Donini LM, Marsili D, Graziani MP, et al. Orthorexia nervosa: validation of a diagnosis questionnaire. Eat Weight Disord - Stud Anorex Bulim Obes 2005;10: e28–32.

16. Guo Y-B, Zhuang K-M, Kuang L, et al. Association between diet and lifestyle habits and irritable bowel syndrome: a case-control study. Gut Liver 2015;9. https://doi.org/10.5009/gnl13437.

17. Okami Y, Kato T, Nin G, et al. Lifestyle and psychological factors related to irritable bowel syndrome in nursing and medical school students. J Gastroenterol 2011;46:1403–10.

18. Reed-Knight B, Squires M, Chitkara DK, et al. Adolescents with irritable bowel syndrome report increased eating-associated symptoms, changes in dietary composition, and altered eating behaviors: a pilot comparison study to healthy adolescents. Neurogastroenterol Motil 2016;28:1915–20.

19. Sullivan G, Blewett AE, Jenkins PL, et al. Eating attitudes and the irritable bowel syndrome. Gen Hosp Psychiatry 1997;19:62–4.

20. Quick V, McWilliams R, Byrd-Bredbenner C. A case-control study of current psychological well-being and weight-teasing history in young adults with and without bowel conditions. J Hum Nutr Diet 2015;28:28–36.

21. Puhl RM, Wall MM, Chen C, et al. Experiences of weight teasing in adolescence and weight-related outcomes in adulthood: a 15-year longitudinal study. Prev Med 2017;100:173–9.

22. Karwautz A, Wagner G, Berger G, et al. Eating pathology in adolescents with celiac disease. Psychosomatics 2008;49:399–406.

23. Wiklund CA, Kuja-Halkola R, Thornton LM, et al. Prolonged constipation and diarrhea in childhood and disordered eating in adolescence. J Psychosom Res 2019; 126:109797.

24. Kayar Y, Agin M, Dertli R, et al. Eating disorders in patients with irritable bowel syndrome. Gastroenterol Hepatol 2020;43:607–13.

25. Salvioli B, Pellicciari A, Iero L, et al. Audit of digestive complaints and psychopathological traits in patients with eating disorders: a prospective study. Dig Liver Dis 2013;45:639–44.

26. Tang TN, Toner BB, Stuckless N, et al. Features of eating disorders in patients with irritable bowel syndrome. J Psychosom Res 1998;45:171–8.

27. Bardone-Cone AM, Wonderlich SA, Frost RO, et al. Perfectionism and eating disorders: current status and future directions. Clin Psychol Rev 2007;27:384–405.

28. Perkins SJ, Keville S, Schmidt U, et al. Eating disorders and irritable bowel syndrome: is there a link? J Psychosom Res 2005;59:57–64.

29. Wang X, Luscombe GM, Boyd C, et al. Functional gastrointestinal disorders in eating disorder patients: altered distribution and predictors using ROME III compared to ROME II criteria. World J Gastroenterol 2014;20:16293.

30. Abraham S, Luscombe GM, Kellow JE. Pelvic floor dysfunction predicts abdominal bloating and distension in eating disorder patients. Scand J Gastroenterol 2012;47:625–31.

31. Kessler U, Rekkedal GÅ, Rø Ø, et al. Association between gastrointestinal complaints and psychopathology in patients with anorexia nervosa. Int J Eat Disord 2020;53:802–6.

32. DeJong H, Perkins S, Grover M, et al. The prevalence of irritable bowel syndrome in outpatients with bulimia nervosa. Int J Eat Disord 2011;44:661–4.

33. Peat CM, Huang L, Thornton LM, et al. Binge eating, body mass index, and gastrointestinal symptoms. J Psychosom Res 2013;75:456–61.

34. Lenhart A, Ferch C, Shaw M, et al. Use of dietary management in irritable bowel syndrome: results of a survey of over 1500 United States gastroenterologists. J Neurogastroenterol Motil 2018;24:437–51.

35. Makhzoumi SH, Schreyer CC, Hansen JL, et al. Hospital course of underweight youth with ARFID treated with a meal-based behavioral protocol in an inpatient-partial hospitalization program for eating disorders. Int J Eat Disord 2019;52: 428–34.
36. Murray HB, Bailey AP, Keshishian AC, et al. Prevalence and characteristics of avoidant/restrictive food intake disorder in adult neurogastroenterology patients. Clin Gastroenterol Hepatol 2020;18:1995–2002.e1.
37. Harer KN, Baker JR, Reister N, et al. Avoidant/restrictive food intake disorder in the adult gastroenterology population: an under-recognized diagnosis? American Journal of Gastroenterology October 2018;113:S247–8.
38. Thomas JJ, Lawson EA, Micali N, et al. Avoidant/restrictive food intake disorder: a three-dimensional model of neurobiology with implications for etiology and treatment. Curr Psychiatry Rep 2017;19:54.
39. Abraham S, Kellow J. Exploring eating disorder quality of life and functional gastrointestinal disorders among eating disorder patients. J Psychosom Res 2011;70:372–7.
40. Hetterich L, Mack I, Giel KE, et al. An update on gastrointestinal disturbances in eating disorders. Mol Cell Endocrinol 2019;497:110318.
41. Norris ML, Harrison ME, Isserlin L, et al. Gastrointestinal complications associated with anorexia nervosa: a systematic review: gastrointestinal complications in anorexia nervosa. Int J Eat Disord 2016;49:216–37.
42. Mattheus HK, Wagner C, Becker K, et al. Incontinence and constipation in adolescent patients with anorexia nervosa—results of a multicenter study from a German web-based registry for children and adolescents with anorexia nervosa. Int J Eat Disord 2020;53:219–28.
43. Sato Y, Fukudo S. Gastrointestinal symptoms and disorders in patients with eating disorders. Clin J Gastroenterol 2015;8:255–63.
44. Schalla MA, Stengel A. Gastrointestinal alterations in anorexia nervosa - a systematic review. Eur Eat Disord Rev 2019. https://doi.org/10.1002/erv.2679.
45. Benini L, Todesco T, Frulloni L, et al. Esophageal motility and symptoms in restricting and binge-eating/purging anorexia. Dig Liver Dis 2010;42:767–72.
46. Mascolo M, Geer B, Feuerstein J, et al. Gastrointestinal comorbidities which complicate the treatment of anorexia nervosa. Eat Disord 2017;25:122–33.
47. Cremonini F, Camilleri M, Clark MM, et al. Associations among binge eating behavior patterns and gastrointestinal symptoms: a population-based study. Int J Obes 2009;33:342–53.
48. Halmos EP, Power VA, Shepherd SJ, et al. A diet low in FODMAPs reduces symptoms of irritable bowel syndrome. Gastroenterology 2014;146:67–75.e5.
49. Faresjo A, Grodzinsky E, Foldevi M, et al. Patients with irritable bowel syndrome in primary care appear not to be heavy healthcare utilizers. Aliment Pharmacol Ther 2006;23:807–14.
50. Mari A, Hosadurg D, Martin L, et al. Adherence with a low-FODMAP diet in irritable bowel syndrome: are eating disorders the missing link? Eur J Gastroenterol Hepatol 2019;31:178–82.
51. Chumpitazi BP, Alfaro-Cruz L, Zia JK, et al. Commentary: adherence with a low-FODMAP diet in irritable bowel syndrome: are eating disorders the missing link? Front Nutr 2019;6:136.
52. Faresjö Å, Johansson S, Faresjö T, et al. Sex differences in dietary coping with gastrointestinal symptoms. Eur J Gastroenterol Hepatol 2010;22:327–33.
53. Werlang ME, Sim LA, Lebow JR, et al. Assessing for eating disorders: a primer for gastroenterologists. Am J Gastroenterol 2021;116:68–76.

54. van Tilburg MAL, Fortunato JE, Squires M, et al. Impact of eating restriction on gastrointestinal motility in adolescents with IBS. J Pediatr Gastroenterol Nutr 2014;58:491–4.

55. Harer K, Jagielski C, Riehl M, et al. Avoidant/restrictive food intake disorder (AR-FID) in the adult GI behavioral health population: demographic and clinical characteristics. San Antonio, Texas: American College of Gastroenterology Annual Conference; October 2019.

56. Sweeting H, Walker L, MacLean A, Patterson C, Räisänen U, Hunt K. Prevalence of eating disorders in males: a review of rates reported in academic research and UK mass media. Int J Mens Health 2015;14. https://doi.org/10.3149/jmh.1402.86.

57. Eddy KT, Thomas JJ, Hastings E, et al. Prevalence of DSM-5 avoidant/restrictive food intake disorder in a pediatric gastroenterology healthcare network. Int J Eat Disord 2015;48:464–70.

# Medical Therapies for Diarrhea-Predominant Irritable Bowel Syndrome

Gregory S. Sayuk, MD, MPH[a,b,c],*

## KEYWORDS

- Irritable bowel syndrome • Diarrhea • Treatment • Pharmacotherapy
- Over-the-counter • Supplement • Emerging therapy

## KEY POINTS

- Diarrhea-predominant irritable bowel syndrome is a symptom-based diagnosis resulting from multiple etiopathologic pathways; this mechanistic heterogeneity provides for diverse treatment strategies in its management.
- Pharmacologic agents currently US Food and Drug Administration approved for the diarrhea-predominant irritable bowel syndrome treatment are the minimally absorbed antibiotic rifaximin, a mixed opioid receptor agonist/antagonist, eluxadoline, and the serotonin 5-HT$_3$ receptor antagonist, alosetron.
- Several nonapproved drug therapies, such as antidiarrheals and antispasmodics, often are used in the management of diarrhea-predominant irritable bowel syndrome, but are limited by their incomplete impact on global irritable bowel syndrome symptoms.
- A growing number of supplemental treatments and emerging therapies offer the prospect of an enhanced armamentarium to apply in the management of the patient with diarrhea-predominant irritable bowel syndrome.

## INTRODUCTION

Irritable bowel syndrome (IBS) is a common functional bowel disorder defined by chronic abdominal pain and altered bowel habits.[1] Prevalence studies estimate that approximately 9% to 14% of adults worldwide are affected by the disorder.[2–4] The diagnosis of IBS using Rome IV criteria relies on the presence of recurrent abdominal pain in association with defecation, alterations in stool frequency, and/or form. IBS is further subclassified by the predominant stool pattern, and in the case of diarrhea-

---

[a] Division of Gastroenterology, Washington University School of Medicine, St Louis, MO, USA;
[b] Department of Psychiatry, Washington University School of Medicine, 915 North Grand Boulevard, St Louis, MO 63106, USA; [c] St. Louis Veterans Affairs Medical Center, St Louis, MO, USA
* Washington University School of Medicine, 915 North Grand Boulevard, St Louis, MO 63106.
*E-mail address:* gsayuk@wustl.edu

Gastroenterol Clin N Am 50 (2021) 611–637
https://doi.org/10.1016/j.gtc.2021.04.003
0889-8553/21/© 2021 Elsevier Inc. All rights reserved.

predominant IBS (IBS-D) the predominance (>25%) of diarrheal stools (Bristol stool form scale [BSFS] type 6 or 7: loose, mushy, watery) and infrequent constipated stools (BSFS 1–2, hard, lumpy, pellet like).[1] The IBS-D is the most common, comprising upwards of 45% of all cases.[2] Many patients with IBS-D endorse additional symptoms including bloating, abdominal distention, urgency with defecation, and a sense of incomplete evacuation, although these symptoms are not requisite in making the diagnosis.[1] Collectively, IBS-D symptoms impart a major negative impact on the health-related quality of life of affected individuals, including engagement in social activities and work productivity.[5,6]

As a disorder defined by symptoms, IBS-D is a heterogeneous condition likely resulting from multiple distinct pathophysiologic pathways, including perturbations in the gut microbiota, alterations in gastrointestinal secretion and motility, dysregulation of enteric–central nervous system function, and gut microinflammation.[7] In some patients, more than 1 factor may be relevant to the development of symptoms. Accordingly, treatment strategies with diverse mechanisms of action have been demonstrated to be beneficial in the management of IBS-D, without a clear gold standard of treatment.[8,9] Optimal IBS-D treatment options address the global symptom profile of the disorder, rather than individual symptoms. Although some newer pharmacologic treatment options have come to be available within the last few years, without exception these treatments are effective in only a subset of IBS-D sufferers, leading to a great need for additional treatment options. The purpose of this review is to summarize the currently available pharmacologic and over-the-counter agents for the management of IBS-D and to highlight some emerging strategies that may augment the armamentarium of IBS-D therapeutic agents in the coming years.

## THERAPIES FOR DIARRHEA-PREDOMINANT IRRITABLE BOWEL SYNDROME APPROVED BY THE US FOOD AND DRUG ADMINISTRATION

Currently there are 3 prescription pharmacotherapies that are approved by the US Food and Drug Administration (FDA) for the treatment of IBS-D, including rifaximin, eluxadoline, and alosetron.[9,10] All of these agents have been subjected to multiple randomized, double-blinded placebo-controlled clinical trials using standard IBS-D end points to establish efficacy. Though calculation of numbers needed to treat (NNT) to improve 1 patient with IBS-D can be generated for each of these therapies, a lack of head-to-head trials and differing primary outcomes across these studies preclude the ability to make statements regarding the comparative effectiveness of these agents.[11,12]

### Rifaximin

Rifaximin is a minimally systemically absorbed, broad spectrum antibiotic indicated for the treatment of both men and women with IBS-D, using a 2-week course of 550 mg 3 times daily.[13] The 2 pivotal studies (TARGET 1 and 2) included more than 1200 nonconstipated patients with IBS who received 2 weeks of rifaximin or placebo, with a primary end point of adequate relief of global IBS symptoms for at least 2 of the first 4 weeks after treatment.[14] This end point was achieved to a significantly greater level as compared with placebo (40.7% of rifaximin treated patient's compared with 31.7% of placebo-treated patients; pooled P<.001). These effects seemed to be durable in the intermediate term, with maintenance of global IBS symptom response as well as bloating improvement through 12 weeks of treatment (pooled P<.001 for each).

TARGET 3 was an IBS-D retreatment trial wherein patients first received rifaximin 550 mg 3 times daily for 2 weeks open-label fashion.[15] Treatment responders were defined by combined end point ($\geq$30% reduction in baseline weekly abdominal pain and $\geq$50% improvement in days per week with a BSFS type 6 or 7 stool for $\geq$2 weeks of the first month after rifaximin treatment). Of 2438 patients with IBS enrolled in the trial, 1074 (44.1%) met this efficacy end point, very similar to the response seen in the 2 earlier RCTs. A full one-third of the patients who initially responded to open-label rifaximin did not experience recurrence of symptoms during 18 weeks of follow-up. Those patients with relapse of symptoms (median time to symptom return, 10 weeks; range, 6–24 weeks) were then randomized in a double-blinded fashion to either a 2-week retreatment with rifaximin or placebo. A significantly greater percentage of the rifaximin retreated patients with IBS-D (n = 328) reported sustained efficacy response compared with those assigned to placebo (n = 308) (38.1% vs 31.5%; $P$ = .03). This study led to the approval of rifaximin IBS-D re-treatment for up to 2 additional courses should symptoms recur. A collective analysis of the published rifaximin randomized controlled trials (RCTs) yielded an NNT of 9.[16] The American College of Gastroenterology (ACG) IBS Monograph, ACG IBS Clinical Guideline, and America Gastroenterological Association (AGA) Clinical Guidelines all recommend the use of rifaximin for the management of IBS-D (**Table 1**).[8,9,17]

A pooled analysis of the phase II and phase III trials demonstrated rifaximin to be very well-tolerated by patients with IBS-D without an increase in adverse events (AEs) or serious AEs compared with placebo.[16] Importantly no cases of *Clostridium difficile* colitis were observed in TARGET 1 and 2.[14] There was 1 case of *C difficile* infection in TARGET 3, although this came in close association with the use of a cephalosporin antibiotic for urinary tract infection in a patient who was no longer taking rifaximin.[15] A cumulative number needed to harm of 8971 has been calculated for rifaximin IBS-D treatment trials, underscoring the favorable safety profile of this medication.[18]

### Eluxadoline

Eluxadoline is an agonist of $\mu$- and $\kappa$-opioid receptors, and an antagonist of the $\delta$-opioid receptor in the bowel, and is FDA approved as a twice daily medication for the treatment of IBS-D in men and women.[19] The $\mu$-opioid receptor effects on the gut mucosa and enteric nervous system reduce intestinal transit and secretion, whereas the $\delta$-opioid effects may balance the $\mu$-effects, decreasing the potential for constipation or tachyphylaxis, and in combination with the $\kappa$-agonism may convey pain benefit and modulation of visceral hypersensitivity.[20] The typical dose is 100 mg 2 times per day, with the 75 mg dose reserved for those who experience constipation or have potential medication interactions (organic anion transporting polypeptide 1B1, OATP1B1 inhibitors, such as cyclosporine or gemfibrozil) or relevant medical comorbidities (eg, Child's A/B cirrhosis). In the 2 pivotal phase 3 IBS-D trials (studies 3001 and 3002, 52 and 26 weeks, respectively) including more than 2400 patients, eluxadoline treatment achieved significantly greater rates of combined response ($\geq$30% reduction in baseline abdominal pain and BSFS <5 or no bowel movement for $\geq$50% of treatment days) at both the 75 and 100 mg doses compared with placebo (26.2%–27.0% vs 16.7%, respectively; $P$<.001 for both).[21] Individual symptom improvement in stool consistency and frequency were achieved with both the 75 and 100 mg doses, and abdominal pain and bloating improvements were significantly greater only with 100 mg dose. Collectively, the RCTs of eluxadoline in IBS-D have a pooled NNT of 12.5 (95% confidence interval [CI], 8–33), although with significant heterogeneity across studies.[8] Although eluxadoline has a similar $\mu$-opioid agonist effect to that of loperamide, both a post hoc analysis of the phase III RCTs, and a prospective phase IV RCT (RELIEF) of patients who had reported inadequate

**Table 1**
Summary of medical therapies for IBS-D

| IBS-D Treatment Option | IBS-D Symptom Impact | | | Expert Recommendations | | | Comments |
|---|---|---|---|---|---|---|---|
| | Abdominal Pain | Diarrhea | Global Symptoms | ACG IBS Monograph [2018] Ref.[8] (Recommendation/ Evidence) | ACG IBS Management Clinical Guideline [2020] Ref.[9] (Recommendation/ Evidence) | AGA IBS Guideline [2014] Ref.[17] (Recommendation/ Evidence) | |
| FDA-approved pharmacotherapies | | | | | | | |
| Rifaximin (Xifaxan) | + | + | + | Weak, moderate quality | Strong, moderate level | Conditional, moderate quality | 36% of patients sustain symptom relief at 6 mo follow-up (mean time to symptom recurrence = 10 wk); approved for up to 2 retreatment courses |
| Eluxadoline (Viberzi) | + | + | + | Weak, moderate quality | Conditional, moderate quality | n/a | Rare serious adverse events of pancreatitis and SOD; contraindicated in patients status post cholecystectomy or with pancreatitis risk factors |
| Alosetron (Lotronex) | + | + | + | Weak, low quality | Conditional, low quality | Conditional, moderate quality | Rare serious adverse events of constipation and ischemic colitis; indicated for women with severe symptoms who have failed traditional therapies |
| Non-FDA approved pharmacotherapies | | | | | | | |

|  |  |  |  |  |  |  |
|---|---|---|---|---|---|---|
| Loperamide | – | + | Strong (against), very low quality | n/a | Conditional, very low quality | Indicated for short-term use, tachyphylaxis can develop with continued use; risk of cardiac events with overuse/misuse |
| Diphenoxylate/atropine | – | + | n/a | n/a | n/a | Indicated for short-term use, may induce constipation |
| Antispasmodics (eg, dicyclomine) | +/– | + | Weak, very low quality | Conditional (against), low quality | Conditional, low quality | Anticholinergic side effects may be limiting |
| TCAs (eg, amitriptyline) | + | +/– | Strong, high quality | Strong, moderate quality | Conditional, low quality [TCA]; Conditional (against), low quality [selective serotonin reuptake inhibitors] | Anticholinergic/antihistaminergic side effects may be limiting; tertiary amine TCAs (such as amitriptyline) may have greater antidiarrheal effects |
| Ramosetron | + | + | n/a | n/a | n/a | Approved in Japan/Asia for IBS-D treatment |
| **Herbal and Supplement Therapies** |  |  |  |  |  |  |
| Probiotics | +/– | + | Weak, low quality | Conditional (against), very low level | n/a | Best evidence with combination probiotics and Lactobacillus planarium DSM 9843 preparatiions |
| Prebiotics | +/– | + | Weak (against), very low quality | n/a | n/a | Galacto-oligosaccharide preparation best studied: may lead to sustained symptom improvements after discontinuation, also increase stool Bifidobacterium levels |

(continued on next page)

**Table 1**
*(continued)*

| IBS-D Treatment Option | IBS-D Symptom Impact | | | Expert Recommendations | | | Comments |
|---|---|---|---|---|---|---|---|
| | Abdominal Pain | Diarrhea | Global Symptoms | ACG IBS Monograph [2018] Ref.[8] (Recommendation/ Evidence) | ACG IBS Management Clinical Guideline [2020] Ref.[9] (Recommendation/ Evidence) | AGA IBS Guideline [2014] Ref.[17] (Recommendation/ Evidence) | |
| Synbiotics | +/– | +/– | + | Weak (against), very low quality | n/a | n/a | Small studies with significant heterogeneity across trials |
| Peppermint | +/– | – | +/– | Weak, low quality | Conditional, low quality | n/a | Results of individual studies may not extrapolate to all peppermint supplements |
| STW 5 (Iberogast) | + | – | +/– | n/a | n/a | n/a | Popular in Europe, available via e-commerce |
| Serum derived bovine immunoglobulin (Enteragam) | +/– | + | +/– | n/a | n/a | n/a | Prescription medical food |
| Glutamine | + | + | + | n/a | n/a | n/a | Safe, additional clinical trials needed |
| Novel and emerging therapies for IBS-D | | | | | | | |
| Bile acid sequestrants (eg, colestipol, colesevelam) | – | +/– | +/– | n/a | Conditional (do not suggest), very low quality | n/a | Serum markers (FGF-19 and C4) may inform use in near future; caution in taking at same time as other medications (may bind and inactivate) |

| | | | | | | |
|---|---|---|---|---|---|---|
| Ondansetron (Zofran) | − | + | +/− | n/a | n/a | n/a |
| Endocannabinoids (eg, dronabinol, olorinab [APD371]) | ? | ? | ? | n/a | n/a | Great potential for future use; additional studies needed in IBS-D |
| Melatonin | + | − | + | n/a | n/a | Safe and well-tolerated; actions may be independent of effect on sleep/mood |

*Abbreviations:* +, beneficial in IBS-D clinical trials; -, not beneficial in IBS-D clinical trials; +/−, mixed results in IBS-D clinical trials; ?, not studied in IBS-D; AE, adverse event; FGF, fibroblast growth factor; n/a, not reported or available; SOD, sphincter of Oddi dysfunction; TCA, tricyclic antidepressant.

symptom control with loperamide observed significantly higher rates of response with eluxadoline compared with placebo.[22,23] The ACG IBS Monograph and ACG Clinical Guidelines suggest the use of eluxadoline for the treatment of global IBS-D symptoms.[8,9]

From a safety perspective, the most common AEs experienced with eluxadoline were constipation (7.4%–8.6%), nausea (7.5%–8.1%), and abdominal pain (5.8%–7.2%).[24] In a pooled safety analysis, rare, but serious AEs of sphincter of Oddi spasm (0.5%) and acute pancreatitis (0.4%) were detected in eluxadoline-treated patients, most often in individuals who were status post cholecystectomy or reported other pancreatitis risk factors (eg, excess alcohol consumption or a prior history of pancreatitis). These AE signals were confirmed in a postmarketing review of the FDA Adverse Event Reporting System.[25] Hence, eluxadoline now is contraindicated in patients with a medical history of these risk factors, as well as patients with advanced liver disease (Child's C cirrhosis).[26] It is imperative that clinicians screen for these risk factors and discuss these potential risks and the associated symptoms with patients before initiating eluxadoline, with an emphasis on the need to immediately discontinue the medication should the patient experience such symptoms. The number needed to harm from the eluxadoline clinical trials was 23.3 and 25.2 for the 100 mg and 75 mg 2 times per day regimens, respectively.[21]

### Alosetron and Other 5-Hydroxytryptamine Receptor Type 3 Antagonists

#### Alosetron

Alosetron is a 5-HT$_3$ antagonist indicated at a dose of 0.5 to 1.0 mg twice daily for the treatment of IBS-D in women with chronic, severe symptoms that have been refractory to other treatments.[27] Alosetron effects on the 5-HT$_3$ receptors decrease secretion and gastrointestinal (GI) motility, and improve abdominal pain.[28] It is restricted to use under a US FDA modified Risk Evaluation and Mitigation Strategy program.[29] Alosetron has been evaluated for the management of IBS-D in several different studies implementing a spectrum of end points. However, in 2 RCTs assessing global IBS-D response, a significant improvement with alosetron was observed compared with placebo (Lembo and colleagues[30] [n = 801; 76% vs 44%; P<.001] and Krause and colleagues[31] [n = 705; 42.9%–50.8% vs 30.7% in placebo]; P≤.02 for each). Most recently, an open-label, prospective study of women with IBS-D (n = 105) treated with alosetron 0.5 to 1.0 mg twice daily revealed an FDA composite end point response of 45% after 12 weeks of treatment.[32] Overall, the NNT for alosetron across the 8 available trials is 7.5 (95% CI, 5–16). The ACG IBS Clinical Guideline (conditional recommendation, low quality of evidence), ACG IBS Monograph (weak recommendation, low quality of evidence), and AGA Guideline on IBS (conditional recommendation, moderate evidence) recommend use of alosetron for global symptom improvement in women with severe symptoms who have failed "traditional" IBS-D treatments.[8,9,17]

Postmarketing safety data of alosetron raised some concerns relating to potential complications of ischemic colitis (1.03 cases per 1000 patient-years) and severe constipation (associated with obstruction and/or perforation; 0.25 cases per 1000 patient-years), and death, leading to initial voluntarily manufacturer removal from the US market (November 2000) followed by reintroduction under a modified Risk Evaluation and Mitigation Strategy program requiring prescriber registration and prescription stickers (June 2002), and most recently a modified Risk Evaluation and Mitigation Strategy (January 2016) requiring completion of a informational program to prescribe alosetron. The number needed to harm across available clinical trials of alosetron is 10 (95% CI, 6–20).[8]

*Ondansetron*

Ondansetron is a familiar 5-HT$_3$ receptor antagonist commonly used as an antiemetic initially developed for chemotherapy-induced nausea and vomiting. Given the similar receptor action to the FDA-approved IBS-D treatment alosetron, small studies have evaluated the use of immediate release ondansetron in IBS-D.[33,34] The largest of these studies included 120 patients with IBS-D who were randomized to ondansetron (4 mg with dose titration up to 8 mg 3 times daily) versus placebo in a double-blinded, placebo-controlled crossover study.[35] The trial found that ondansetron significantly improved IBS symptoms severity and adequate relief compared with placebo ($P \leq .001$ for each), and also improved the individual symptoms of stool consistency, defecation frequency, and urgency. However, abdominal pain scores were not significantly impacted by ondansetron treatment. These data inspired the evaluation of a novel bimodal release ondansetron formulation (RHB-102) in 126 patients with IBS-D.[36] The primary end point of overall stool consistency response was achieved at a significantly greater rate with RHB-102 (56% vs 35%; $P = .036$) during the 8-week trial. However, overall pain response and composite (pain and stool consistency) responses were numerically, but not statistically, improved with the bimodal release ondansetron. The only AE experience at a greater rate with active treatment was constipation, which resolved upon withholding treatment.

*Ramosetron*

Ramosetron is a potent, selective serotonin 5-HT$_3$ receptor antagonist that has previously been used for chemotherapy-related and postoperative nausea and vomiting.[37,38] It has also been studied in the treatment of IBS-D, and although not currently approved for use in the United States, ramosetron has received an IBS-D indication in Japan and parts of Asia. A total of 5 RCTs including more than 1900 nonconstipated patients with IBS have demonstrated relief of overall IBS symptoms, abdominal discomfort, and improvements in stool consistency compared with placebo. A recent systemic review and network meta-analysis found that ramosetron 2.5 µg once daily ranked first for effect on abdominal pain among currently licensed pharmacologic therapies.[39] Ramosetron seems to be effective in both male and female patients, and active treatment and his trials occurred without serious AEs (eg, ischemic colitis), although more hard stools and constipation were observed in the ramosetron groups.[39]

## OTHER PHARMACOTHERAPIES FOR DIARRHEA-PREDOMINANT IRRITABLE BOWEL SYNDROME NOT APPROVED BY THE US FOOD AND DRUG ADMINISTRATION

Although 3 FDA-approved pharmacotherapies now are available for IBS-D management, the recognition that only a portion of patients respond to individual trials of these treatments, potentially serious AE profiles, the observation that some patients may experience relapse or recurrence of their symptoms with these medications, and the reality that these branded therapies are more expensive than generic treatment options all drive the use of additional medication options in the management of IBS-D.

*Loperamide*

Loperamide is a widely available over-the-counter antidiarrheal agent indicated for use in the management of acute, nonspecific diarrhea. The recommended adult dose is 4 mg peroral initially, and 2 mg after each loose stool, up to 16 mg/d.[40] As a peripherally restricted µ-opioid receptor agonist, loperamide has been demonstrated to decrease intestinal transit and subsequently enhance fluid reabsorption, making it an effective option for short-term use in controlling diarrheal symptoms.[41,42] As a result, loperamide is one of the most commonly used agents for the management of IBS-D symptoms.[8,43] Yet, loperamide has limited efficacy in addressing the abdominal symptoms of this disorder (eg, pain, discomfort, and bloating) and is not indicated for long-term use.[44] Patients using loperamide often experience difficulties in balancing the control of their diarrhea without inducing constipation. To date, there are only a few very small clinical trials published evaluating loperamide treatment in IBS.[44–47] These studies collectively fail to demonstrate statistical improvement of global IBS symptoms with loperamide and, as a result, the ACG Monograph on IBS recommends against loperamide use in the management of IBS-D.[8] The AGA Guideline suggests using loperamide over no drug treatment and IBS-D as a conditional recommendation based on a very low quality of evidence.[17] Although it is available without a prescription, and is generally regarded as a safe agent when used as directed, US FDA post-marketing safety surveillance has detected a cardiotoxicity signal, including arrhythmias (ventricular tachycardia and torsades de pointes), syncope, and cardiac arrest when misused at higher doses than indicated.[48] More recently, these observations led the FDA to publish a loperamide safety alert relating to these cardiac AEs.[49] As an opioid receptor agonist, a theoretic concern for the development of pancreatitis exists with the use of loperamide. There have been rare cases of pancreatitis reported in association with loperamide, particularly with overdose.[50,51]

### Diphenoxylate and Atropine

Diphenoxylate/atropine is a prescription antidiarrheal preparation consisting of a synthetic μ-opioid receptor agonist coupled with the anticholinergic agent, atropine.[52] The latter component has minimal direct receptor effects in the gut and is combined with diphenoxylate to elicit intolerable systemic effects in the event of misuse or excessive use of the agent. Excess doses of the agent will potentially result in systemic anticholinergic effects (eg, flushing, dry mouth, tachycardia, and sedation). Regardless, there are reports in the literature of diphenxylate abuse and dependence.[53] Its main effects are the inhibition of gastric intestinal motility and secretion, with minimal modulation of pain, despite the μ-opioid receptor effect of the agent.[54] Like loperamide, diphenoxylate/atropine is only indicated for the short-term management of acute diarrhea at a dose of diphenoxylate 5 mg/atropine 0.025 mg up to 4 times daily. Although sometimes prescribed for IBS-D, diphenoxylate/atropine has few limited data in this patient population, and may be less effective than loperamide.[55]

### Antispasmodics

As a class, the antispasmodic agents are very frequently prescribed for the management of IBS-D. These medications generally induce relaxation of smooth muscle within the gastrointestinal tract, decreasing contractility and peristalsis. Many of these agents also have an antisecretory effect. From a pharmacodynamic perspective, antispasmodic medications include anticholinergics, antimuscarinics, calcium antagonists, and compounds with direct effects on smooth muscle. In the United States, dicyclomine (20 mg orally up to 4 times daily), hyoscyamine (0.125–0.250 mg orally or sublingually 3–4 times daily), scopolamine (hyoscine; 1–1.5 mg transdermally every 3 days), methscopolamine (2.5–5 mg orally up to 3 times daily), and glycopyrrolate (1–2 mg orally up to twice daily) are the only antispasmodic agents commercially available.[56] Although commonly used in this setting, there are few clinical trial data to support the use of these agents in IBS-D. With dicyclomine, there are 2 clinical trials including fewer than 200 patients[57,58]; 3 RCTs have studied hyoscine in patients with IBS[59–61] and a single study reported 25 patients randomized to hyoscyamine or placebo.[62] Studies of the other noted agents have not been reported in IBS. The trials examining dicyclomine and hyoscine specifically have demonstrated statistically significant improvement in IBS symptoms, with a NNT in the 3 to 4 range.[8] Although antispasmodics are often prescribed and used on an as as-needed basis, all of these trials examined these medications under a scheduled regimen. The 2 best studied antispasmodics, otilinium (5 RCTs, 791 patients), and pinaverium (4 RCTs, 615 patients) unfortunately are not available for use in the United States. Collectively, the antispasmodic literature does demonstrate significant improvement in global IBS symptoms.[8] However, these studies encompass a multitude of different agents and contain potential methodologic limitations, significant heterogeneity, and funnel plot asymmetry, suggesting potential publication bias or effects of small studies, leading to a dampened enthusiasm for the use of these agents (ACG IBS Monograph: weak recommendation based on very low quality of evidence[8]; ACG IBS Clinical Guidelines: recommend against the use of antispasmodics, low quality of evidence[9]; AGA guideline: use antispasmodics over no drug treatment, low quality of evidence.)[17] The main side effects of these agents based on their mechanisms of action are anticholinergic, including sedation, dry mouth, and difficulties with urination. These AEs are experienced at a statistically higher rate compared with placebo, and are the main limitation in the use of these medications for the treatment of IBS-D.

### Neuromodulators

Neuromodulators (antidepressants, antipsychotics, and other medications targeting the central nervous system) are a mainstay in the management of IBS and other disorders of gut–brain interaction.[63] The use of antidepressants for the treatment of disorders with a chronic, functional pain component has long been recognized as a potentially beneficial treatment strategy not just in IBS, but also in other somatic and extraintestinal disorders such as fibromyalgia, interstitial cystitis, and headaches.[64,65] The 2 main classes of antidepressant agents used in IBS are the tricyclic antidepressants (TCAs) and the selective serotonin reuptake inhibitors. Although in IBS-D there is a high prevalence of psychiatric comorbidity, including depression and anxiety, the antidepressant agents are thought to primarily exert a benefit in neuromodulation of perturbations in the function of the brain–gut axis,[66] rather than a primary effect on mood.[31,63] In the case of IBS-D, the anticholinergic and antihistaminergic effects of the TCAs, particularly prominent with the tertiary amines (imipramine, amitriptyline, and doxepin), may be exploited in improving the diarrheal symptoms via decreases and intestinal transit and secretion.[67] In contrast, the enhanced bowel motility associated with the selective serotonin reuptake inhibitors may be less desirable in the patient with IBS-D. Across all IBS subtypes, the TCAs have demonstrated very favorable NNTs in meta-analysis, leading to a strong recommendations for their use in the management of global IBS symptoms in the ACG IBS Monograph (strong recommendation, high quality of evidence),[8] ACG Clinical Guideline (strong recommendation, moderate quality of evidence),[9] and AGA Guideline (conditional recommendation, low quality of evidence).[68] Other neuromodulators with some evidence in support of their use in IBS have included antipsychotics such as quetiapine,[69] and more recently a study of the calcium channel $\alpha 2\delta$ ligand pregabalin demonstrating beneficial effects on abdominal pain, bloating, and diarrhea.[70] For an in-depth review of neuromodulator therapy and IBS, see Hans Törnblom and Douglas A. Drossman's article, "Psychopharmacological Therapies for Irritable Bowel Syndrome," in this issue of Gastroenterology Clinics of North America.

## HERBAL AND SUPPLEMENT THERAPIES FOR DIARRHEA-PREDOMINANT IRRITABLE BOWEL SYNDROME

Complementary and alternative therapeutic approaches, including supplements and herbals, are used by as many as one-half of patients with IBS-D.[71,72] These preparations often can be used in conjunction with prescription IBS-D pharmacotherapy, and in some cases will be sufficient for the control of IBS-D symptoms as monotherapies. On the whole, these agents have not been subjected to the scrutiny of multiple, rigorous RCTs, resulting in weaker evidence in support of their use. Nevertheless, supplemental therapies generally are well-tolerated and overall are regarded as safe. From a cost perspective, few of these agents will be covered by insurance prescription programs, potentially resulting in a greater out-of-pocket costs to the patient.

### Probiotics

Probiotic preparations consist of either live or attenuated micro-organisms (generally bacteria or nonpathogenic yeasts) that are thought to be beneficial in terms of their potential to positively modulate the gut microflora, with positive changes in intestinal metabolomics, permeability, and low-grade inflammation.[73] An increased interest in probiotic strategies to manage IBS-D symptoms has resulted from a greater recognition that the intestinal microbiota is closely linked to the development of IBS symptoms and, moreover, that alterations in the gut microbiome profile can be detected in patients with IBS compared with healthy controls.[74,75] (For more details, see Prashant Singh and Anthony Lembo's article, "Emerging Role of the Gut Microbiome in IBS," in this issue.) There have been a large number of trials that have examined the use of probiotics in IBS; a recent meta-analysis identified 37 RCTs enrolling more than 4400 patients with IBS reporting on the efficacy of probiotics on the persistence of IBS symptoms.[16] Few studies focused specifically on the management of IBS-D. More than one-half of the trials in this meta-analysis examined a probiotic preparation containing a combination of strains. When examined collectively, combination probiotics demonstrated significant IBS symptom improvements with an NNT of 7 (95% CI, 5–19), although significant between-study heterogeneity and funnel plot asymmetry were detected, suggesting possible small study effects or publication bias. In terms of single strain probiotics, 3 RCTs including 314 patients used *Lactobacillus plantarum DSM 9843*, and found that the relative risk of IBS symptoms persisting was significantly lower with probiotic therapy (NNT = 3; 95% CI, 2–8), although again with significant heterogeneity across studies.[76–78] Other significant single strain studies included *Streptococcus faecium* and *Escherichia coli DSM 7252*, and a trend toward significance was observed with *Bifidobacterium* in 3 RCT.[16] Conversely, several other single strain probiotics studies, including *Lactobacillus* species and *Saccharomyces cerevisiae*, failed to demonstrate superiority over placebo.

With regard to a decrease in global IBS symptoms or abdominal pain scores, again patients treated with combination probiotics in 19 trials including 1341 patients suggested active treatment lead to modest, significant improvement in IBS symptoms, although no single strain study demonstrated ineffective probiotic on global IBS or abdominal pain symptoms.[16] Similarly, combination probiotic preparations significantly decreased flatulence scores and trended toward decreasing abdominal bloating.

Given the considerable variety of individual strains and combination probiotics available, the suggestion of only modest benefits with some of the preparations, and the overall lack of larger, well-designed studies focusing specifically on IBS-D, it is extremely challenging to interpret this literature and provide informed guidance for probiotic use to the patient with IBS-D. Accordingly, inconsistencies exist in the expert guidance relating to probiotic use, with the recent ACG Clinical Guideline suggesting against the use of probiotics for the treatment of global IBS symptoms (very low level of evidence),[9] whereas the earlier ACG IBS Monograph endorses the use of probiotics to improve global IBS symptoms, bloating, and flatulence (weak recommendation based on a low quality of evidence).[8] A recent AGA Clinical Practice Guideline recommends the use of probiotics for IBS only in the context of a clinical trial.[68]

Regardless, recognizing IBS patients' interest in nonpharmacologic approaches to the management of their symptoms, probiotics remain an attractive IBS-D treatment option. Further, surveys of gastroenterologist and primary care providers indicate that the majority of these physicians regard probiotics to be safe, and nearly all of the physicians in 1 survey indicated recommending probiotics for patients with IBS.[79] Indeed, a meta-analysis of the available RCTs has failed to demonstrate any signal for greater risk of AEs with probiotics compared with placebo.[16] However, caution should be exercised in patients who may have greater susceptibility to rare AEs (eg, systemic infection in immunocompromised or acutely ill individuals).[80]

## Prebiotics

Prebiotics are a nonviable food component believed to convey health benefits to the patient based on its potential to modulate the gut microbiota. Prebiotics may be classified as disaccharides (eg, lactulose), oligosaccharides (eg, fructo-oligosaccharide, galacto-oligosaccharide [GOS], and transgalacto-oligosaccharides) or polysaccharides (eg, inulin, cellulose, or pectin).[81] Prebiotics are naturally occurring in cereals, fruits, and vegetables, but may also be synthetically derived. Prebiotics are minimally digested or absorbed within the small intestine, and thus exert their beneficial effects on the gut microbiota primarily in the colon. Specific prebiotics have been shown to promote the growth of particular strains and species of bacterial organisms.[82,83] There have been a few trials of prebiotics and IBS patient populations.[16,84] One such study of 44 patients with IBS (23 with IBS-D) using a transgalacto-oligosaccharide prebiotic demonstrated significant improvements in a composite IBS symptom score as well as a subjective global assessment after 4 weeks of treatment.[85] Individual symptoms were also improved in this study, including stool consistency, flatulence, and bloating ($P<.05$ for each compared with baseline). These symptom improvements were associated with enhanced levels of Bifidobacterium in the stool, a finding also observed in other prebiotic studies,[86–88] and of potential importance particularly in IBS where Bifidobacterium levels have been observed to be reduced in patients compared with healthy controls.[89] A more recent study comparing a GOS prebiotic to a low fermentable oligosaccharides, disaccharides, monosaccharides and polyols (FODMAP) diet found that both groups experienced significant reductions in IBS symptom scores, although the sustained benefit beyond the active treatment period was observed only with the prebiotic but not with the low FODMAP diet.[90] This study also demonstrated an increase in abundance of stool Bifidobacterium with the GOS prebiotic.

Human milk oligosaccharides are a functional component of breast milk, composed of structurally diverse, complex glycans found in high concentrations that are believed to have positive prebiotic-like effect on intestinal Bifidobacterium abundance in adults.[91] In a randomized, double-blind, controlled study of 61 patients with IBS (26 IBS-D, 20 mixed IBS [IBS-M]), a 4:1 mix of 2'-O-fucosyllactose and Lacto-N-neotetraose (2'FL/LNnT) or placebo were administered for 4 weeks. The severity of overall or individual GI symptoms remained stable in both study arms, and no symptom deterioration was seen in any of the groups. However, the 2'FL/LNnT influenced the overall fecal microbiota composition and increased the Bifidobacterium spp.

abundance, suggesting that human milk oligosaccharides could potentially be used to reestablish a healthy microbiota profile in patients with IBS.[89]

Other studies of prebiotics in IBS have failed to demonstrate a positive benefit.[92] Proper dosing of prebiotics is important, because low doses may favorably modulate the gut microbiota and decrease symptoms, and higher doses may have neutral or even negative impact on IBS symptoms.[84] Although prebiotics remain a treatment strategy of considerable promise, based on the available data the ACG IBS Monograph suggested against the use of prebiotics for overall symptom improvement and IBS (weak recommendation, quality of evidence very low).[8]

### Synbiotics

Synbiotics are a form of dietary supplement that provides a combination of probiotics and prebiotics, intended to function in a synergistic fashion wherein this supplement stimulates selective growth and activation of a beneficial intestinal microbiota, leading to positive symptom effects on the patient's health.[93] This strategy, although first described many years ago, remains in the early stages of application to IBS. A study by Min and colleagues[94] evaluated a yogurt/acacia fiber preparation enriched with *Bifidobacterium lactis* compared with a placebo yogurt drink among 130 patients with IBS, found a significant benefit in IBS symptoms and satisfaction with bowel habits in patients with IBS, irrespective of the predominant bowel pattern. Another study of 68 patients with IBS evaluated a combination probiotic including *Lactobacillus acidophilus*, *Lactobacillus helveticus*, and *Bifidobacterium spp.* coupled with a vitamin and phytoextract-enriched medium, and compared this preparation with a heat-inactivated symbiotic. The active synbiotic led to patient reports of improved symptoms compared with baseline in nearly 80% of individuals after 12 weeks.[95] These small studies, although individually positive, collectively do not demonstrate a significant effect in decreasing symptoms in meta-analysis, owing to significant between-study heterogeneity.[16] Several additional studies in adults and children with IBS have suggested a positive effect of synbiotics on improvement in abdominal pain and diarrhea,[96,97] as well as numeric improvements in IBS-QOL, bloating severity, and satisfaction with bowel movements.[98] In an attempt to understand the mechanisms of benefit of synbiotics, 1 study of 72 patients with IBS-D randomized to *Saccharomyces boulardii* or placebo in combination with ispaghula husk, demonstrated decreases in proinflammatory cytokines, tumor necrosis factor-$\alpha$, and IL-8, along with increases in the anti-inflammatory cytokine IL-10, with the synbiotic.[99] Given these limited data in IBS populations, a diversity of preparations, and significant heterogeneity in the existing literature, the ACG IBS Monograph suggests against the use of synbiotics at the current time (weak recommendation based on a very low quality of evidence).[8]

### Peppermint

Mint plants have a long history of perceived medical benefits and descriptions of their potential to soothe the stomach date back to ancient Egypt and Rome.[100] Peppermint oil is extracted from the plant leaves via steam distillation and has been demonstrated to exert multiple effects in the GI tract, including relaxation of smooth muscle (via calcium channel blockade and/or modulation of the enteric nervous system function), downregulation of visceral sensory afferents (effects on transient receptor potential cation channels), and perhaps even antimicrobial and anti-inflammatory effects. The physiologic effects of peppermint oil have been reported to involve the entire luminal gastrointestinal tract, from the esophagus to the colon.[101] Collectively, peppermint preparations have been studied in IBS in more than 800 patients enrolled in more than a dozen RCTs worldwide. However, the majority of these studies were small, and did not specifically focus on IBS-D. In a meta-analysis, peppermint oil yielded improvement in overall IBS symptoms (NNT = 3), as well as abdominal pain specifically (NNT = 4), although it must be acknowledged that the results of the clinical trials of peppermint and IBS are mixed, and examine a variety of different preparations and definitions of response.[102,103] A larger, double-blinded trial randomized 190 patients with IBS to receive peppermint oil preparations targeting a small intestinal release, ileocolonic release, or placebo for 8 weeks.[104] Using the US FDA/European Medicines Agency recommended end point of at least a 30% decrease in weekly average of worst abdominal pain compared with baseline, none of the peppermint preparations were superior to placebo. However, some of the secondary end points, including a decrease in discomfort, abdominal pain, and IBS severity, were achieved at a statistically significant level.[104] Another notable study examining a proprietary blend of triple-coated peppermint oil microspheres was studied in a small cohort of nonconstipated patients with IBS at a dose of 180 mg orally 3 times daily compared with placebo over 4 weeks. This peppermint oil preparation significantly improved the Total IBS Symptom Score, as well as individual symptoms of abdominal pain and discomfort, bloating, distention, and pain at evacuation ($P<.05$ for each). Overall, peppermint oil seems to be well-tolerated, with the main AEs relating to the development of heartburn or dyspeptic symptoms. Particularly low rates of dyspepsia (2.9%) were observed with the triple-coated formulation.[105] The ACG IBS Guideline and Monograph both recommend the use of peppermint to provide relief of global IBS symptoms, albeit based on lower quality evidence.

### STW 5 (Iberogast)

The herbal medicinal preparation STW 5 (Iberogast) has been used for decades in the management of functional gastrointestinal disorders, and is a popular option with patients in Europe.[106] It is readily available in the United States via mainstream e-commerce. STW 5 is believed to exert its benefit through spasmolytic, anti-inflammatory, and mucosal barrier effects on the small bowel and colon.[107,108] Although it has been studied more carefully in patients with functional dyspepsia (efficacy superior to placebo in 7 controlled, randomized, double-blinded studies),[109] it has also been shown to be beneficial in patients with IBS.[110] A large observational study of more than 2500 patients with IBS found that global symptom improvement was rated as very good or good by 78% of patients.[110] A 4-week, placebo-controlled RCT of 208 patients (57 IBS-D, 86 IBS-M) observed significant improvements in IBS abdominal symptoms compared with placebo, without any serious AEs.[111] Further appropriately powered studies using modern clinical trial end points would be of considerable interest.

### Glutamine

Glutamine is an essential amino acid that serves as a major energy substrate for rapidly dividing cells, such as in the gut epithelium, and may restore intestinal permeability after injury.[112,113] Previous detection of increased intestinal permeability in patients with IBS-D,[114] the suggestion that glutamine mucosal content may be decreased in these patients,[115] and the in vitro demonstration that glutamine enhances expression of the tight junction proteins responsible for the maintenance of intestinal permeability in the colonic biopsies of patients with IBS-D inspired a clinical trial of dietary glutamine supplementation.[116] One hundred six patients with postinfection IBS-D were randomized to glutamine 5 g 3 times daily or placebo for 8 weeks; a high percentage of the glutamine-treated patients (79.6%) achieved the primary end point ($\geq$50 point decrease on the IBS Symptom Severity Score), compared with only 5.8% of the placebo group (NNT of <2).[117] Secondary end points including stool frequency, abdominal pain, and quality of life also were improved, as was intestinal permeability (lactulose/mannitol ratio) in the glutamine group. Although these data are compelling, some have criticized the per-protocol rather than intention-to-treat analysis, the low placebo response, and likely underpowering of the study.[117] Regardless, glutamine supplementation is likely safe and the mild side effect profile (dizziness, heartburn, and stomach pain) make glutamine a reasonable treatment option, particularly in patients with postinfection IBS-D while larger RCTs are awaited to confirm these findings.

### Serum-Derived Bovine Immunoglobulin/Protein Isolate

Serum-derived bovine immunoglobulin/protein isolate (SBI, EnteraGam) is a prescription "medical food" believed to have a positive effect on GI mucosal barrier integrity by decreasing intestinal permeability, decreasing intestinal inflammation, and optimizing nutrient absorption.[118–121] A survey conducted in patients with IBS-D or IBS-M taking SBI found that more than 90% of patients reported significant improvements in bowel frequency and the majority also reported that it "helped them manage their condition" (66.9%) and "return to activities they enjoyed" (59.1%).[122] Another study of patients with IBS-D (n = 66) receiving SBI 10 g/d or placebo for 6 weeks demonstrated significant within-group decreases with SBI in abdominal pain, loose stools, bloating, and urgency ($P<.05$ for each), although no statistical differences were observed between the SBI group and placebo for any of the symptoms.[123] Although intriguing, the present level of evidence in support of SBI use in the treatment of IBS-D is insufficient to enthusiastically recommend this product to patients. Additional trials examining more rigorous end points (FDA combined response) and a standard study duration ($\geq$12 weeks) are required to more convincingly establish SBI efficacy in IBS-D.

## NOVEL AND EMERGING THERAPIES FOR DIARRHEA-PREDOMINANT IRRITABLE BOWEL SYNDROME
### Bile Acid Sequestrants

Under normal circumstances, approximately 5% of the bile acids secreted by the liver are unabsorbed by the terminal ileum and reach the colon. The delivery of excess bile acids to the colon results in the production of secondary bile acids through deconjugation by colonic bacteria.[124] In the colon, these bile acids have the potential to enhance fluid secretion, alter permeability and inflammation, and promote high amplitude propagated contractions.[125] As a result, bile acid malabsorption classically leads to diarrheal symptoms, but also commonly is associated with abdominal pain and urgency, all prototypical symptoms of IBS-D. Type 2, or "idiopathic" bile acid diarrhea has been suggested to be present in upwards of 30% of patients with functional diarrhea or IBS-D, making bile acid diarrhea an attractive treatment target in patients with IBS-D.[126] Although traditional tests for bile acid diarrhea, including [75]Se-homocholic acid taurine retention testing is not readily accessible in clinical practice, 48-hour stool collection can be performed to quantify total and individual bile acids, and serum testing for 2 markers, fibroblast growth factor-19 and C4, are on the horizon and should facilitate clinical recognition of bile acid diarrhea in the near future.[124,127]

Bile acid sequestrants (eg, colestipol, colesevelam, and cholestyramine), nonabsorbed resins designed as lipid-lowering agents to bind and inactivate bile acids, thus have a clear mechanistic rationale as a treatment of patients with IBS-D with bile acid diarrhea. In open-label fashion, the use of colestipol led to significant improvements in IBS symptoms severity, and more than one-half of the 27 patients with IBS-D achieved adequate relief of their symptoms.[128] Another small, open-label study of colesevelam demonstrated improvements in stool consistency on the BSFS.[129] However, a recent placebo-controlled IBS-D study found that although patients randomized to colesevelam experienced significant sequestration of fecal bile acid, this finding did not translate into significant improvements in stool frequency and consistency, nor did it significantly affect colonic transit or intestinal permeability.[130] A meta-analysis of earlier studies suggested that responses to cholestyramine may relate to the documented severity of the bile acid malabsorption.[131] Bile acid sequestrants are generally well-tolerated, but must not be taken at the same time as other medications to minimize the potential of unintended binding and impairment of absorption of other drugs.

At present, an empiric trial of a bile sequestrant is a viable treatment option in patients with suspected IBS-D, though this strategy would benefit from additional large RCTs. In the meanwhile, the ACG IBS Guidelines do not suggest the use of bile acid sequestrants to treat global IBS-D symptoms (conditional recommendation based on very low level of evidence).[9]

### Cannabinoids

The endogenous cannabinoid system has been identified within the GI tract, including the cannabinoid receptors $CB_1$ and $CB_2$, endocannabinoids, and the enzymes involved in endocannabinoid biosynthesis and degradation (eg, fatty acid amide hydrolase).[132,133] $CB_1$ receptors are primarily located in enteric neurons and the cell bodies of extrinsic sensory neurons (eg, dorsal root ganglia and vagal afferents) and modulate neurotransmitter release, such as acetylcholine, resulting in a variety of physiologic effects, including attenuation of visceral pain[134] and decreases in intestinal contractility.[135] $CB_2$ receptors are mainly involved with immune functions (eg, lamina propria macrophages and plasma cells), and their activation primarily affects visceral pain and inflammation.[136]

Dronabinol, a synthetic tetrahydrocannabinol analog that activates both $CB_1$ and $CB_2$, has been studied in volunteers with IBS-D. A short course of dronabinol compared with placebo failed to significantly effect gut transit (gastric, small bowel, and colon), but did slow colonic transit in the subset of patients with a CNR1 rs806378 CT/TT genotype.[137] Another single-dose study by the same group in 75 patients with IBS (35 with IBS-D) found dronabinol to decrease colonic motility indices and increase colonic compliance with more prominent effects among patients with IBS-D. However, dronabinol was not found to alter colonic sensation or tone significantly.[138]

Patients with IBS-D have been shown to have higher plasma levels of the endogenous cannabinoid ligands, 2-arachidonylglycerol and lower levels the biolipids oleoylethanolamide and palmitoylethanolamine (PEA). Lower PEA levels were associated with cramping and abdominal pain.[139] An RCT study of N-PEA found that it decreased IBS pain severity and frequency.[140]

Olorinab (APD371) is a highly selective, peripherally active $CB_2$ agonist that is thought to carry minimal potential for misuse or dependence. In an open-label phase IIa study in Crohn's disease, olorinab improved abdominal pain scores compared with baseline (>30% improvement in 11/13 [84.6%]) and a significant improvement in pain-free days and quality of life.[141]

Although patients often inquire about the use of cannabis (medical marijuana) to address their IBS symptoms, cannabis contains multiple cannabinoids including the psychoactive compound, tetrahydrocannabinol, leading to central effects and the potential for dependence, as well unintended off-target effects. The future of endocannabinoid-based therapies is promising and likely will rely on peripherally active agents that can exploit the recognized receptor-specific functions of this system within the GI tract.

### Melatonin

Melatonin (N-acetyl-5-methoxytryptamine) is a pineal gland hormone best recognized for its potential benefit and regulation of circadian rhythm disorders and sleep. However, the enterochromaffin cells the gastrointestinal tract also produce melatonin, and contain levels 1 to 2 log orders higher than in the plasma.[142] Melatonin also has the potential to improve depression and anxiety, comorbidities common to IBS and recognized to potentially exacerbate IBS symptoms.[143] It is thus speculated that melatonin may have an important role in gut function, although understanding this relationship is complex given the association of sleep disturbances with the development of visceral hyperalgesia and increased IBS symptoms.[144,145] A small study in patients with IBS demonstrated that 8 weeks of melatonin improved overall IBS and extracolonic symptoms, as well as quality of life improvements that were statistically significant compared with placebo.[146] A larger, RCT study of 40 patients with IBS (18 IBS-D, 8 IBS-M) with sleep disturbances found that melatonin 3 mg at bedtime decreased the mean abdominal pain scores and led to an objective increase in mean rectal pain thresholds, without significant improvements in sleep disturbance parameters, suggesting an effective melatonin on the bowel, independent of actions on sleep or psychological comorbidities.[147]

## SUMMARY

The treatment of IBS-D requires the clinician to develop a familiarity with the use of a variety of prescription and nonprescription options, including herbals and supplements. Although prescription antidiarrheal and antispasmodic agents remain a mainstay of therapy, they are limited by their potential to impact primarily the bowel symptoms of the disorder (stool frequency and consistency), with lesser effects on the bothersome abdominal symptoms (pain, discomfort, and bloating). Neuromodulators, including the TCAs and selective serotonin reuptake inhibitors, have the potential to impact global IBS-D symptoms, but require clinician insights to proper selection, dosing, and adjustments of these agents. The 3 FDA-approved medications—rifaximin, eluxadoline, and alosetron—have clearly demonstrated efficacy in the management of both the bowel and abdominal symptoms of IBS-D, but may come at a higher cost to the patient, and in some cases (alosetron, eluxadoline) are associated with rare, but serious potential AEs. Prescription options with promise are emerging from a more sophisticated understanding of IBS pathogenesis, and include the bile acid sequestrants and the cannabinoid agents, as well as the $5-HT_3$ antagonists, ondansetron and ramosetron. Modulation of the gut microbiota using probiotics, prebiotics, and synbiotics has a strong rationale for use in IBS-D, but currently lacks definitive evidence of benefit. Strategies for their use will continue to be refined through further study. Other supplements with evolving evidence in support of their use in IBS-D include peppermint oil, STW 5, and melatonin. IBS-D treatment is not amenable to a one size fits all approach; the recognition of multiple mechanistic factors, and variation in patient symptoms and responses to therapy necessitate a multimodal strategy that implements the full complement of prescription medications, herbals, and supplements to optimize symptom outcomes for patients with IBS-D.

## CLINICS CARE POINTS

- Antidepressants, in particular the tricyclic agents, are very effective therapeutic options for IBS-D.
- Evidence-based prescription therapies for IBS-D include rifaximin and eluxadoline, and in treatment-refractory women alosetron can be considered.
- Alternative therapies with emerging evidence for use in IBS-D include bile acid sequestrants, ondansetron, and peppermint preparations.
- Antidiarrheals, such as loperamide or diphenoxylate/atropine, are useful for acute diarrhea management, but are ineffective in IBS-D as a maintenance therapy.
- Antispasmodics (anticholinergic) medications do not impact global IBS symptoms and thus generally are not recommended in IBS-D treatment.

## DISCLOSURE

Dr G.S. Sayuk is a speaker and consultant for Salix, Allergan, Ironwood, and Alnylam, and is a speaker for the GI Health Foundation.

## REFERENCES

1. Mearin F, Lacy BE, Chang L, et al. Bowel disorders. Gastroenterology; section ii: fgids: diagnostic groups bowel 2016;150(6):1393–407.
2. Lovell RM, Ford AC. Global prevalence of and risk factors for irritable bowel syndrome: a meta-analysis. Clin Gastroenterol Hepatol 2012;10(7):712–21.e4.
3. Sperber AD, Dumitrascu D, Fukudo S, et al. The global prevalence of IBS in adults remains elusive due to the heterogeneity of studies: a Rome Foundation working team literature review. Gut 2017;66(6):1075–82.
4. Simren M, Palsson OS, Whitehead WE. Update on Rome IV criteria for colorectal disorders: implications for clinical practice. Curr Gastroenterol Rep 2017; 19(4):15.
5. Sayuk GS, Wolf R, Chang L. Comparison of symptoms, healthcare utilization, and treatment in diagnosed and undiagnosed individuals with diarrhea-predominant irritable bowel syndrome. Am J Gastroenterol 2017;112(6):892–9.
6. Buono JL, Carson RT, Flores NM. Health-related quality of life, work productivity, and indirect costs among patients with irritable bowel syndrome with diarrhea. Health Qual Life Outcomes 2017;15(1):35.
7. Ford AC, Lacy BE, Talley NJ. Irritable bowel syndrome. N Engl J Med 2017; 376(26):2566–78.
8. Ford AC, Moayyedi P, Chey WD, et al. American College of Gastroenterology Monograph on management of irritable bowel syndrome. Am J Gastroenterol 2018;113(Suppl 2):1–18.
9. Lacy BE, Pimentel M, Brenner DM, et al. ACG clinical guideline: management of irritable bowel syndrome. Am J Gastroenterol 2021;116(1):17–44.
10. Brenner DM, Sayuk GS. Current US Food and Drug Administration-Approved Pharmacologic therapies for the treatment of irritable bowel syndrome with diarrhea. Adv Ther 2020;37(1):83–96.
11. Nuovo J, Melnikow J, Chang D. Reporting number needed to treat and absolute risk reduction in randomized controlled trials. JAMA 2002;287(21):2813–4.

12. Christensen PM, Kristiansen IS. Number-needed-to-treat (NNT)–needs treatment with care. Basic Clin Pharmacol Toxicol 2006;99(1):12–6.
13. Rifaximin (Xifaxan) Prescribing Information. Available at: https://shared.salix. com/shared/pi/xifaxan550-pi.pdf. Accessed January 1, 2021.
14. Pimentel M, Lembo A, Chey WD, et al. Rifaximin therapy for patients with irritable bowel syndrome without constipation. N Engl J Med 2011;364(1):22–32.
15. Lembo A, Pimentel M, Rao SS, et al. Repeat treatment with rifaximin is safe and effective in patients with diarrhea-predominant irritable bowel syndrome. Gastroenterology 2016;151(6):1113–21.
16. Ford AC, Harris LA, Lacy BE, et al. Systematic review with meta-analysis: the efficacy of prebiotics, probiotics, synbiotics and antibiotics in irritable bowel syndrome. Aliment Pharmacol Ther 2018;48(10):1044–60.
17. Weinberg DS, Smalley W, Heidelbaugh JJ, et al. American Gastroenterological Association Institute Guideline on the pharmacological management of irritable bowel syndrome. Gastroenterology 2014;147(5):1146–8.
18. Shah E, Kim S, Chong K, et al. Evaluation of harm in the pharmacotherapy of irritable bowel syndrome. Am J Med 2012;125(4):381–93.
19. Eluxadoline (Viberzi) Prescribing Information. Available at: https://media. allergan.com/actavis/actavis/media/allergan-pdf-documents/product-prescribing/viberzi_pi.pdf. Accessed January 1, 2021.
20. Wade PR, Palmer JM, McKenney S, et al. Modulation of gastrointestinal function by MuDelta, a mixed micro opioid receptor agonist/micro opioid receptor antagonist. Br J Pharmacol 2012;167(5):1111–25.
21. Lembo AJ, Lacy BE, Zuckerman MJ, et al. Eluxadoline for irritable bowel syndrome with diarrhea. N Engl J Med 2016;374(3):242–53.
22. Lacy BE, Chey WD, Cash BD, et al. Eluxadoline efficacy in IBS-D patients who report prior loperamide use. Am J Gastroenterol 2017;112(6):924–32.
23. Brenner DM, Sayuk GS, Gutman CR, et al. Efficacy and safety of eluxadoline in patients with irritable bowel syndrome with diarrhea who report inadequate symptom control with loperamide: RELIEF phase 4 study. Am J Gastroenterol 2019;114(9):1502–11.
24. Cash BD, Lacy BE, Schoenfeld PS, et al. Safety of eluxadoline in patients with irritable bowel syndrome with diarrhea. Am J Gastroenterol 2017;112(2):365–74.
25. Liu R, Staller K. Update on eluxadoline for the treatment of irritable bowel syndrome with diarrhea: patient selection and perspectives. Drug Des Devel Ther 2020;14:1391–400.
26. FDA warns about an increased risk of serious pancreatitis with irritable bowel drug Viberzi (eluxadoline) in patients without a gallbladder. Available at: https://www.fda.gov/media/103593/download. Accessed January 1, 2021.
27. Alosetron (Lotronex) Prescribing Information. Available at: https://www.lotronex. com/hcp/_docs/PI%20v.Sebela_Final.pdf. Accessed January 1, 2021.
28. Cremonini F, Nicandro JP, Atkinson V, et al. Randomised clinical trial: alosetron improves quality of life and reduces restriction of daily activities in women with severe diarrhoea-predominant IBS. Aliment Pharmacol Ther 2012;36(5):437–48.
29. Alosetron (Lotronex) Risk Evaluation and Mitigation Strategy (REMS) program. Available at: https://www.lotronexrems.com/Prescribers.html. Accessed January 1, 2021.
30. Lembo T, Wright RA, Bagby B, et al. Alosetron controls bowel urgency and provides global symptom improvement in women with diarrhea-predominant irritable bowel syndrome. Am J Gastroenterol 2001;96(9):2662–70.

31. Krause R, Ameen V, Gordon SH, et al. A randomized, double-blind, placebo-controlled study to assess efficacy and safety of 0.5 mg and 1 mg alosetron in women with severe diarrhea-predominant IBS. Am J Gastroenterol 2007; 102(8):1709–19.

32. Lacy BE, Nicandro JP, Chuang E, et al. Alosetron use in clinical practice: significant improvement in irritable bowel syndrome symptoms evaluated using the US Food and Drug Administration composite endpoint. Therap Adv Gastroenterol 2018;11. 1756284818771674.

33. Steadman CJ, Talley NJ, Phillips SF, et al. Selective 5-hydroxytryptamine type 3 receptor antagonism with ondansetron as treatment for diarrhea-predominant irritable bowel syndrome: a pilot study. Mayo Clin Proc 1992;67(8):732–8.

34. Maxton DG, Morris J, Whorwell PJ. Selective 5-hydroxytryptamine antagonism: a role in irritable bowel syndrome and functional dyspepsia? Aliment Pharmacol Ther 1996;10(4):595–9.

35. Garsed K, Chernova J, Hastings M, et al. A randomised trial of ondansetron for the treatment of irritable bowel syndrome with diarrhoea. Gut 2014;63(10): 1617–25.

36. Plasse TF, Barton G, Davidson E, et al. Bimodal release ondansetron improves stool consistency and symptomatology in diarrhea-predominant irritable bowel syndrome: a randomized, double-blind, trial. Am J Gastroenterol 2020;115(9): 1466–73.

37. Fujii Y, Saitoh Y, Tanaka H, et al. Ramosetron vs granisetron for the prevention of postoperative nausea and vomiting after laparoscopic cholecystectomy. Can J Anaesth 1999;46(10):991–3.

38. Kim HJ, Shin SW, Song EK, et al. Ramosetron versus ondansetron in combination with aprepitant and dexamethasone for the prevention of highly emetogenic chemotherapy-induced nausea and vomiting: a multicenter, randomized phase III trial, KCSG PC10-21. Oncologist 2015;20(12):1440–7.

39. Qi Q, Zhang Y, Chen F, et al. Ramosetron for the treatment of irritable bowel syndrome with diarrhea: a systematic review and meta-analysis of randomized controlled trials. BMC Gastroenterol 2018;18(1):5.

40. Hanauer SB. The role of loperamide in gastrointestinal disorders. Rev Gastroenterol Disord 2008;8(1):15–20.

41. Ruppin H. Review: loperamide–a potent antidiarrhoeal drug with actions along the alimentary tract. Aliment Pharmacol Ther 1987;1(3):179–90.

42. Baker DE. Loperamide: a pharmacological review. Rev Gastroenterol Disord 2007;7(Suppl 3):S11–8.

43. Chang L, Lembo A, Sultan S. American Gastroenterological Association Institute Technical Review on the pharmacological management of irritable bowel syndrome. Gastroenterology 2014;147(5):1149–72.e2.

44. Efskind PS, Bernklev T, Vatn MH. A double-blind placebo-controlled trial with loperamide in irritable bowel syndrome. Scand J Gastroenterol 1996;31(5):463–8.

45. Hovdenak N. Loperamide treatment of the irritable bowel syndrome. Scand J Gastroenterol Suppl 1987;130:81–4.

46. Lavo B, Stenstam M, Nielsen AL. Loperamide in treatment of irritable bowel syndrome–a double-blind placebo controlled study. Scand J Gastroenterol Suppl 1987;130:77–80.

47. Adami CE, Gobato RC, Gestic MA, et al. Correlations of HOMA2-IR and HbA1c with algorithms derived from bioimpedance and spectrophotometric devices. Obes Surg 2012;22(12):1803–9.

48. Swank KA, Wu E, Kortepeter C, et al. Adverse event detection using the FDA post-marketing drug safety surveillance system: cardiotoxicity associated with loperamide abuse and misuse. J Am Pharm Assoc (2003) 2017;57(2S):S63–7.

49. FDA warns about serious heart problems with high doses of the antidiarrheal medicine loperamide (Imodium), including from abuse and misuse. Available at: https://www.fda.gov/media/98335/download. Accessed January 1, 2021.

50. Gawron AJ, Bielefeldt K. Risk of pancreatitis following treatment of irritable bowel syndrome with eluxadoline. Clin Gastroenterol Hepatol 2018;16(3): 378–84.e2.

51. Epelde F, Boada L, Tost J. Pancreatitis caused by loperamide overdose. Ann Pharmacother 1996;30(11):1339.

52. Jain M, Wylie WP. Diphenoxylate and atropine. Treasure Island (FL): StatPearls; 2020.

53. Firoozabadi A, Mowla A, Farashbandi H, et al. Diphenoxylate hydrochloride dependency. J Psychiatr Pract 2007;13(4):278–80.

54. Gattuso JM, Kamm MA. Adverse effects of drugs used in the management of constipation and diarrhoea. Drug Saf 1994;10(1):47–65.

55. Palmer KR, Corbett CL, Holdsworth CD. Double-blind cross-over study comparing loperamide, codeine and diphenoxylate in the treatment of chronic diarrhea. Gastroenterology 1980;79(6):1272–5.

56. Saad RJ. Peripherally acting therapies for the treatment of irritable bowel syndrome. Gastroenterol Clin North Am 2011;40(1):163–82.

57. Matts SG. An assessment of dicyclomine hydrochloride ('Merbentyl') in the irritable colon syndrome. Br J Clin Pract 1967;21(11):549–51.

58. Page JG, Dirnberger GM. Treatment of the irritable bowel syndrome with Bentyl (dicyclomine hydrochloride). J Clin Gastroenterol 1981;3(2):153–6.

59. Ritchie JA, Truelove SC. Treatment of irritable bowel syndrome with lorazepam, hyoscine butylbromide, and ispaghula husk. Br Med J 1979;1(6160):376–8.

60. Schafer E, Ewe K. [The treatment of irritable colon. Efficacy and tolerance of buscopan plus, buscopan, paracetamol and placebo in ambulatory patients with irritable colon]. Fortschr Med 1990;108(25):488–92.

61. Nigam P, Kapoor KK, Rastog CK, et al. Different therapeutic regimens in irritable bowel syndrome. J Assoc Physicians India 1984;32(12):1041–4.

62. Carling L, Svedberg LE, Hulten S. Short term treatment of the irritable bowel syndrome: a placebo-controlled trial of peppermint oil against hyoscyamine. Opuscula Medica 1989;34(3):55–7.

63. Drossman DA, Tack J, Ford AC, et al. Neuromodulators for functional gastrointestinal disorders (disorders of gut-brain interaction): a Rome Foundation Working Team report. Gastroenterology 2018;154(4):1140–71.e1.

64. O'Malley PG, Jackson JL, Santoro J, et al. Antidepressant therapy for unexplained symptoms and symptom syndromes. J Fam Pract 1999;48(12):980–90.

65. Clouse RE, Lustman PJ. Use of psychopharmacological agents for functional gastrointestinal disorders. Gut 2005;54(9):1332–41.

66. Mayer EA, Naliboff BD, Craig AD. Neuroimaging of the brain-gut axis: from basic understanding to treatment of functional GI disorders. Gastroenterology 2006;131(6):1925–42.

67. Gorard DA, Libby GW, Farthing MJ. Effect of a tricyclic antidepressant on small intestinal motility in health and diarrhea-predominant irritable bowel syndrome. Dig Dis Sci 1995;40(1):86–95.

68. Su GL, Ko CW, Bercik P, et al. AGA clinical practice guidelines on the role of probiotics in the management of gastrointestinal disorders. Gastroenterology 2020; 159(2):697–705.

69. Grover M, Dorn SD, Weinland SR, et al. Atypical antipsychotic quetiapine in the management of severe refractory functional gastrointestinal disorders. Dig Dis Sci 2009;54(6):1284–91.

70. Saito YA, Almazar AE, Tilkes KE, et al. Randomised clinical trial: pregabalin vs placebo for irritable bowel syndrome. Aliment Pharmacol Ther 2019;49(4): 389–97.

71. van Tilburg MA, Palsson OS, Levy RL, et al. Complementary and alternative medicine use and cost in functional bowel disorders: a six month prospective study in a large HMO. BMC Complement Altern Med 2008;8:46.

72. Hussain Z, Quigley EM. Systematic review: complementary and alternative medicine in the irritable bowel syndrome. Aliment Pharmacol Ther 2006;23(4): 465–71.

73. Hill C, Guarner F, Reid G, et al. Expert consensus document. The International Scientific Association for Probiotics and Prebiotics consensus statement on the scope and appropriate use of the term probiotic. Nat Rev Gastroenterol Hepatol 2014;11(8):506–14.

74. Vaga S, Lee S, Ji B, et al. Compositional and functional differences of the mucosal microbiota along the intestine of healthy individuals. Sci Rep 2020; 10(1):14977.

75. Hugerth LW, Andreasson A, Talley NJ, et al. No distinct microbiome signature of irritable bowel syndrome found in a Swedish random population. Gut 2020; 69(6):1076–84.

76. Ducrotte P, Sawant P, Jayanthi V. Clinical trial: Lactobacillus plantarum 299v (DSM 9843) improves symptoms of irritable bowel syndrome. World J Gastroenterol 2012;18(30):4012–8.

77. Nobaek S, Johansson ML, Molin G, et al. Alteration of intestinal microflora is associated with reduction in abdominal bloating and pain in patients with irritable bowel syndrome. Am J Gastroenterol 2000;95(5):1231–8.

78. Niedzielin K, Kordecki H, Birkenfeld B. A controlled, double-blind, randomized study on the efficacy of Lactobacillus plantarum 299V in patients with irritable bowel syndrome. Eur J Gastroenterol Hepatol 2001;13(10):1143–7.

79. Williams MD, Ha CY, Ciorba MA. Probiotics as therapy in gastroenterology: a study of physician opinions and recommendations. J Clin Gastroenterol 2010; 44(9):631–6.

80. Doron S, Snydman DR. Risk and safety of probiotics. Clin Infect Dis 2015; 60(Suppl 2):S129–34.

81. Markowiak P, Slizewska K. Effects of probiotics, prebiotics, and synbiotics on human health. Nutrients 2017;9(9):1021.

82. Gibson GR, Probert HM, Loo JV, et al. Dietary modulation of the human colonic microbiota: updating the concept of prebiotics. Nutr Res Rev 2004;17(2): 259–75.

83. Roberfroid M, Gibson GR, Hoyles L, et al. Prebiotic effects: metabolic and health benefits. Br J Nutr 2010;104(Suppl 2):S1–63.

84. Wilson B, Whelan K. Prebiotic inulin-type fructans and galacto-oligosaccharides: definition, specificity, function, and application in gastrointestinal disorders. J Gastroenterol Hepatol 2017;32(Suppl 1):64–8.

85. Silk DB, Davis A, Vulevic J, et al. Clinical trial: the effects of a trans-galactooligosaccharide prebiotic on faecal microbiota and symptoms in irritable bowel syndrome. Aliment Pharmacol Ther 2009;29(5):508–18.
86. Vogt L, Meyer D, Pullens G, et al. Immunological properties of inulin-type fructans. Crit Rev Food Sci Nutr 2015;55(3):414–36.
87. Vulevic J, Juric A, Walton GE, et al. Influence of galacto-oligosaccharide mixture (B-GOS) on gut microbiota, immune parameters and metabonomics in elderly persons. Br J Nutr 2015;114(4):586–95.
88. Mego M, Manichanh C, Accarino A, et al. Metabolic adaptation of colonic microbiota to galactooligosaccharides: a proof-of-concept-study. Aliment Pharmacol Ther 2017;45(5):670–80.
89. Zhuang X, Xiong L, Li L, et al. Alterations of gut microbiota in patients with irritable bowel syndrome: a systematic review and meta-analysis. J Gastroenterol Hepatol 2017;32(1):28–38.
90. Huaman JW, Mego M, Manichanh C, et al. Effects of prebiotics vs a diet low in FODMAPs in patients with functional gut disorders. Gastroenterology 2018; 155(4):1004–7.
91. Ray C, Kerketta JA, Rao S, et al. Human milk oligosaccharides: the journey ahead. Int J Pediatr 2019;2019:2390240.
92. Wilson B, Rossi M, Dimidi E, et al. Prebiotics in irritable bowel syndrome and other functional bowel disorders in adults: a systematic review and meta-analysis of randomized controlled trials. Am J Clin Nutr 2019;109(4):1098–111.
93. Gibson GR, Roberfroid MB. Dietary modulation of the human colonic microbiota: introducing the concept of prebiotics. J Nutr 1995;125(6):1401–12.
94. Min YW, Park SU, Jang YS, et al. Effect of composite yogurt enriched with acacia fiber and Bifidobacterium lactis. World J Gastroenterol 2012;18(33): 4563–9.
95. Tsuchiya J, Barreto R, Okura R, et al. Single-blind follow-up study on the effectiveness of a symbiotic preparation in irritable bowel syndrome. Chin J Dig Dis 2004;5(4):169–74.
96. Rogha M, Esfahani MZ, Zargarzadeh AH. The efficacy of a synbiotic containing Bacillus Coagulans in treatment of irritable bowel syndrome: a randomized placebo-controlled trial. Gastroenterol Hepatol Bed Bench 2014;7(3):156–63.
97. Saneian H, Pourmoghaddas Z, Roohafza H, et al. Synbiotic containing Bacillus coagulans and fructo-oligosaccharides for functional abdominal pain in children. Gastroenterol Hepatol Bed Bench 2015;8(1):56–65.
98. Bogovic Matijasic B, Obermajer T, Lipoglavsek L, et al. Effects of synbiotic fermented milk containing Lactobacillus acidophilus La-5 and Bifidobacterium animalis ssp. lactis BB-12 on the fecal microbiota of adults with irritable bowel syndrome: a randomized double-blind, placebo-controlled trial. J Dairy Sci 2016;99(7):5008–21.
99. Basturk A, Artan R, Yilmaz A. Efficacy of synbiotic, probiotic, and prebiotic treatments for irritable bowel syndrome in children: a randomized controlled trial. Turk J Gastroenterol 2016;27(5):439–43.
100. Ulbricht C, Costa D, Grimes Serrano JM, et al. An evidence-based systematic review of spearmint by the natural standard research collaboration. J Diet Suppl 2010;7(2):179–215.
101. Chumpitazi BP, Kearns GL, Shulman RJ. Review article: the physiological effects and safety of peppermint oil and its efficacy in irritable bowel syndrome and other functional disorders. Aliment Pharmacol Ther 2018;47(6):738–52.

102. Alammar N, Wang L, Saberi B, et al. The impact of peppermint oil on the irritable bowel syndrome: a meta-analysis of the pooled clinical data. BMC Complement Altern Med 2019;19(1):21.
103. Khanna R, MacDonald JK, Levesque BG. Peppermint oil for the treatment of irritable bowel syndrome: a systematic review and meta-analysis. J Clin Gastroenterol 2014;48(6):505–12.
104. Weerts Z, Masclee AAM, Witteman BJM, et al. Efficacy and safety of peppermint oil in a randomized, double-blind trial of patients with irritable bowel syndrome. Gastroenterology 2020;158(1):123–36.
105. Cash BD, Epstein MS, Shah SM. A novel delivery system of peppermint oil is an effective therapy for irritable bowel syndrome symptoms. Dig Dis Sci 2016; 61(2):560–71.
106. Ottillinger B, Storr M, Malfertheiner P, et al. STW 5 (Iberogast(R))–a safe and effective standard in the treatment of functional gastrointestinal disorders. Wien Med Wochenschr 2013;163(3–4):65–72.
107. Ammon HP, Kelber O, Okpanyi SN. Spasmolytic and tonic effect of Iberogast (STW 5) in intestinal smooth muscle. Phytomedicine 2006;13(Suppl 5):67–74.
108. Allescher HD, Abdel-Aziz H. Mechanism of action of STW 5 in functional dyspepsia and IBS: the origin of multi-target. Dig Dis 2017;35(Suppl 1):18–24.
109. Melzer J, Iten F, Reichling J, et al. Iberis amara L. and Iberogast–results of a systematic review concerning functional dyspepsia. J Herb Pharmacother 2004; 4(4):51–9.
110. Malfertheiner P. STW 5 (Iberogast) therapy in gastrointestinal functional disorders. Dig Dis 2017;35(Suppl 1):25–9.
111. Madisch A, Holtmann G, Plein K, et al. Treatment of irritable bowel syndrome with herbal preparations: results of a double-blind, randomized, placebo-controlled, multi-centre trial. Aliment Pharmacol Ther 2004;19(3):271–9.
112. Klimberg VS, Souba WW. The importance of intestinal glutamine metabolism in maintaining a healthy gastrointestinal tract and supporting the body's response to injury and illness. Surg Annu 1990;22:61–76.
113. De-Souza DA, Greene LJ. Intestinal permeability and systemic infections in critically ill patients: effect of glutamine. Crit Care Med 2005;33(5):1125–35.
114. Bertiaux-Vandaele N, Youmba SB, Belmonte L, et al. The expression and the cellular distribution of the tight junction proteins are altered in irritable bowel syndrome patients with differences according to the disease subtype. Am J Gastroenterol 2011;106(12):2165–73.
115. Zhou Q, Souba WW, Croce CM, et al. MicroRNA-29a regulates intestinal membrane permeability in patients with irritable bowel syndrome. Gut 2010;59(6): 775–84.
116. Zhou Q, Verne ML, Fields JZ, et al. Randomised placebo-controlled trial of dietary glutamine supplements for postinfectious irritable bowel syndrome. Gut 2019;68(6):996–1002.
117. Ford AC, Gibson PR. Efficacy of glutamine in postinfection IBS. Gut 2019; 68(10):1905–6.
118. Bosi P, Casini L, Finamore A, et al. Spray-dried plasma improves growth performance and reduces inflammatory status of weaned pigs challenged with enterotoxigenic Escherichia coli K88. J Anim Sci 2004;82(6):1764–72.
119. Asmuth DM, Ma ZM, Albanese A, et al. Oral serum-derived bovine immunoglobulin improves duodenal immune reconstitution and absorption function in patients with HIV enteropathy. AIDS 2013;27(14):2207–17.

120. Peace RM, Campbell J, Polo J, et al. Spray-dried porcine plasma influences intestinal barrier function, inflammation, and diarrhea in weaned pigs. J Nutr 2011; 141(7):1312–7.

121. Enteragam Product Information. Available at: https://enteragam.com/assets/lib/EnteraGam_Product_Information.pdf. Accessed January 1, 2021.

122. Shaw AL, Tomanelli A, Bradshaw TP, et al. Impact of serum-derived bovine immunoglobulin/protein isolate therapy on irritable bowel syndrome and inflammatory bowel disease: a survey of patient perspective. Patient Prefer Adherence 2017;11:1001–7.

123. Wilson D, Evans M, Weaver E, et al. Evaluation of serum-derived bovine immunoglobulin protein isolate in subjects with diarrhea-predominant irritable bowel syndrome. Clin Med Insights Gastroenterol 2013;6:49–60.

124. Vijayvargiya P, Camilleri M. Current practice in the diagnosis of bile acid diarrhea. Gastroenterology 2019;156(5):1233–8.

125. Kirwan WO, Smith AN, Mitchell WD, et al. Bile acids and colonic motility in the rabbit and the human. Gut 1975;16(11):894–902.

126. Valentin N, Camilleri M, Altayar O, et al. Biomarkers for bile acid diarrhoea in functional bowel disorder with diarrhoea: a systematic review and meta-analysis. Gut 2016;65(12):1951–9.

127. Vijayvargiya P, Camilleri M. Update on bile acid malabsorption: finally ready for prime time? Curr Gastroenterol Rep 2018;20(3):10.

128. Bajor A, Tornblom H, Rudling M, et al. Increased colonic bile acid exposure: a relevant factor for symptoms and treatment in IBS. Gut 2015;64(1):84–92.

129. Camilleri M, Acosta A, Busciglio I, et al. Effect of colesevelam on faecal bile acids and bowel functions in diarrhoea-predominant irritable bowel syndrome. Aliment Pharmacol Ther 2015;41(5):438–48.

130. Vijayvargiya P, Camilleri M, Carlson P, et al. Effects of colesevelam on bowel symptoms, biomarkers, and colonic mucosal gene expression in patients with bile acid diarrhea in a randomized trial. Clin Gastroenterol Hepatol 2020; 18(13):2962–70.e6.

131. Wedlake L, A'Hern R, Russell D, et al. Systematic review: the prevalence of idiopathic bile acid malabsorption as diagnosed by SeHCAT scanning in patients with diarrhoea-predominant irritable bowel syndrome. Aliment Pharmacol Ther 2009;30(7):707–17.

132. D'Argenio G, Petrosino S, Gianfrani C, et al. Overactivity of the intestinal endocannabinoid system in celiac disease and in methotrexate-treated rats. J Mol Med (Berl) 2007;85(5):523–30.

133. Izzo AA, Camilleri M. Emerging role of cannabinoids in gastrointestinal and liver diseases: basic and clinical aspects. Gut 2008;57(8):1140–55.

134. Sanson M, Bueno L, Fioramonti J. Involvement of cannabinoid receptors in inflammatory hypersensitivity to colonic distension in rats. Neurogastroenterol Motil 2006;18(10):949–56.

135. Storr MA, Sharkey KA. The endocannabinoid system and gut-brain signalling. Curr Opin Pharmacol 2007;7(6):575–82.

136. Izzo AA. The cannabinoid CB(2) receptor: a good friend in the gut. Neurogastroenterol Motil 2007;19(9):704–8.

137. Wong BS, Camilleri M, Eckert D, et al. Randomized pharmacodynamic and pharmacogenetic trial of dronabinol effects on colon transit in irritable bowel syndrome-diarrhea. Neurogastroenterol Motil 2012;24(4):358-e169.

138. Wong BS, Camilleri M, Busciglio I, et al. Pharmacogenetic trial of a cannabinoid agonist shows reduced fasting colonic motility in patients with nonconstipated irritable bowel syndrome. Gastroenterology 2011;141(5):1638–47.e1-7.
139. Fichna J, Wood JT, Papanastasiou M, et al. Endocannabinoid and cannabinoid-like fatty acid amide levels correlate with pain-related symptoms in patients with IBS-D and IBS-C: a pilot study. PLoS One 2013;8(12):e85073.
140. Cremon C, Stanghellini V, Barbaro MR, et al. Randomised clinical trial: the analgesic properties of dietary supplementation with palmitoylethanolamide and polydatin in irritable bowel syndrome. Aliment Pharmacol Ther 2017;45(7):909–22.
141. Maselli DB, Camilleri M. Pharmacology, clinical effects, and therapeutic potential of cannabinoids for gastrointestinal and liver diseases. Clin Gastroenterol Hepatol 2020;13. https://doi.org/10.1016/j.cgh.2020.04.020. S1542-3565(20)30504-8.
142. Srinivasan V, Pandi-Perumal SR, Trahkt I, et al. Melatonin and melatonergic drugs on sleep: possible mechanisms of action. Int J Neurosci 2009;119(6):821–46.
143. Srinivasan V, Smits M, Spence W, et al. Melatonin in mood disorders. World J Biol Psychiatry 2006;7(3):138–51.
144. Patel A, Hasak S, Cassell B, et al. Effects of disturbed sleep on gastrointestinal and somatic pain symptoms in irritable bowel syndrome. Aliment Pharmacol Ther 2016;44(3):246–58.
145. Schey R, Dickman R, Parthasarathy S, et al. Sleep deprivation is hyperalgesic in patients with gastroesophageal reflux disease. Gastroenterology 2007;133(6):1787–95.
146. Lu WZ, Gwee KA, Moochhalla S, et al. Melatonin improves bowel symptoms in female patients with irritable bowel syndrome: a double-blind placebo-controlled study. Aliment Pharmacol Ther 2005;22(10):927–34.
147. Song GH, Leng PH, Gwee KA, et al. Melatonin improves abdominal pain in irritable bowel syndrome patients who have sleep disturbances: a randomised, double blind, placebo controlled study. Gut 2005;54(10):1402–7.

# Focus on Pharmacotherapy for Irritable Bowel Syndrome with Constipation

Joy J. Liu, MD, Darren M. Brenner, MD*

## KEYWORDS

- Irritable bowel syndrome • IBS-C • Constipation • Treatment • Pharmacotherapy

## KEY POINTS

- Irritable bowel syndrome with constipation (IBS-C) is a disorder characterized by abdominal pain associated with the passage of hard, lumpy stools.
- Multiple effective FDA-approved therapies are now available for treating global IBS-C symptoms.
- Some national gastroenterology societies suggest that over-the-counter laxatives should not be used to treat IBS-C given their lack of ability to improve abdominal symptoms.

## INTRODUCTION

Irritable bowel syndrome (IBS) with constipation (IBS-C) is a disorder of gut-brain interaction currently defined by the Rome IV criteria as abdominal pain occurring greater than or equal to 1 d/wk associated with alterations in pain perception with defecation, and/or changes in stool form, and/or frequency.[1] IBS is further categorized by predominant stool texture using the Bristol Stool Form Scale (BSFS). Patients with IBS-C report that greater than one-quarter of their stools are BSFS 1 to 2 (hard/lumpy) in texture and less than 25% are BSFS 6 to 7 (loose/watery) (**Fig. 1**). Recent studies suggest that IBS affects 4.6% of the US population and IBS-C accounts for approximately 30% of these diagnoses.[2–4]

IBS-C is distinguished from functional constipation (FC) by the Rome IV definitions because most experts now consider them to be similar disorders along a spectrum of symptoms.[5] Rome IV concedes that individuals with IBS or FC can experience pain; however, pain serves as the sine qua non symptom of the former but is not predominant in the latter. Furthermore, individuals diagnosed with FC should not meet criteria for IBS-C. There is substantial clinical overlap and individuals may alternate between

Division of Gastroenterology/Hepatology, Department of Medicine, Northwestern University, 676 North St Clair Street, Suite 1400, Chicago, IL 60611, USA
* Corresponding author.
*E-mail address:* darren.brenner@nm.org

Gastroenterol Clin N Am 50 (2021) 639–653
https://doi.org/10.1016/j.gtc.2021.04.004
0889-8553/21/© 2021 Elsevier Inc. All rights reserved.

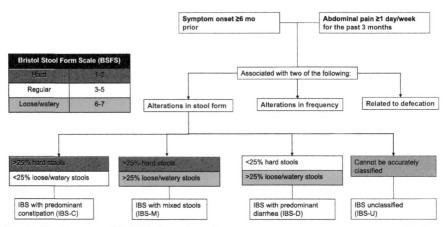

**Fig. 1.** Classification of irritable bowel syndrome.

IBS-C and FC at different points in their lives.[5] As such, it is not surprising that many recently Food and Drug Administration (FDA)-approved therapeutics for constipation are approved and have proven effective for both disorders.[6]

The methodology used in randomized controlled trials (RCTs) to evaluate the efficacy of pharmaceuticals for treating IBS-C has evolved over the past two decades.[7] More recent trials have consistently used Rome criteria for inclusion, and in 2012, the FDA provided guidance on specific end points. Currently, patients must meet an overall responder end point defined as a weekly average of greater than or equal to 30% improvement in abdominal pain plus an increase of at least one complete spontaneous bowel movement (CSBM) per week compared with baseline during the same week for greater than or equal to 50% of a 12-week trial.[8] Although this end point may seem arbitrary, it correlates well with a positive clinical response.[9,10] Data on primary end points, outcomes, and adverse effects from phase III trials for FDA-approved agents to treat IBS-C are found in **Table 1**.

Multiple over-the-counter (OTC) laxatives are used to treat constipation associated with IBS-C; however, data supporting their efficacy are limited or lacking. Whereas many of these agents may improve bowel function (stool frequency, texture, straining) they have minimal impact on abdominal symptoms, such as bloating and pain. Consequently, major gastrointestinal societies are now suggesting against their use and instead recommending other agents with more robust data.[11,12] These include the secretagogues (lubiprostone, linaclotide, prucalopride, tenapanor) and prokinetics (tegaserod). This article reviews the efficacy, safety, and tolerability profiles for each of these agents with a focus on results from their pivotal trials.

## OVER-THE-COUNTER LAXATIVES

OTC therapies have been a mainstay of treatment of constipation because they are generally safe, well-tolerated, and cost-effective. Multiple classes of OTCs exist including bulking agents (methylcellulose, psyllium, bran), osmotic laxatives (polyethylene glycol [PEG]), magnesium-containing compounds (magnesium oxide, sulfate, hydroxide), stimulant laxatives (senna, bisacodyl, cascara), and stool softeners (docusate). Although there are varying levels of evidence supporting the use of OTC laxatives for FC, data for IBS-C are sparse.

**Table 1**
Phase III trial data for agents used to treat IBS-C

| Drug | Year of FDA Approval for IBS-C | Primary End Points Studied for IBS-C in Phase III Trials | Primary Outcome | Adverse Effects in Treatment Group |
|---|---|---|---|---|
| Polyethylene glycol | NA | No data to report | NA | NA |
| Lubiprostone | 2008 in women | Moderate relief in 4/4 wk or significant relief in 2/4 wk per mo in ≥ 2/3 mo of study | 17.9% (8 μg BID lubiprostone) vs 10.1% (placebo) (P = .001)[20] | Nausea (8%), diarrhea (6%), abdominal distention (2%) |
| Linaclotide | 2012 | Combined ≥30% reduction from baseline in worst abdominal pain + an increase of at least 1 CSBM/wk from baseline during the same week for ≥6/12 wk (FDA overall responder end point) | 33.7% (290 μg daily linaclotide) vs 13.9% (placebo) (P < .001)[21] 3.6% (290 μg daily linaclotide) vs 21.0% (placebo) (P < .0001)[27] 60% (290 μg daily linaclotide) vs 48.8% (placebo) (P = .001)[28] | Diarrhea (19.7%)[21] Diarrhea (19.5%)[27] Diarrhea (9.4%)[28] |
| Plecanatide | 2018 | Combined ≥30% reduction from baseline in worst abdominal pain + an increase of at least 1 CSBM/wk from baseline during the same week for ≥6/12 wk (FDA overall responder end point) | 26% (3 mg daily plecanatide) vs 16% (placebo) (P≤.009)[30] | Diarrhea (4.3%) |
| Tenapenor | 2019 | Combined ≥30% reduction from baseline in worst abdominal pain + an increase of at least 1 CSBM/wk from baseline during the same week for ≥6/12 wk (FDA overall responder end point) | 27% (50 mg BID tenapenor) vs 18.7% (placebo) (P = .02)[35] 36.5% (50 mg BID tenapenor) vs 23.7% (placebo) (P < .001)[36] | Diarrhea (14.66%)[35] Diarrhea (16.04%)[36] |

(continued on next page)

**Table 1**
*(continued)*

| Drug | Year of FDA Approval for IBS-C | Primary End Points Studied for IBS-C in Phase III Trials | Primary Outcome | Adverse Effects in Treatment Group |
|---|---|---|---|---|
| Tegaserod | 2002 in women, 2019 reapproved in women <65 y of age without a history of cardiovascular ischemic events | Subjective global assessment: Some relief 100% of the time or considerable or complete relief ≥ 50% of the time at the end of 1st and 3rd mo<br>≥ 30% reduction from baseline in worst abdominal pain + ≥50% increase in SBM frequency (≥1/ wk) for ≥6/12 wk | End of 1st mo: 34% (6 mg BID tegaserod) vs 21.3% (placebo) (P < .001)<br>End of 3rd mo: 44.1% (6 mg BID tegaserod) vs 36.5% (placebo) (P < .001)[40]<br>36% (6 mg BID tegaserod) vs 24.3% (placebo) (P < .001)[40] | Headache (14.2%), abdominal pain (12.3%), diarrhea (8.6%) |

*Abbreviation:* SBM, spontaneous bowel movement.

Although not a medication per se, dietary fiber has proven somewhat effective for treating constipation-related symptoms. Specifically, fibers found in such foods as oat bran, kiwifruit, prunes, mangos, and ficus carica, and the supplement psyllium, can increase stool bulk, decrease colonic transit time, and may have prebiotic effects.[13,14] A 2018 American College of Gastroenterology systematic review concluded that soluble fiber provides overall symptom relief in IBS and the recently published American College of Gastroenterology Clinical Guideline on the management of IBS also suggested the use of soluble, viscous, poorly fermentable fibers (psyllium) as first-line agents for IBS-C.[11,15]

PEG is an osmotic laxative that increases intraluminal water content and is FDA-approved for treating occasional constipation. Two RCTs assessing PEG in IBS-C were small (combined n = 181), heterogeneous, and associated with high risks of bias.[16,17] Neither study evaluated a global symptom end point as its primary outcome. Although data from the larger of the two studies revealed that PEG increased spontaneous bowel movement (SBM) frequency and improved stool texture, it did not improve abdominal pain or bloating.[17] In fact, PEG has the potential to worsen bloating and abdominal discomfort in patients with IBS-C.[18] Based on the current evidence, the American College of Gastroenterology and the Canadian Association of Gastroenterology suggest against using PEG to treat global IBS symptoms. The American Gastroenterological Association and the Mexican Association of Gastroenterology continue to recommend its use; however, the American Gastroenterological Association guideline was last updated in 2014 before FDA approval of many the secretagogue and prokinetic agents (**Table 2**).[19,20]

## SECRETAGOGUES
### Lubiprostone

Lubiprostone was the first secretagogue approved by the FDA (8 µg twice daily) for the treatment of IBS-C in women greater than or equal to 18 years of age. Lubiprostone is a locally acting prostaglandin $E_1$ derivative that activates type 2 chloride channels on intestinal epithelial cells resulting in increased intestinal fluid secretion and peristalsis.[21] Animal studies have further suggested that lubiprostone improves visceral hyperalgesia via restoration of the intestinal epithelial barrier and reductions in intestinal permeability, but the precise mechanism of its analgesic effects remains unknown.[22–24]

The most robust data supporting the use of lubiprostone for patients with IBS-C comes from two large phase III studies.[25] In aggregate, 1171 patients who met Rome II criteria for IBS-C were randomized to receive lubiprostone (n = 783), 8 µg, or placebo (n = 388) twice daily for 12 weeks. The primary end point was a predecessor to the current FDA-recommended end point for IBS-C studies. Specifically, to be considered a responder, patients had to endorse either significant or moderate relief of their IBS symptoms for 2/4 or 4/4 weeks of a month, respectively, and maintain this response through at least 2 months of the 3-month study. Furthermore, responders could at no time endorse more than mild worsening of symptoms, discontinue treatment because of a lack of efficacy, or increase consumption of rescue laxatives beyond the amount received at baseline. Overall, a significantly higher percentage of patients consuming lubiprostone met this rigorous primary end point (17.9%) compared with placebo (10.1%) ($P = .001$). There was a delay, however, in achieving this significance until the second (Study 0431; $P = .016$) and third months (Study 0432; $P = .026$) of the individual studies. Lubiprostone also significantly improved multiple secondary outcomes including abdominal pain/discomfort, bloating, stool frequency,

**Table 2**
Comparison of guidelines for the treatment of IBS-C from North American gastrointestinal societies

| | American College of Gastroenterology (2020) | American Gastroenterological Association (2014) | Asociación Mexicana de Gastroenterología (2016) | Canadian Association of Gastroenterology (2019) |
|---|---|---|---|---|
| Polyethylene glycol | Conditional recommendation against use, low-quality evidence | Conditional recommendation for use, low-quality evidence | Strong recommendation for use, moderate-quality evidence | Conditional recommendation against use, very low-quality evidence |
| Lubiprostone | Strong recommendation for use, moderate-quality evidence | Conditional recommendation for use, moderate-quality evidence | Strong recommendation for use, moderate-quality evidence (not available in Mexico for IBS-C) | Conditional recommendation for use, moderate-quality evidence |
| Linaclotide | Strong recommendation for use, high-quality evidence | Strong recommendation for use, high-quality evidence | Strong recommendation for use, high-quality evidence | Strong recommendation for use, high-quality evidence |
| Plecanatide | Strong recommendation for use, strong-quality evidence | NA | NA | NA |
| Tenapenor | NA | NA | NA | NA |
| Tegaserod | Strong/conditional recommendation for use, low-quality evidence (for women <65 y and <1 cardiovascular risk factor who have not responded to secretagogues) | NA | NA | NA |

and constipation severity compared with placebo ($P < .001$ for all secondary outcomes). There was a trend toward improvement in overall quality of life (Irritable Bowel Syndrome-Quality of Life; $P = .066$) with significant improvements identified in the subcategories of "body image" and "health worry" by Week 12 ($P \leq .025$). The most common treatment-emergent adverse event (TEAE) reported by patients in the lubiprostone cohort was nausea (8% vs 4% placebo) and serious adverse events were rare. Because more than 90% of the subjects in the pivotal studies were female, FDA approval was only granted for females greater than or equal to 18 years of age.

A subsequent 36-week open-label extension study validated the durability of response and safety profile of lubiprostone.[26] Using the same primary responder definition, response rates to lubiprostone were maintained or increased over time to a maximum 37% to 44% after 10 to 13 months. The significant improvements in secondary end points were also maintained. Lubiprostone remained safe and tolerable with diarrhea (11%) and nausea (11%) most commonly leading to cessation of therapy. No serious adverse events were reported during this extension period.

For purposes of comparisons with other secretagogues, a post hoc analysis was more recently completed, defining "responders" as those experiencing an average weekly pain reduction of greater than or equal to 30% and an increase of at least one SBM per week compared with baseline for greater than or equal to 6 of 12 treatment weeks.[27] This end point is slightly less rigorous than the current FDA-recommended CSBM end point because the latter also accounts for the sensation of incomplete evacuation. However, when the lubiprostone data were collected more than a decade ago, CSBM responses were not recorded. Of the 505 participants included in this analysis (n = 325 lubiprostone, n = 180 placebo), a significantly greater percentage of individuals receiving lubiprostone met the composite end point compared with placebo (26.3% vs 15.3%, respectively; $P = .008$). There were also significant improvements in abdominal pain (36.7% vs 25.5%; $P = .005$) and bloating (32.0% vs 20.4%; $P = .012$), but changes in stool features were not reported.

In a recent high-quality systematic review/meta-analysis, lubiprostone proved more effective than placebo for global IBS-C symptom relief with a number needed to treat (NNT) of 12.5 and relative risk of symptom persistence of 0.91 (95% confidence interval [CI], 0.87–0.95).[12] Rates of treatment-emergent nausea have also been analyzed with a significantly greater number of events reported by individuals receiving twice-daily lubiprostone compared with placebo (10.9% vs 6.4%, respectively; $P<.01$). Rates of nausea may be higher when patients do not take lubiprostone with food. Discontinuation because of nausea, however, was similar between groups.[28] Overall, there is current consensus across North American societal guidelines that lubiprostone, 8 µg twice daily, is effective for relieving global IBS-C symptoms (see **Table 2**).

### Guanylate Cyclase-C Receptor Agonists

Guanylate cyclase-C receptor agonists represent a second class of secretagogues that are FDA-approved to treat patients with IBS-C. There are currently two therapeutics in this class (linaclotide and plecanatide), and both have similar mechanisms of action. These small peptides target cuanylate cyclase-C receptors found on the brush border membranes of intestinal epithelial cells. Activation of these receptors leads to downstream production of a secondary mediator, cGMP, which functions intracellularly to induce fluid secretion and accelerate intestinal transit and extracellularly (based on animal model data) to reduce the activity of visceral nociceptive neurons.[29,30] Whereas linaclotide is a pH-independent molecule and functions nonpreferentially in the small intestine and colon, plecanatide is a pH-dependent uroguanylin analogue that exerts its primary effects in the acidic environment of the small intestine.

Three North American phase IIb[31] and phase III trials[26,32] and one multinational study (North America, Oceania, China)[33] have substantiated the efficacy of a once-daily 290-$\mu$g dose of linaclotide for treating IBS-C. In each of these trials, linaclotide proved superior to placebo for an array of abdominal and bowel symptoms. The most robust data were captured in two parallel North American phase III randomized, double-blind, placebo-controlled studies.[26,32] In these trials, overall responders were defined using the current FDA guidance end point for IBS-C. Specifically, participants were considered weekly responders if they experienced a greater than or equal to 30% reduction in abdominal pain and an increase of greater than or equal to one CSBM during the same week and an overall responder if the weekly response was met for at least 50% of treatment weeks. In the first study, 33.6% of linaclotide-treated patients (n = 405) achieved this response compared with 21% of the 395 patients receiving placebo ($P<.0001$).[32] Patients who completed all 12 weeks were subsequently eligible to enter a 4-week double-blind randomized withdrawal period. The efficacy of linaclotide was further supported because those remaining on linaclotide (n = 158) maintained their initial response, whereas those rerandomized from placebo to linaclotide (n = 335) experienced improvements in abdominal pain and CSBMs, and those rerandomized from linaclotide to placebo (n = 154) experienced recurrence of their symptoms without evidence of rebound. The results of the second study were comparable, with 33.7% of 402 linaclotide-treated patients achieving the FDA responder end point compared with 13.9% of 403 placebo patients receiving placebo ($P<.0001$).[26] In contrast to the first study, patients in this trial were enrolled a priori to continue double-blinded treatment for 26 weeks and there was no evidence of a decay in response over time. Significant improvements were also noted across a spectrum of predefined secondary abdominal (pain, bloating, discomfort, fullness, cramping) and stool (SBMs, CSBMs, straining, and stool consistency) symptoms and an adequate relief assessment, across both studies. Importantly, these changes were maintained throughout the initial 12-week double-blinded periods in both studies and 26 weeks in the second trial.

The benefits of plecanatide have been established in three high-quality phase IIb/III studies.[34,35] In two identical phase III trials, 2189 individuals were randomized to receive placebo (n = 733), 3-mg plecanatide (n = 728), or 6-mg plecanatide (n = 728) once daily for 12 weeks.[35] Given that 3 mg once daily is the FDA-approved dose, the subsequent data focus on those results. The primary end point in these studies was identical to the FDA responder end point used in the linaclotide trials and was met by 26% of patients receiving 3 mg of plecanatide compared with 16% receiving placebo ($P\leq.009$). Furthermore, a sustained efficacy responder end point not assessed in any previous IBS-C therapeutic trials was established a priori. To be considered a sustained responder, individuals had to qualify as overall responders plus experience improvement in the weekly responder end point during greater than or equal to 2 of the last 4 weeks of the trial. Overall, 24.5% and 15.5% of plecanatide- and placebo-treated patients, respectively, were considered sustained responders ($P < .015$). Similar to linaclotide, significant improvements were recognized for multiple abdominal (pain, bloating cramping, discomfort, fullness) and bowel (CSBMs, SBMs, stool consistency, straining) symptoms with significance compared with placebo achieved during weeks 1 to 2 for all end points and maintained through all subsequent weeks of both trials.

Multiple systematic reviews/meta-analysis have attempted to differentiate the efficacy, safety, and tolerability of these two therapeutics. Compared with placebo, use of linaclotide, 290 $\mu$g, yielded a relative risk of failure to respond to therapy of 0.80 (95% CI, 0.76–0.85; NNT = 6)[15,36] and an odds ratio (OR) of response of 2.43

(95% CI, 1.48–3.98; NNT = 6)[37] based on the current FDA composite responder end point. Similarly, plecanatide, 3 mg, had a likelihood of symptom persistence of 0.88 (95% CI, 0.84–0.92; NNT = 10) and an OR of response to treatment of 1.87 (95% CI, 1.47–2.38; NNT = 9).[32,34] Diarrhea was the most common TEAE experienced by patients across the phase III studies. Diarrhea occurred in 20% of individuals receiving 290 μg of linaclotide per day in comparison with 4.3% of those taking 3 mg of plecanatide. There were increased odds of diarrhea with use of either product compared with placebo (linaclotide, 290 μg: OR, 8.02 [95% CI, 5.20–12.37]; plecanatide, 3 mg: OR, 5.55 [95% CI, 1.62–19.00]); however, no significant differences in the rates of diarrhea or withdrawal because of diarrhea have been identified between these two agents.[34] As such, both seem comparably safe, well tolerated, and received strong recommendations for use across US gastrointestinal society guidelines.[11,15,19]

## *Tenapanor*

Tenapanor is a first-in-class sodium-hydrogen ion exchanger-3 receptor inhibitor that reduces sodium absorption from the small intestine and colon secondarily increasing water secretion and decreasing intestinal transit time. In preclinical studies, tenapanor seemed to mediate visceral hypersensitivity via inhibition of TRPV1 receptors. This presumed mechanism requires further validation.[38] Although actively approved for IBS-C it has yet to become commercially available, and clinical trials are ongoing to determine its effect in phosphate management in patients with chronic kidney disease on hemodialysis.

Tenapenor was recently assessed for use in IBS-C in two large phase III studies: T3MPO-1 and T3MPO-2. In both, individuals were randomized to receive 50 mg of tenapanor twice daily or placebo. Similar to the linaclotide trials, patients completing the initial 12-week portion of T3MPO-1 were subsequently transitioned into a 4-week randomized withdrawal period, whereas those enrolled in T3MPO-2 continued to receive blinded therapy for 26 weeks. The primary end point was identical to the FDA end point used in the previous secretagogue studies. In T3MPO-1, 27.0% of those receiving tenapenor (n = 307) achieved this end point compared with 18.7% of those receiving placebo (n = 299) (P = .020).[39] These results were echoed in T3MPO-2 (tenapenor n = 293 [36.5%] vs placebo n = 300 [23.7%]; P < .001), with persistence noted at 26 weeks.[40] Durable responder analyses were also reported in both studies with significant improvements favoring tenapanor for individuals meeting the FDA composite weekly end point for greater than or equal to 9 out of 12 weeks plus greater than or equal to 3 of the last 4 weeks of treatment (P < .001). During the 4-week randomized withdrawal period of T3MPO-1, expected improvements, reductions, and maintenance of responses were witnessed in the placebo to tenapenor, tenapenor to placebo, and continuation of tenapenor cohorts, respectively. With the exception of straining, significant improvements were achieved in abdominal (pain, discomfort, bloating, cramping, fullness) and bowel symptoms (SBMs, CSBMs, stool consistency) across 12 weeks in T3MPO-1 and 26 weeks in T3MPO-2. Similar to other agents in this class, diarrhea was the most commonly reported adverse event, occurring in 14.6% of tenapanor and 1.7% of placebo-treated patients in T3MPO-1, and 16% and 3.7% of patents in T3MPO-2. One case of diarrhea in T3MPO-2 was defined as serious and believed to be "possibly related" to treatment. T3MPO-3, a single-arm, long-term safety study (52 weeks) comprised of patients from T3MPO-1 and T3MPO-2, validated the initial safety findings with only 2.1% of patients discontinuing therapy for any reason.[41,42]

## PROKINETICS
### Tegaserod

Tegaserod is the first and only prokinetic agent currently FDA approved for treating IBS-C, specifically women less than 65 years of age with no prior history of cardiovascular ischemic events (angina, myocardial infarction, transient ischemic attack, stroke). It is also the only IBS-C-approved therapeutic with demonstrated symptom improvement in an RCT enrolling individuals with IBS mixed subtype, although it is not approved for this indication.[43]

Prucalopride, a second prokinetic agent, has also been approved, but for the treatment of chronic idiopathic constipation rather than IBS-C.[44] To date, there have been no clinical trials evaluating its efficacy in IBS-C. Tegaserod is a serotonin subtype-4 (5-$HT_4$) specific agonist that exerts its effects in the enteric nervous system. Activation of 5-$HT_4$ receptors on neurons in the submucosal and myenteric plexuses directly stimulates secretion and propulsion, and animal studies have suggested that activation of the afferent submucosal neurons may reduce visceral sensitivity. Thus, tegaserod exerts prosecretory and prokinetic effects.

Tegaserod was initially approved in 2002 for treating women with IBS-C but was voluntarily withdrawn from the market in 2007 after it was associated with a small but statistically significant increase in cardiovascular events. It was reapproved in early 2019 at a dose of 6 mg twice daily after two independent adjudications of 29 clinical trials determined that it was safe for use in the currently restricted population.[45]

The initial phase III studies were completed almost two decades ago and based on FDA guidance at that time, the primary end point was a subjective global assessment whereby individuals were considered responders if they rated themselves "considerably" or "completely" relieved greater than or equal to 50% or "somewhat relieved" 100% of the time during the first and last months of the 12-week studies. The results were recently updated post hoc using the same primary outcomes adapted in accordance with the current FDA-approved population.[46] In pooled analyses of four studies, 1386 women less than 65 years of age with no history of cardiovascular ischemic events who received 6 mg of tegaserod twice daily were more likely to experience significant global improvements in symptoms compared with 1366 women who received placebo during both the first 4 weeks and last month of the trials (pooled OR, 1.95 [$P < .001$]; pooled OR, 1.38 [$P < .001$], respectively). In an attempt to draw comparisons with other IBS-C therapies using the current FDA guidance end point, the same data were also reanalyzed using a composite of abdominal pain and stool frequency. Responders were defined as those experiencing a greater than or equal to 30% reduction in weekly abdominal pain intensity and a greater than or equal to 50% increase in stool frequency ($\geq 1$/wk) for greater than or equal to 6 of 12 weeks of treatment, and 36.0% of tegaserod-treated patients attained this response in contrast to 24.3% of those receiving placebo ($P < .001$).[45,46]

Given concerns regarding the cardiovascular safety of tegaserod, a pooled safety analysis of 2749 individuals from the aforementioned four trials was also completed.[45] The most common TEAE was headaches occurring in 14.2% of patients receiving 6 mg of tegaserod twice daily compared with 12.1% of control subjects. Importantly, only one (0.1%) patient in the tegaserod cohort experienced a cardiovascular ischemic event TEAE. This patient had preexisting severe three-vessel coronary artery disease and the investigator involved did not believe this event was related to tegaserod. More detailed analyses have further validated the safety of tegaserod. In a population of 9547 tegaserod-treated women less than or equal to 65 years without a history of cardiovascular ischemic disease, the rates of major adverse cardiovascular

**Table 3**
**Prescribing considerations for IBS-C agents**

| Drug | FDA-Approved Dose for IBS-C | When to Consume |
|------|------------------------------|-----------------|
| Lubiprostone | 8 μg BID | With food and water |
| Linaclotide | 290 μg daily | On empty stomach at least 30 min before first meal of day |
| Plecanatide | 3 mg daily | Any time of day with or without food |
| Tenapenor | 50 mg BID | Immediately before breakfast and dinner |
| Tegaserod | 6 mg BID | At least 30 min before breakfast and dinner |

events ranged from 0.1% to 0.3%. In an even more limited population comprised of 7785 of the 9547 women meeting the previous criteria who also had less than or equal to one cardiovascular risk factor (age $\geq$ 55, active tobacco use, body mass index greater than 30 kg/m$^2$, diabetes mellitus, current hypertension/hyperlipidemia or history of antihypertensive/hyperlipidemic use) the rate of major adverse cardiovascular events approached 0.01%.[47,48]

Tegaserod is currently being marketed as a second-line agent for IBS-C. That said, a high percentage of patients with IBS-C still qualify to use it because a recent US population-based survey revealed that 91% of patients with IBS-C are less than 65 years of age and more than two-thirds are female.[5] Importantly, tegaserod works differently than the secretagogues, affording potential benefits via an alternative mechanism of action for refractory patients.

*Comparison of Therapies*

Despite the proven efficacy of the agents previously discussed, a paucity of comparative effectiveness trials limits the ability to derive stepwise treatment algorithms. Until such time as these studies are completed, we rely on meta-analyses and clinical guidelines to assist in directing treatment decisions. In a recent meta-analysis of 18 RCTs comparing lubiprostone, linaclotide, plecanatide, tenapanor, and tegaserod with placebo using the current FDA guidance end point, linaclotide, 290 μg once daily, was deemed to be the most effective.[49] However, all of the therapeutics seemed more effective than placebo and no single agent was clearly superior to the others. These findings must still be interpreted with caution because the primary end point in this analysis was consistent with primary end points of the linaclotide, plecanatide, and tenapenor studies but required retrofitting of the data for lubiprostone and tegaserod. Furthermore, the response estimate for tegaserod may have been overestimated because the surrogate end point used in this study, SBM, not CSBMs, is less robust.

The American College of Gastroenterology (2020),[11] American Gastroenterological Association[19] (currently undergoing updating with presumed publication in 2021), Canadian Association of Gastroenterology (2019),[12] and Mexican Association of Gastroenterology (2016)[20] guideline committees have all provided guidance on products available in their respective countries. Overall, there do not seem to be major differences in recommendations (see **Table 2**). Until better comparisons are made, real-world prescribing habits will likely continue to be influenced by prescribing and dosing considerations (**Table 3**), anecdotal success, cost, and third-party payer coverage.

**SUMMARY**

IBS-C is a common condition that causes significant distress and impairs quality of life. The Rome IV criteria outlined in 2016 provide a more consistent and specific definition of IBS-C, and trials for IBS-C therapeutics have largely adopted the FDA standardized definition of "responder." OTC laxatives are often used as first-line agents, but they are falling out of favor given their inability to improve abdominal symptoms. Lubiprostone, linaclotide, plecanatide, tenapenor, and tegaserod seem effective for treating abdominal and bowel symptoms. Although gastroenterology societal guidelines (see **Table 2**) provide valuable assessments as to the strength of evidence supporting recommendations, they are of limited utility given the lack of variability separating these products. The choice of appropriate medication depends on patient goals, tolerability of adverse effects, cost, and insurance coverage.

## CLINICS CARE POINTS

- Multiple international society guidelines have recommended against PEG as a first-line option for IBS-C, because it does not reduce global IBS symptoms.
- The secretagogues (lubiprostone, linaclotide, plecanatide) are all effective compared with placebo and side effects are generally mild, the two most common of which are nausea (lubiprostone) and diarrhea (linaclotide, plecanatide).
- Tegaserod has been reapproved for treating women with IBS-C less than 65 years with no history of cardiovascular ischemic events.
- There are no head-to-head trials directly comparing IBS-C therapies, but systematic reviews and meta-analyses suggest that all FDA-approved agents are effective.

## DISCLOSURE

J.J. Liu does not have any disclosures to report. D.M. Brenner has served as an advisor, consultant, or speaker for the following: Allergan (AbbVie), Ironwood, Salix, Takeda, Alphasigma, Arena, and Alynlam Pharmaceuticals. He is also supported in research by an unrestricted gift from the Irene D. Pritzker Foundation.

## REFERENCES

1. Lacy BE, Mearin F, Chang L, et al. Bowel disorders. Gastroenterology 2016; 150(6):1393–407.e5.
2. Palsson OS, Whitehead W, Törnblom H, et al. Prevalence of Rome IV functional bowel disorders among adults in the United States, Canada, and the United Kingdom. Gastroenterology 2020;158(5):1262–73.e3.
3. Ford AC. Commentary: estimating the prevalence of IBS globally—past, present and future. Aliment Pharmacol Ther 2020;51(1):198–9.
4. Shin A, Lembo A. IBS in America. American Gastroenterological Association; 2015. p. 45. Available at: https://www.multivu.com/players/English/7634451-aga-ibs-in-america-survey/. Accessed December 10, 2020.
5. Heidelbaugh JJ, Stelwagon M, Miller SA, et al. The spectrum of constipation-predominant irritable bowel syndrome and chronic idiopathic constipation: US survey assessing symptoms, care seeking, and disease burden. Am J Gastroenterol 2015;110(4):580–7.
6. Cash BD. Understanding and managing IBS and CIC in the primary care setting. Gastroenterol Hepatol 2018;14(5 Suppl 3):3–15.
7. Miller LE. Study design considerations for irritable bowel syndrome clinical trials. Ann Gastroenterol Q Publ Hell Soc Gastroenterol 2014;27(4):338–45.

8. U.S. Department of Health and Human Services Food and Drug Administration. Guidance for industry irritable bowel syndrome—clinical evaluation of drugs for treatment 2012. p. 1–14. Available at: www.fda.gov.

9. Lacy BE, Lembo AJ, MacDougall JE, et al. Responders vs clinical response: a critical analysis of data from linaclotide phase 3 clinical trials in IBS-C. Neurogastroenterol Motil 2014;26(3):326–33.

10. Macdougall JE, Johnston JM, Lavins BJ, et al. An evaluation of the FDA responder endpoint for IBS-C clinical trials: analysis of data from linaclotide phase 3 clinical trials. Neurogastroenterol Motil 2013;25(6):481–6.

11. Lacy B, Pimentel M, Brenner D, et al. ACG clinical guideline: management of irritable bowel syndrome. Am J Gastroenterol 2020;116(1):17–44. Available at: https://journals.lww.com/ajg/Fulltext/9000/00000/acg_clinical_guideline__management_of_irritable.98972.aspx. Accessed December 15, 2020.

12. Moayyedi P, Andrews CN, MacQueen G, et al. Canadian Association of Gastroenterology clinical practice guideline for the management of irritable bowel syndrome (IBS). J Can Assoc Gastroenterol 2019;2(1):6–29.

13. Chang C-C, Lin Y-T, Lu Y-T, et al. Kiwifruit improves bowel function in patients with irritable bowel syndrome with constipation. Asia Pac J Clin Nutr 2010;19(4):451–7.

14. Muir J. An overview of fiber and fiber supplements for irritable bowel syndrome. Gastroenterol Hepatol 2019;15(7):387–9.

15. Ford AC, Moayyedi P, Chey WD, et al. American College of Gastroenterology monograph on management of irritable bowel syndrome. Am J Gastroenterol 2018;113(Suppl 2):1–18.

16. Awad RA, Camacho S. A randomized, double-blind, placebo-controlled trial of polyethylene glycol effects on fasting and postprandial rectal sensitivity and symptoms in hypersensitive constipation-predominant irritable bowel syndrome. Colorectal Dis 2010;12(11):1131–8.

17. Chapman RW, Stanghellini V, Geraint M, et al. Randomized clinical trial: macrogol/PEG 3350 plus electrolytes for treatment of patients with constipation associated with irritable bowel syndrome. Am J Gastroenterol 2013;108(9):1508–15.

18. Bharucha AE, Pemberton JH, Locke GR. American Gastroenterological Association Technical Review on Constipation. Gastroenterology 2013;144(1):218–38.

19. Weinberg DS, Smalley W, Heidelbaugh JJ, et al. American Gastroenterological Association Institute guideline on the pharmacological management of irritable bowel syndrome. Gastroenterology 2014;147(5):1146–8.

20. Carmona-Sánchez R, Icaza-Chávez ME, Bielsa-Fernández MV, et al. The Mexican consensus on irritable bowel syndrome. Rev Gastroenterol Mex 2016;81(3):149–67.

21. Cuppoletti J, Malinowska DH, Tewari KP, et al. SPI-0211 activates T84 cell chloride transport and recombinant human ClC-2 chloride currents. Am J Physiol Cell Physiol 2004;287(5):C1173–83.

22. Moeser AJ, Nighot PK, Engelke KJ, et al. Recovery of mucosal barrier function in ischemic porcine ileum and colon is stimulated by a novel agonist of the ClC-2 chloride channel, lubiprostone. Am J Physiol Gastrointest Liver Physiol 2007;292(2):G647–56.

23. Creekmore AL, Hong S, Zhu S, et al. Chronic stress-associated visceral hyperalgesia correlates with severity of intestinal barrier dysfunction. Pain 2018;159(9):1777–89.

24. Sweetser S, Busciglio IA, Camilleri M, et al. Effect of a chloride channel activator, lubiprostone, on colonic sensory and motor functions in healthy subjects. Am J Physiol - Gastrointest Liver Physiol 2009;296(2):G295–301.

25. Drossman DA, Chey WD, Johanson JF, et al. Clinical trial: lubiprostone in patients with constipation-associated irritable bowel syndrome: results of two randomized, placebo-controlled studies. Aliment Pharmacol Ther 2009;29(3):329–41.

26. Chey WD, Lembo AJ, Lavins BJ, et al. Linaclotide for irritable bowel syndrome with constipation: a 26-week, randomized, double-blind, placebo-controlled trial to evaluate efficacy and safety. Am J Gastroenterol 2012;107(11):1702–12.

27. Chang L, Chey WD, Drossman D, et al. Effects of baseline abdominal pain and bloating on response to lubiprostone in patients with irritable bowel syndrome with constipation. Aliment Pharmacol Ther 2016;44(10):1114–22.

28. Cryer B, Drossman DA, Chey WD, et al. Analysis of nausea in clinical studies of lubiprostone for the treatment of constipation disorders. Dig Dis Sci 2017;62(12): 3568–78.

29. Currie MG, Fok KF, Kato J, et al. Guanylin: an endogenous activator of intestinal guanylate cyclase. Proc Natl Acad Sci U S A 1992;89(3):947–51.

30. Forte LR. Uroguanylin and guanylin peptides: pharmacology and experimental therapeutics. Pharmacol Ther 2004;104(2):137–62.

31. Johnston JM, Kurtz CB, Macdougall JE, et al. Linaclotide improves abdominal pain and bowel habits in a phase IIb study of patients with irritable bowel syndrome with constipation. Gastroenterology 2010;139(6):1877–86.e2.

32. Rao S, Lembo AJ, Shiff SJ, et al. A 12-week, randomized, controlled trial with a 4-week randomized withdrawal period to evaluate the efficacy and safety of linaclotide in irritable bowel syndrome with constipation. Am J Gastroenterol 2012; 107(11):1714–24 [quiz p.1725].

33. Yang Y, Fang J, Guo X, et al. Linaclotide in irritable bowel syndrome with constipation: a phase 3 randomized trial in China and other regions. J Gastroenterol Hepatol 2018;33(5):980–9.

34. Miner P, DeLuca R, La Portilla M, et al. Plecanatide, a novel uroguanylin analog: a 12-week, randomized, double-blind, placebo-controlled, dose-ranging trial to evaluate efficacy and safety in patients with irritable bowel syndrome with constipation (IBS-C): 1831. Off J Am Coll Gastroenterol ACG 2014;109:S541.

35. Brenner DM, Fogel R, Dorn SD, et al. Efficacy, safety, and tolerability of plecanatide in patients with irritable bowel syndrome with constipation: results of two phase 3 randomized clinical trials. Am J Gastroenterol 2018;113(5):735–45.

36. Atluri DK, Chandar AK, Bharucha AE, et al. Effect of linaclotide in irritable bowel syndrome with constipation (IBS-C): a systematic review and meta-analysis. Neurogastroenterol Motil 2014;26(4):499–509.

37. Shah ED, Kim HM, Schoenfeld P. Efficacy and tolerability of guanylate cyclase-C agonists for irritable bowel syndrome with constipation and chronic idiopathic constipation: a systematic review and meta-analysis. Am J Gastroenterol 2018; 113(3):329–38.

38. Li Q, King AJ, Liu L, et al. Tenapanor reduces IBS pain through inhibition of TRPV1-dependent neuronal hyperexcitability in vivo: 484. Off J Am Coll Gastroenterol ACG 2017;112:S255.

39. Chey WD, Lembo AJ, Rosenbaum DP. Efficacy of Tenapanor in treating patients with irritable bowel syndrome with constipation: a 12-week, placebo-controlled phase 3 trial (T3MPO-1). Am J Gastroenterol 2020;115(2):281–93.

40. Chey WD, Lembo AJ, Yang Y, et al. Efficacy of tenapanor in treating patients with irritable bowel syndrome with constipation: a 26-week, placebo-controlled phase 3 trial (T3MPO-2). Am J Gastroenterol 2020;115(2):281–93.

41. Lembo A, Chey WD, Rosenbaum DP. An open label long-term safety trial (T3MPO-3) of tenapanor in patients with irritable bowel syndrome with constipation (IBS-C): presidential poster award: 430. Off J Am Coll Gastroenterol ACG 2018;113:S252.

42. Markham A. Tenapanor: first approval. Drugs 2019;79(17):1897–903.

43. Chey WD, Paré P, Viegas A, et al. Tegaserod for female patients suffering from IBS with mixed bowel habits or constipation: a randomized controlled trial. Am J Gastroenterol 2008;103(5):1217–25.

44. Shire US Inc. Motegrity (Prucalopride). U.S. Food and Drug Administration Website. 2018. Available at: https://www.accessdata.fda.gov/drugsatfda_docs/label/2018/210166s000lbl.pdf. Accessed January 19, 2021.

45. Shah ED, Lacy BE, Chey WD, et al. S0495 The safety profile of tegaserod 6 Mg BID in irritable bowel syndrome with constipation in women <65 years of age without cardiovascular disease history. Off J Am Coll Gastroenterol ACG 2020; 115:S247.

46. Shah ED, Lacy BE, Chey WD, et al. S0492 Tegaserod 6 Mg BID for treating abdominal pain and bloating in women with irritable bowel syndrome with constipation but without cardiovascular risk factors: a pooled analysis of 4 clinical trials. Off J Am Coll Gastroenterol ACG 2020;115:S246.

47. NDA/BLA Multi-Disciplinary review and evaluation: Zelnorm (tegaserod). FDA; 2019. Available at: https://www.accessdata.fda.gov/drugsatfda_docs/nda/2019/021200Orig1s015MultidisciplineR.pdf. Accessed December 10, 2020.

48. Zelnorm (tegaserod) [package insert]. Covington, LA: Alfasigma USA, Inc; 2019. Available at: https://www.accessdata.fda.gov/drugsatfda_docs/label/2019/021200Orig1s015lbl.pdf.

49. Black CJ, Burr NE, Ford AC. Relative efficacy of tegaserod in a systematic review and network meta-analysis of licensed therapies for irritable bowel syndrome with constipation. Clin Gastroenterol Hepatol 2020;18(5):1238–9.e1.

# Psychopharmacologic Therapies for Irritable Bowel Syndrome

Hans Törnblom, MD, PhD[a],*, Douglas A. Drossman, MD[b,c]

## KEYWORDS

- Irritable bowel syndrome • Disorders of gut brain interaction
- Multidimensional clinical profile • Treatment • Antidepressants • Neuromodulator

## KEY POINTS

- Psychopharmacologic therapies are justified based on their capability to reregulate a disordered neurologic communication pattern that involves disorders of gut-brain interaction (DGBI), including irritable bowel syndrome (IBS).
- Serotonin and noradrenalin activation are key mechanisms to modulate chronic abdominal pain in IBS.
- Psychopharmacologic therapies used to treat DGBIs are better labeled as central neuromodulators, as they are scientifically based and reduce stigma.
- Tricyclic antidepressants are supported by the greatest weight of evidence for improving IBS symptoms among the central neuromodulators. Other classes like serotonin-norepinephrine reuptake inhibitors show empiric value in treating chronic pain and appear to have fewer side effects but require further study in IBS.
- Augmentation therapy, that is, combining 2 or more neuromodulators, or other treatments, is useful when monotherapy is unsuccessful, is partially successful, or produces side effects. It is helpful in IBS with multiple somatic and psychological symptoms.

## INTRODUCTION

Irritable bowel syndrome (IBS)[1] is the most well-known disorder of gut-brain interaction (DGBI),[2] formerly known as functional gastrointestinal (GI) disorders, and as such, the most described in terms of pathophysiologic mechanisms. The symptoms relate to dysregulation of the gut-brain axis involving multiple central and peripheral mechanisms associated with visceral and central hypersensitivity; altered microbiota, gut motility disturbance, and altered gut-brain signaling. The human ability to adapt and

[a] Department of Molecular and Clinical Medicine, Institute of Medicine, Sahlgrenska Academy, University of Gothenburg, Gothenburg SE-41345, Sweden; [b] Drossman Center for the Education and Practice of Biopsychosocial Care, UNC Center for Functional GI and Motility Disorders, University of North Carolina at Chapel Hill, Chapel Hill, NC 27517, USA; [c] The Rome Foundation, Raleigh, NC, USA, and Drossman Gastroenterology, Durham NC, USA
* Corresponding author.
*E-mail address:* hans.tornblom@gu.se

Gastroenterol Clin N Am 50 (2021) 655–669
https://doi.org/10.1016/j.gtc.2021.04.005
0889-8553/21/© 2021 Elsevier Inc. All rights reserved.

learn from stress and other perturbations on this system is most often beneficial. Still, it sometimes becomes a burden when maladaptive neuromodulation, or even neural degeneration, occurs, and patients with these disorders may experience disabling symptoms and poor quality of life that persist over long periods of time.

This article uses 3 clinical cases to illustrate the role of gut-brain interaction mechanisms underlying common and uncommon IBS presentations and the rationale and evidence for using psychopharmacologic therapies to reduce symptoms. Consistent with the Rome Foundation's new definitional guidelines, the authors relabel agents working in both the brain and the gut as "gut-brain neuromodulators." This term includes the primarily central neuromodulators (eg, antidepressants, and antipsychotics) and the primarily peripheral neuromodulators. This new terminology is more scientifically based and avoids the stigma of being considered "psychiatric" when treating patients with these disorders. These medications act on central neurotransmitters: noradrenaline (NA), serotonin (5-HT), and to some extent dopamine, to affect pain regulation. The reader can review the recent Rome Foundation working team report[3] for a detailed review of these treatments' pharmacologic, clinical, and treatment aspects for IBS and other DGBIs. As a general rule of thumb, central neuromodulators are recommended when IBS-associated abdominal pain is moderate to severe or persistent. Also, it will often complement peripheral neuromodulators acting on the enteric nervous system, covered in other parts of this issue. The peripheral neuromodulators include the antispasmodics, the guanylate cyclase C receptor agonists linaclotide[4] and plecanatide,[5] the peripheral opioid receptor agonist/antagonist eluxadoline,[6] and the serotonin receptor (5-HT4) agonist prucalopride[7] and antagonists (5-HT3) alosetron,[8] ramosetron,[9] and ondansetron.[10] Their putative place in the treatment of IBS, either alone or in combination with central neuromodulators, can also be found elsewhere.[11]

## CENTRAL NEUROMODULATORS IN IRRITABLE BOWEL SYNDROME
### First-Line Treatment Options

When abdominal pain dominates in patients with DGBI, the *tricyclic antidepressants* *(TCA)* have the best evidence for efficacy.[12,13] They have a complex mode of action whereby 5-HT and NA reuptake inhibition help downregulate incoming visceral signals from the gut. Additional receptor antagonistic properties (5-HT2A and 2C, muscarinic 1, histamine 1) can be useful, for example, for sedation and to treat insomnia and increase transit time in IBS with diarrhea. It is also responsible for side effects, including dizziness, dry mouth and eyes, and constipation. Amitriptyline and imipramine (tertiary amines) more commonly produce side effects because of their greater antimuscarinic and antihistaminic actions than desipramine and nortriptyline (secondary amines). The recommended dose range is 25 to 100 mg/d (up to 150 mg/d), where the balance between treatment benefit and side effects helps determine the final dose.

The *serotonin noradrenaline reuptake inhibitors* *(SNRIs)* have empiric value for the treatment of abdominal pain in the context of a DGBI. Studies of neuropathic pain in diabetes, fibromyalgia, back pain, and headache justify this,[3] which is particularly useful when many of these symptoms coexist with IBS. SNRIs have fewer side effects than TCAs and are an alternative when patients cannot tolerate the TCAs' side effects. The serotonergic effect on gut transit and lack of antimuscarinic effects makes them an alternative when constipation or comorbid depression is part of the illness. Based on different noradrenergic properties, the SNRIs have individual optimal dose ranges to treat abdominal pain: duloxetine 30 to 90 mg/d, venlafaxine at least 225 mg/d. Milnacipran is indicated for fibromyalgia and widespread body pain, and although not marketed for depression in the United States, it is available for that in several countries worldwide. It is an alternative treatment option if other SNRIs are not helpful or produce side effects that are limiting. Nausea is the most common side effect that can be reduced if the medication is taken with food and attenuates after 1 to 2 weeks of treatment.

Finally, *selective serotonin reuptake inhibitors (SSRIs)* are alternative treatments when the core symptoms of IBS are driven by anxiety, depression, and obsessive or phobic features. They should be used within the same dose ranges as their psychiatric indications, and benefits are gauged mainly on global improvement reports. These agents are not helpful for abdominal pain in IBS.[3]

### Second-Line Treatment Options

*Atypical antipsychotics*, particularly olanzapine and quetiapine, are add-on treatment options to consider for refractory abdominal pain in IBS.[14] They are less prone to produce extrapyramidal side effects than the first-generation antipsychotics. *Quetiapine* has multiple receptor effects: D2, 5-HT2A, H1 receptor antagonism, partial 5-HT1A receptor antagonism, and affinity for $\alpha$1 and $\alpha$2 receptors. It is also an NA reuptake inhibitor mediated by one of its metabolites.[3] Quetiapine has effects on fibromyalgia-related pain,[15] and it has a sedative effect that can improve a disturbed sleep pattern in a patient with chronic pain. It is used in the low-dose range (25–200 mg/d) when treating DGBIs and can improve pain and global scores.[16] Among the atypical antipsychotics, *Olanzapine* has been most studied and provides the best evidence for improving chronic pain, particularly in fibromyalgia and headaches.[17] The olanzapine dose for this indication most often is 2.5 to 10 mg/d. There are potentially serious side effects when treating with atypical antipsychotics. There is a risk of initiating a metabolic syndrome, including weight gain and increased blood lipid and glucose levels. There is also risk of QT interval prolongation and *torsade des pointes* with the potential for sudden cardiac death. However, QT interval prolongation is rare and is related to high-dose regimens in the treatment of psychosis.[18] The doses used to treat GI symptoms are much lower than those used for psychiatric patients and involve younger patients with fewer comorbidities. There are guidelines recommending monitoring routines for early detection of these adverse effects. The *delta-ligand agents gabapentin and pregabalin* are peripheral neuromodulators that block the $\alpha 2\delta$ subunit of voltage-sensitive calcium channels on neurons. They have experimental evidence to reduce visceral hypersensitivity in IBS.[19] Also, pregabalin in a randomized trial using 225 mg twice a day for 12 weeks showed benefit in relieving abdominal pain, bloating, and diarrhea in IBS.[20] The delta-ligand agents also help comorbid fibromyalgia[21] or abdominal wall pain, which can further justify its use when also present in IBS patients.

*Low-dose naltrexone*, 4.5 mg/d, is a possible second-line treatment for chronic pain in geographic areas where this formulation is available. It can be extrapolated for IBS by having some evidence from treatment of pain in fibromyalgia, complex regional pain syndromes, and abdominal pain in Crohn disease. The analgesic effects do not appear to be mediated by its opioid-receptor antagonism, but rather by its anti-inflammatory and neuroprotective effects via microglial cells.[22]

In **Fig. 1**, the general use of central neuromodulators in the context of IBS is summarized and can be used as a guide for clinical treatment decisions. Dose ranges and common side effects for neuromodulators are summarized in **Table 1**.

### THE MULTIDIMENSIONAL CLINICAL PROFILE

The multidimensional clinical profile (MDCP)[23] provides case-based examples that help the clinician understand the full dimensionality of the patient's symptom

**Central neuromodulator treatment in IBS**

**SSRIs**

Anxiety, depression, phobic features prominent and pain is not dominant (paroxetine, fluoxetine, sertraline, citalopram, escitalopram)

**TCAs**

**First-line treatment** when pain predominates (amitriptyline, nortriptyline, trimipramine, imipramine, desipramine)

**SNRIs**

**First-line treatment** when pain predominates and/or when side effects from TCAs preclude treatment (duloxetine, venlafaxine, milnacipran)

**Augmentation**

When insufficient effect or dosage restricted by side effects

**Delta ligand agents** (gabapentin, pregabalin) Comorbid fibromyalgia, abdominal wall pain
**SSRIs** When anxiety and phobic features dominant

**Atypical antipsychotics**
Pain with disturbed sleep (olanzapine, quetiapine), anxiety, nausea (olanzapine, sulpiride), additional somatic symptoms ("side effects"), comorbid fibromyalgia
**Low-dose naltrexone**
Second-line treatment for poorly treated pain. Comorbid fibromyalgia

**Psychological Treatment**
**CBT** when maladaptive cognitions and catastrophizing present
**DBT, EMDR** with history of PTSD or trauma
**Hypnosis, Mindfulness, Relaxation** as alternative treatments

**Fig. 1.** The most common classes of medications used to modulate a disordered gut-brain interaction in patients with IBS. Central neuromodulators are most often used as monotherapy or in cases with insufficient treatment effects in combination. The combined clinical assessment according to a MDCP guide choice of medications. Nonpharmacologic treatment options should also be considered (not covered in this article) as augmentation where this could be given also as an adjunct to central neuromodulators. DBT, dialectical behavior therapy; EMDR, eye movement desensitization and reprocessing; PTSD, posttraumatic stress disorder. (Data from Drossman, D.A., et al., Neuromodulators for Functional Gastrointestinal Disorders (Disorders of Gut-Brain Interaction): A Rome Foundation Working Team Report. Gastroenterology, 2018. 154(4): p. 1140-1171).

**Table 1**
**Dose range and common side effects among the major classes of neuromodulators used in the treatment of abdominal pain in irritable bowel syndrome**

| First-Line Treatment | TCA | SSRI | SNRI |
|---|---|---|---|
| Daily dose | 25–100 (−150) mg | Regular psychiatric dose range | Duloxetine 30–90 mg Venlafaxine 225 mg Milnacipran 100 mg |
| Side effects | Sedation, constipation, hypotension, dry mouth, arrhythmias, weight gain, sexual dysfunction | Agitation, diarrhea, insomnia, night sweats, headache, weight loss, sexual dysfunction | Nausea, agitation, dizziness, sleep disturbance, fatigue, liver dysfunction |
| Second-line treatment | Atypical antipsychotics | Delta ligand agents | Low-dose naltrexone |
| Daily dose | Quetiapine 25–100 mg Olanzapine 2.5–10 mg | Pregabalin 450 mg | 4.5 mg |
| Side effects | Sedation, somnolence, dry mouth Metabolic syndrome (weight ↑, glucose ↑, hyperlipidemia) Cardiac arrythmias, abnormal liver function tests | Sleepiness, weight gain, dry mouth, constipation Swelling of hands or feet, irritability, dizziness | More vivid dreams, headache |

experiences. It guides the clinician toward targeted treatments and helps promote a good patient-physician relationship. The MDCP also provides information on the central and peripheral mechanisms that lead to symptom benefit.[11] The MDCP relies on the following 5 parameters:

A. *Categorical diagnosis*: The DGBI diagnosis for this category is based on Rome IV criteria. It is usually symptom based but may include physiologic data for some diagnoses. The additional categories in later discussion help optimize clinical care by providing more detailed features that may direct treatment.

B. *Clinical modifiers*: These are additional symptoms or features related and additive to the categorical diagnoses, such as stool pattern, postprandial symptoms, food intolerances. Their presence can help understand the putative pathophysiologic mechanism even if they require a portion of clinical judgment not purely based on evidence. They also help identify more specific treatments targeted to the modifiers (eg, treatment of IBS with diarrhea or with constipation).

C. *Impact on daily activities*: This provides some dimension to the overall effect on patient illness perceptions, behaviors, and daily functioning. It offers a biopsychosocial composite of patient-reported GI and extraintestinal symptoms, degree of disability, and illness-related perceptions and behaviors. The severity is defined primarily by the patient's judgment as mild, moderate, or severe and reconciles with physician judgment. At times, there can be a difference between the patient report and the clinician's observation that needs to be clarified when planning treatment.

D. *Psychosocial modifiers*: These include psychiatric and psychological symptoms or syndromes, such as comorbid anxiety, depression, excessive worry, and major stressors, such as traumatic life events. The Rome IV psychosocial flags can be used to identify an indication for psychopharmacologic agents or referral to a mental health professional (**Table 2**).

E. *Physiologic modifiers of visceral function and biomarkers*: Examples include the presence of slow transit constipation, delayed gastric emptying, or anti-vinculin antibodies in IBS.

**Table 2**
**Rome IV Psychosocial Flags that can be used to identify an indication for psychopharmacologic agents or referral to a mental health professional**

| Psychosocial Flag | Characteristics |
| --- | --- |
| Anxiety | Tense or wound up most of the time |
| Depression | Downhearted or low most of the time |
| Suicidal ideation | Often or occasionally felt like hurting or killing oneself |
| Abuse and trauma history | Distress from having been emotionally, physically, or sexually victimized |
| Partner abuse | Afraid for personal safety in one's intimate relationship |
| Pain severity | Severe bodily pain in last 4 wk |
| Somatic symptoms associated with distress and health concerns | Worries about physical symptoms for the last 6 mo that the clinician believes are serious |
| Impairment/disability | Pain or other symptoms interfere with normal activities over last 4 wk quite a bit or more |
| Drug/alcohol use | Excess alcohol use, prescription drugs for nonmedical reasons, and/or frequent illegal drug use |

## IMPLEMENTING TREATMENT WITH CENTRAL NEUROMODULATORS IN IRRITABLE BOWEL SYNDROME

In the 3 cases that follow, the patient-doctor relationship is the essential starting point. It is characterized by the following: (1) active listening to identify the patients concerns and expectations, (2) an explanation of IBS and the current situation with agreement on mutual understanding, (3) offering treatments based on this under-standing, and (4) including realistic short- and long-term goals patients can follow. The stigma connected to central neuromodulators' use should be dealt with by conveying basic knowledge about the gut-brain axis related to dysregulation of pain control and the DGBI, such as IBS.[24] A video explaining gut-brain axis and pain control with a patient is seen here: https://romedross.video/3b8jcVz. Sharing this in the context of peripheral and central neurologic pain mechanisms is helpful, including understanding neurotransmitter modulation. There are tutorials available online (https://romedross.video/Q_ANeuromod4) and in a recent book addressing this issue.[25] The doctor should tell the patient that the use of a neuromodulator is connected to a long-term treatment commitment monitored by the patient and doc-tor in collaboration.

After mutually selecting the patient's medication and explaining the expected symptom-reducing effects, interpreting potential side effects are essential. One reason for treatment failure is the risk for nocebo effects soon after initiation of treatment. This negative expectation can be reduced if the wrongful preconceptions about central neu-romodulators are discussed and clarified. A lower than effective starting dose can be prescribed for patients claiming they are sensitive to medications in general. It also helps to offer information about how to recognize the nocebo effect: symptoms appear early after the start of treatment, are often intense, and are often identified by the patient as already present before starting treatment, although with milder intensity.[26] At times, it may help to undertake pharmacogenomic testing if this is available. Here, the profile indicates the medications' metabolic profile, so those with rapid or slow metabolism and degradation can be reviewed and used in treatment planning.[27]

If an insufficient treatment effect is evident on the follow-up visit, increasing the medication dose is the first option as long as the maximum dose is not achieved. If the patient develops agitation, anxiety, diaphoresis, hyperreflexia, or mental status changes, after starting or raising the dose of a central neuromodulator, serotonin syn-drome should be considered. In this case, the medication should be stopped or reduced, and if severe, psychiatric consultation may be considered. However, IBS's dosages, even in combination with other neuromodulators, is usually much lower than occurs with psychiatric dosages, and serotonin syndrome is much less com-mon.[3] If other side effects restrict dosage, consider combination with an appropriate augmenting drug at the tolerated dose. Remember not to switch medication too soon based on side effects unless they represent an obvious pharmacologic effect (eg, anti-cholinergic symptoms with TCA) that has not resolved after 1 or 2 weeks. It is also important to consider behavioral or brain-gut treatments. There is good evidence for reducing IBS symptoms with cognitive behavioral therapy, gut-directed hypnother-apy, multicomponent psychological therapy, and dynamic psychotherapy.[13]

Finally, with a successful response to treatment, the treatment length to achieve relapse prevention needs to be considered. Although there are no formal trials to address relapse prevention in IBS, we can extrapolate the data from major depressive disorders.[11,28,29] In line with these studies, tapering or stopping treatment with a cen-tral neuromodulator should not begin until 6 to 12 months after reaching a clinical response. The taper is conducted over several weeks to avoid withdrawal effects.

## CASE 1. POSTINFECTION IRRITABLE BOWEL SYNDROME WITH DIARRHEA, DISTURBING ABDOMINAL PAIN, AND PSYCHOSOCIAL COMORBIDITIES

A 23-year-old woman presents with a 1-year history of intermittent lower-abdominal pain accompanied with and relieved by loose, frequent stools. The symptoms started after an acute salmonella infection during a holiday trip abroad. The trip was a treat to herself after a saddening break-up from a 4-year relationship. Her primary care physician diagnosed her with IBS, and loperamide has helped to control diarrhea. However, in addition to the abdominal pain, she also developed epigastric pain unrelated to meals. These pains have remained nagging and in the background. The persisting unpredictable episodes of abdominal pain have become increasingly embarrassing and difficult to manage. Intermittent use of hyoscyamine, eluxadoline, and a course of rifaximin while helping to reduce the diarrhea has been of little benefit for the pain, and she has started to limit her social life and managing her university studies in economics. She makes efforts to limit speaking in front of people. On one occasion, she developed severe abdominal pain and had to hand over the presentation to another person. She now reports anticipatory fear when confronted with similar situations where she needs to present to a group. She worries that her symptoms will continue to worsen, and she will never function normally. She had a 2-year history of a bulimic eating disorder during high school, where dieting to lose a few pounds of weight "went out of control," leading her to vomit and purge. These symptoms resolved after several years, but she still worries about gaining weight, so she carefully watches her diet. In general, she looks upon herself as "nervous." She has not previously sought health care for any of these issues. She asks for painkillers to have at hand "in case of an emergency."

### *Multidimensional Clinical Profile*

A. Categorical diagnosis: IBS. Functional dyspepsia.
B. *Clinical modifiers:* Post-infection (PI) IBS with diarrhea; PI epigastric pain syndrome (EPS).
C. Impact on daily activities: Moderate.
D. *Psychosocial modifiers:* Anticipatory anxiety, catastrophizing, history of bulimia nervosa.
E. Physiologic modifiers of visceral function and biomarkers: None.

This patient developed PI-IBS and functional dyspepsia, and her symptoms progressed to moderate daily function impairment and concurrent psychological distress. The PI-IBS diagnosis was confirmed by a positive stool culture during acute infectious gastroenteritis, in a previously healthy young woman. The symptoms of pain and diarrhea became chronic, thereby fulfilling Rome IV criteria for PI (PI-IBS).[30] If stool cultures are not obtained or are not positive, the criteria for PI-IBS can still be met providing the patient has $\geq 2$ of fever, diarrhea, or vomiting during the acute infection-like event. The most common IBS subtype as in this case of PI-IBS is IBS with diarrhea.

Breaking up after a long-term relationship was a significant life event that occurred in conjunction with and after the infectious episode; this increases the risk for developing PI-IBS.[31,32] Furthermore, the symptom-associated anticipatory anxiety and catastrophizing thoughts have further restricted her social life. Her fear and shame related to her symptoms produce maladaptive cognitions that affect her studies, leading to impairment in her daily activities.

Patients with IBS have an increased risk of concurrent anxiety compared with otherwise healthy individuals,[33] and in those with overlapping DGBI diagnoses, the prevalence of anxiety is further increased[34] and associated with increased health care use, medication use, and risk for undergoing GI surgery.[35]

In sum, this is a patient with predisposing factors (GI infection at the time of a life event, being "nervous," with history of bulimic eating disorder), developed PI-IBS, which increased the risk for visceral and later central sensitization, psychological co-morbidity, and functional impairment. Treatment must address the brain and gut.

**CENTRAL NEUROMODULATORS: THERAPEUTIC OPTIONS**

Because abdominal pain is the predominant symptom, and peripheral treatments although helping diarrhea have not helped the pain, central neuromodulators can be used:

1. A TCA is a preferred treatment for IBS, with pain as the chief complaint.[3] The efficacy of a TCA in treating IBS symptoms was demonstrated most recently in a 2019 meta-analysis. The study showed a reduced relative risk of no improvement in symptoms compared with a placebo of 0.65 (95% confidence interval, 0.55–0.77).[13] TCAs also ranked first among the therapeutic options when addressing IBS-associated abdominal pain effects using a network meta-analysis methodology.[12] In this particular patient, treatment of the EPS with a TCA is also favored based on a large multicenter study.[36] The drawback of using at least higher dosages of a TCA is the risk of side effects, where drowsiness and dry mouth are common.[13] One specific side effect, constipation mediated by anticholinergic mechanisms, makes TCAs the preferred option in IBS with diarrhea like in this case. The clinician can choose either a tertiary or a secondary amine based on whether the antimuscarinic (reduce diarrhea) or an antihistaminic (improve disturbed sleep) effect is preferred. If the patient tolerates treatment well, increasing the dose up to full antidepressant doses, 100 to 150 mg/d, is useful if improvement of significant psychiatric comorbidity is also a treatment goal.[37]

2. An SNRI is the alternative to a TCA. It can be prescribed as monotherapy to treat abdominal pain if the TCA is not tolerated or provides insufficient benefit. The risk for constipation is much less than a TCA, and nausea, the main side effect, tends to diminish over a week or 2 and can improve when taken with a meal.

3. Augmentation treatment refers to combining treatments when individual therapeutic effects are either insufficient or complicated by side effects that restrict dosage.[3] In this example, using a low-dose SSRI combined with a low-dose TCA or SNRI treatment can be considered if the anxiety is a dominant clinical feature. When anxiety or depression coexists with IBS, they can intensify the GI symptoms.[38] Thus, there are dual effects of treating pain with the TCA (or SNRI) and treating anxiety with a low-dose SSRI. Also, brain-gut therapies, such as cognitive-behavioral treatment (CBT), are augmenting methods for pharmacologic agents. This may be of particular value here because of the high level of symptom-related anxiety and catastrophizing behaviors that are amenable to CBT. Further information about these treatments can be found elsewhere.[39]

**CASE 2. IRRITABLE BOWEL SYNDROME WITH CONSTIPATION WORSENED BY USE OF OPIOIDS**

A 41-year old man with IBS diagnosed at age 17 presents for the fourth time in a year to a gastroenterology outpatient clinic. The last 3 occasions over 2 months were at 2 different doctors' offices. The symptoms include cramping lower-abdominal pain and bloating associated with the need to empty his bowel, which worsen when under psychological distress. He has 3 bowel movements a week, and he feels the need to strain; the pain is partially relieved with defecation. The stool form varies from very hard to formed, sometimes on the same day, and there is a sensation of incomplete evacuation. He never has loose stools. Bulking agents and osmotic laxatives have had no meaningful effect on his symptoms. A year ago, he was prescribed linaclotide, but he developed diarrhea, and it was discontinued. An additional problem is lower-back pain, for which he is prescribed tramadol. Occasionally, he takes 50 mg on demand up to 3 times daily during weekdays to stand while at work even if his back is not painful; on those days, he feels it also slightly improves the lower-abdominal pain. However, since taking the tramadol, his constipation symptoms have become worse. He is vague about the dosage and which doctor he sees for the prescription. Over the last 2 years, the intensity of IBS pain and constipation has increased. Over the previous 4 months, he has been on sick leave because of severe postprandial attacks of abdominal pain that severely impact his daily functioning. He also suffers from anxiety, and an irregular sleep pattern, despite zolpidem that his doctor prescribed on the previous visit. He is interested in treatment for constipation that he believes is the reason for the abdominal pain. However, a study with radio-opaque markers showed a normal whole-gut transit time.

### Multidimensional Clinical Profile

A. *Categorical diagnosis:* IBS. Opioid-induced constipation.
B. *Clinical modifiers:* IBS with constipation (IBS-C). Insomnia. Chronic back pain.
C. Impact on daily activities: Severe.
D. *Psychosocial modifiers:* Anxiety, stress sensitivity, insomnia.
E. Physiologic modifiers of visceral function and biomarkers: Normal oroanal transit time.

This patient had IBS-C that worsened with the use of tramadol. The IBS is due to the abdominal pain associated with hard stool and relief with defecation. The clinical modifier, IBS-C, is based on the patient straining, having hard stools, and a sensation of incomplete bowel movements. The concurrent tramadol, prescribed for back pain, worsened his constipation and led to the diagnosis of opioid-induced constipation. However, an exacerbation of constipation symptoms after adding opioids is also often called opioid-exacerbated constipation. Tramadol is not recommended for his IBS pain[40] and aggravates the constipation.[41]

The psychosocial modifiers include sensitivity to stress and comorbid anxiety, which is important to note as problems that could also be addressed by nonpharmacologic, behavioral therapeutic options. Adding to this, he has insomnia, a psychosocial modifier commonly associated with chronic pain.[42] He is unable to work because of IBS symptoms. This may occur short term[43]; however, being on long-term sick leave is a more complex signal of having multiple illness components resulting in the severe impact on daily activities his IBS has.

In this case, the physiologic test using radio-opaque markers that assess whole-gut transit time showed normal transit. Most patients suffering from IBS-C do not have delayed GI transit.[44] From 2 days before and during the days that the transit study is performed, tramadol needs to be discontinued, and most patients can be motivated to do so even if it might result in increased short-term discomfort. In some situations, the improvement in bowel habits might motivate the patients to find other solutions than opioids for the pain, giving an opportunity to explain the value of central neuromodulators.

### Central Neuromodulators: Therapeutic Options

This clinical scenario of long-standing IBS pain with a risk of becoming complicated by opioids leads to considering using one or more of the following central neuromodulators in parallel with stopping tramadol.

1. An SNRI. With IBS-C, a neuromodulator without anticholinergic effects is preferred as a first-line treatment. An SNRI can benefit the low-back pain, and it may also treat the abdominal pain without increasing constipation relative to a TCA.
2. A TCA could be considered as in case 1 based on its value in treating IBS-related abdominal pain. The secondary amines, desipramine and nortriptyline, can be considered in a patient with normal gut transit constipation. The irregular sleep pattern can also benefit from this class of drugs.
3. An atypical antipsychotic, for example, quetiapine, can be considered based on its effects on severe abdominal pain and its ability to help with his sleep difficulties. This option could be added as augmentation to an SNRI if the effects from the initial therapy are insufficient.
4. The treatment of constipation can be reevaluated based on the response to withdrawing tramadol treatment that was needed during the investigation of gut transit. The normal transit study indicates that his constipation probably does not need other than first-line treatment options like a bulking agent or an osmotic laxative. If tramadol cannot be stopped short term, the best option in this case would probably be a peripheral μ-opioid receptor antagonist[45] until sufficient effects from the central neuromodulator treatment have developed.

## CASE 3. IRRITABLE BOWEL SYNDROME MIXED PROGRESSING TO CENTRALLY MEDIATED ABDOMINAL PAIN SYNDROME WITH SEVERE OPIOID COMPLICATIONS

A 36-year-old woman having IBS with mixed bowel habits was diagnosed 8 years ago after 5 years of progressive symptoms. In the last 2 years, abdominal pain has become more intense and constant and is no longer related to her bowel habit. She also had a laparoscopically verified diagnosis of mild endometriosis diagnosed 3 years ago. There are 2 one-year-long episodes of major depression at ages 21 and 27, and she is on continuous SSRI treatment (escitalopram 10 mg/d). Her gynecologist and primary care doctors prescribe oxycodone to treat the endometriosis. The oxycodone doses have progressively escalated from 20 mg/d to more than 80 mg/d in the last year. The patient claims that this medication is the only way to bear the pain. Despite the increase in oxycodone dose, there has been a progression to constant unbearable abdominal pain leading to multiple awakenings at night over the last several years. In addition, she reports progressive constipation that does not respond to bulking agents, osmotic or stimulant laxatives, linaclotide, or prucalopride. She perceives the abdominal pain as being related to her constipation. Life is "black" and "on hold" in the same way she has experienced during the previous depressions. She requests to have her colon removed to cure the constipation. Otherwise, she "might as well be dead." Her social life is in ruins, and she has been unable to work for more than a year.

### Multidimensional Clinical Profile

A. *Categorical diagnosis:* Centrally mediated abdominal pain syndrome. Opioid-induced constipation. Narcotic bowel syndrome.
B. Clinical modifiers: Endometriosis.
C. Impact on daily activities: Severe.
D. *Psychosocial modifiers:* Recurrent major depressive disorder.
E. Physiologic modifiers of visceral function and biomarkers: None.

This patient had IBS with mixed bowel habits, but this categorical diagnosis has progressed to centrally mediated abdominal pain syndrome, which is not related to bowel habits specifically. Instead, the current constipation is related to concurrent use of opioids, thereby fulfilling diagnostic criteria for opioid-induced constipation.[1] A demonstration of how this diagnosis of opioid-induced constipation can be presented to a patient is seen in this video: https://romedross.video/CashOIC. Furthermore, the now chronic, progressive abdominal pain that leads to escalating oxycodone doses is consistent with narcotic bowel syndrome.[46,47] Narcotic bowel syndrome is characterized by the paradoxic development of, or increases in, abdominal pain associated with continuous or increasing dosages of opioids. To make a diagnosis of narcotic bowel syndrome, 2 or more of the following should be present: (a) The pain worsens or incompletely resolves with continued or escalating dosages of narcotics; (b) There is marked worsening of pain when the narcotic dose wanes and improvement when narcotics are reinstituted; (c) There is a progression of the frequency, duration, and intensity of pain episodes. A discussion with a patient having centrally mediated abdominal pain syndrome wanting opioids for pain is seen in this video: https://romedross.video/TackCAPS.

The combined medical history, IBS, endometriosis, and a major depressive disorder, together with the current opioid-related complications, are consistent with severe impact on her daily activities. Her overarching description of the recent life, the reports of the pain severity, suicidal ideation, and severe functional impairment of function, are critical factors relating to a very severe illness experience. A brief discussion of how to explain the approach to management in a patient similar to this can be seen in this video: https://romedross.video/2GRui4U.

### Central Neuromodulators: Therapeutic Options

In the above-described situation, the illness presentation favors central sensitization as an important gut-brain disorder mechanism, along with the development of a narcotic bowel syndrome. Narcotic bowel syndrome is difficult to treat and will involve several steps in parallel with initiating central neuromodulator treatment.

1. A good patient-physician relationship is an essential prerequisite for a successful outcome in a complicated case like this. Initiating any treatment must include ending opioid use. In this case, the patient's misconception regarding colectomy as a cure needs to be addressed respectfully. At times, patients are reluctant to go off opioids fearing there are no other treatments. A good relationship can help to define a treatment plan whereby the use of central neuromodulators can begin, and then with some improvement, the opioids can be eliminated by protocol. An example of negotiating this type of treatment plan can be found at: https://vimeo.com/498198552/7d7f9e6f64.
2. Treatment of *narcotic bowel syndrome and opioid-induced constipation* is needed before most other aspects of DGBI treatment can be successful. There is good evidence that discontinuing opioids through a detoxification protocol is associated with a significant improvement in pain and coping, which is crucial for the patient to understand and have trust in.[47,48] The detoxification protocol that describes this outcome starts with a period of fixed opioid dose reduction (15%–33% per day) calculated on the initial opioid dose until the patient is entirely off the medication. The time period to achieve this was longer when managed in outpatient care ($39 \pm 21$ days) compared with in-patient care ($7 \pm 3$ days). In order to reduce anxiety, benzodiazepine treatment is used during the detoxification. Oral clonidine to counteract withdrawal effects is introduced when the opioid dose is half the initial dosage. During the detoxification period, a PEG solution to treat the opioid-induced constipation or a peripheral μ-opioid receptor antagonist should be used[45] and later stopped after opioid discontinuation.

In parallel with the opioid detoxification, depending on the predominant symptom profile, the following neuromodulator options are used:

### A serotonin noradrenalin reuptake inhibitor
See cases 1 and 2 regarding the dosages and rationale. An SNRI would be the initiating treatment to be used before starting detoxification.

### Atypical antipsychotics
Quetiapine and olanzapine both have an anxiolytic and sleep-inducing effect and augment the pain benefit of the SNRI. They should be added to the SNRI. This addition can be useful when severe abdominal pain is associated with a disturbed sleeping pattern. Sedation is also the most common side effect along with weight gain. The value for this class of drugs is best evidenced by treatment in patients with fibromyalgia and chronic headaches, in a review article treating IBS,[14] and a case-series study in DGBI patients.[16]

### Delta ligand agents (gabapentin, pregabalin)
This class of treatment may be considered as a neuromodulator with peripheral effect, even if there are data to support central effects as well.[49] One recent randomized double-blind, placebo-controlled trial in IBS where pregabalin 225 mg twice daily for 12 weeks was compared with placebo suggested positive effects on the abdominal pain component and bloating and diarrhea.[20] This comparison is in line with the heightened visceral sensory thresholds from pregabalin noted in previous experiments on IBS patients.[19,50] The best evidence for delta ligand agent use comes from treatment of fibromyalgia,[21] a common comorbidity in IBS, that could further justify a trial in patients with complex pain conditions that include IBS. In this case, the risk of contributing to the existing opioid-induced constipation should be kept in mind.

3. Involving a mental health professional is based on the psychosocial red flags (see **Table 2**) and the presence of a major depressive disorder. At this point, a collaborative effort is crucial to achieving a successful outcome. It is necessary to set up the above described protocol in collaboration with a psychiatrist as part of an augmentation program in most cases that also involve a long-term follow-up.

## CLINICS CARE POINTS

- A multidimensional clinical profile guides the clinician toward targeted treatments that incorporate the illness's biopsychosocial and dimensional features.
- Conveying a basic understanding of the gut-brain axis and its relation to chronic GI symptoms helps the patient understand why central neuromodulators are beneficial.
- According to guidelines in this article, explaining both the expected symptom-reducing effects of central neuromodulators and the potential side effects is essential after agreeing on treatment.
- When the initial treatment dose is insufficient, increasing the medication dose is the first option until the maximum dose is achieved.
- To avoid relapse, tapering treatment with a central neuromodulator should not begin until 6 to 12 months after reaching a clinical response.

## DISCLOSURE

Hans Törnblom has nothing to declare, and Douglas A. Drossman has nothing to declare.

## REFERENCES

1. Lacy BE, Mearin F, Chang L, et al. Bowel disorders. Gastroenterology 2016;150: 1393–407.
2. Drossman DA. Functional gastrointestinal disorders: history, pathophysiology, clinical features and Rome IV. Gastroenterology 2016;150:1262–9.
3. Drossman DA, Tack J, Ford AC, et al. Neuromodulators for functional gastrointestinal disorders (disorders of gut-brain interaction): a Rome Foundation working team report. Gastroenterology 2018;154(4):1140–71.e1141.
4. Chey WD, Lembo AJ, Lavins BJ, et al. Linaclotide for irritable bowel syndrome with constipation: a 26-week, randomized, double-blind, placebo-controlled trial to evaluate efficacy and safety. Am J Gastroenterol 2012;107(11):1702–12.
5. Brenner DM, Fogel R, Dorn SD, et al. Efficacy, safety, and tolerability of plecanatide in patients with irritable bowel syndrome with constipation: results of two phase 3 randomized clinical trials. Am J Gastroenterol 2018;113(5):735–45.
6. Lembo AJ, Lacy BE, Zuckerman MJ, et al. Eluxadoline for irritable bowel syndrome with diarrhea. N Engl J Med 2016;374(3):242–53.
7. Camilleri M, Kerstens R, Rykx A, et al. A placebo-controlled trial of prucalopride for severe chronic constipation. N Engl J Med 2008;358(22):2344–54.
8. Lacy BE, Nicandro JP, Chuang E, et al. Alosetron use in clinical practice: significant improvement in irritable bowel syndrome symptoms evaluated using the US Food and Drug Administration composite endpoint. Therap Adv Gastroenterol 2018;11. 1756284818771674.
9. Fukudo S, Kinoshita Y, Okumura T, et al. Ramosetron reduces symptoms of irritable bowel syndrome with diarrhea and improves quality of life in women. Gastroenterology 2016;150(2):358–66.
10. Garsed K, Chernova J, Hastings M, et al. A randomised trial of ondansetron for the treatment of irritable bowel syndrome with diarrhoea. Gut 2014;63(10): 1617–25.
11. Tornblom H, Drossman DA. Psychotropics, antidepressants, and visceral analgesics in functional gastrointestinal disorders. Curr Gastroenterol Rep 2018; 20(12):58.
12. Black CJ, Yuan Y, Selinger CP, et al. Efficacy of soluble fibre, antispasmodic drugs, and gut-brain neuromodulators in irritable bowel syndrome: a systematic review and network meta-analysis. Lancet Gastroenterol Hepatol 2020;5(2): 117–31.
13. Ford AC, Lacy BE, Harris LA, et al. Effect of antidepressants and psychological therapies in irritable bowel syndrome: an updated systematic review and meta-analysis. Am J Gastroenterol 2019;114(1):21–39.
14. Pae CU, Lee SJ, Han C, et al. Atypical antipsychotics as a possible treatment option for irritable bowel syndrome. Expert Opin Investig Drugs 2013;22(5):565–72.
15. McIntyre A, Paisley D, Kouassi E, et al. Quetiapine fumarate extended-release for the treatment of major depression with comorbid fibromyalgia syndrome: a double-blind, randomized, placebo-controlled study. Arthritis Rheumatol 2014; 66(2):451–61.
16. Grover M, Dorn SD, Weinland SR, et al. Atypical antipsychotic quetiapine in the management of severe refractory functional gastrointestinal disorders. Dig Dis Sci 2009;54(6):1284–91.
17. Jimenez XF, Sundararajan T, Covington EC. A systematic review of atypical antipsychotics in chronic pain management: olanzapine demonstrates potential in

central sensitization, fibromyalgia, and headache/migraine. Clin J Pain 2018; 34(6):585–91.

18. Ventriglio A, Gentile A, Stella E, et al. Metabolic issues in patients affected by schizophrenia: clinical characteristics and medical management. Front Neurosci 2015;9:297.

19. Houghton LA, Fell C, Whorwell PJ, et al. Effect of a second-generation alpha2-delta ligand (pregabalin) on visceral sensation in hypersensitive patients with irritable bowel syndrome. Gut 2007;56(9):1218–25.

20. Saito YA, Almazar AE, Tilkes KE, et al. Randomised clinical trial: pregabalin vs placebo for irritable bowel syndrome. Aliment Pharmacol Ther 2019;49(4):389–97.

21. Lee YH, Song GG. Comparative efficacy and tolerability of duloxetine, pregabalin, and milnacipran for the treatment of fibromyalgia: a Bayesian network meta-analysis of randomized controlled trials. Rheumatol Int 2016;36(5):663–72.

22. Younger J, Parkitny L, McLain D. The use of low-dose naltrexone (LDN) as a novel anti-inflammatory treatment for chronic pain. Clin Rheumatol 2014;33(4):451–9.

23. Drossman DA, Ed S, Chang L, et al. Rome IV multidimensional clinical profile for the functional gastrointestinal disorders. 2nd edition. Ralegh, NC: The Rome Foundation; 2016.

24. Feingold JH, Drossman DA. Deconstructing stigma as a barrier to treating DGBI: lessons for clinicians. Neurogastroenterol Motil 2021;33(2):e14080.

25. Drossman DA, Ruddy J. Gut feelings: disorders of gut-brain interaction and the patient-doctor relationship. Chapel Hill NC: DrossmanCare; 2021. p. 1–207.

26. Thiwan S, Drossman DA, Morris CB, et al. Not all side effects associated with tricyclic antidepressant therapy are true side effects. Clin Gastroenterol Hepatol 2009;7(4):446–51.

27. Camilleri M. Implications of pharmacogenomics to the management of IBS. Clin Gastroenterol Hepatol 2019;17(4):584–94.

28. Baldessarini RJ, Lau WK, Sim J, et al. Duration of initial antidepressant treatment and subsequent relapse of major depression. J Clin Psychopharmacol 2015; 35(1):75–6.

29. Sim K, Lau WK, Sim J, et al. Prevention of relapse and recurrence in adults with major depressive disorder: systematic review and meta-analyses of controlled trials. The Int J Neuropsychopharmacol 2016;19(2).

30. Barbara G, Grover M, Bercik P, et al. Rome Foundation working team report on post-infection irritable bowel syndrome. Gastroenterology 2019;156(1):46–58 e47.

31. Neal KR, Barker L, Spiller RC. Prognosis in post-infective irritable bowel syndrome: a six year follow up study. Gut 2002;51(3):410–3.

32. Drossman DA. Mind over matter in the postinfective irritable bowel. Gut 1999; 44(3):306–7.

33. Zamani M, Alizadeh-Tabari S, Zamani V. Systematic review with meta-analysis: the prevalence of anxiety and depression in patients with irritable bowel syndrome. Aliment Pharmacol Ther 2019;50(2):132–43.

34. Pinto-Sanchez MI, Ford AC, Avila CA, et al. Anxiety and depression increase in a stepwise manner in parallel with multiple FGIDs and symptom severity and frequency. Am J Gastroenterol 2015;110(7):1038–48.

35. Aziz I, Palsson OS, Tornblom H, et al. The prevalence and impact of overlapping Rome IV-diagnosed functional gastrointestinal disorders on somatization, quality of life, and healthcare utilization: a cross-sectional general population study in three countries. Am J Gastroenterol 2018;113(1):86–96.

36. Talley NJ, Locke GR, Saito YA, et al. Effect of amitriptyline and escitalopram on functional dyspepsia: a multicenter, randomized controlled study. Gastroenterology 2015;149(2):340–9.e342.
37. Drossman DA, Toner BB, Whitehead WE, et al. Cognitive-behavioral therapy versus education and desipramine versus placebo for moderate to severe functional bowel disorders. Gastroenterology 2003;125(1):19–31.
38. Midenfjord I, Borg A, Tornblom H, et al. Cumulative effect of psychological alterations on gastrointestinal symptom severity in irritable bowel syndrome. Am J Gastroenterol 2020;116(4):769–79.
39. Van Oudenhove L, Crowell MD, Drossman DA, et al. Biopsychosocial aspects of functional gastrointestinal disorders. Gastroenterology 2016;150:1355–67.
40. Szigethy E, Knisely M, Drossman D. Opioid misuse in gastroenterology and non-opioid management of abdominal pain. Nat Rev Gastroenterol Hepatol 2018; 15(3):168–80.
41. Brock C, Olesen SS, Olesen AE, et al. Opioid-induced bowel dysfunction: pathophysiology and management. Drugs 2012;72(14):1847–65.
42. Ballou S, Alhassan E, Hon E, et al. Sleep disturbances are commonly reported among patients presenting to a gastroenterology clinic. Dig Dis Sci 2018; 63(11):2983–91.
43. Frandemark A, Tornblom H, Jakobsson S, et al. Work productivity and activity impairment in irritable bowel syndrome (IBS): a multifaceted problem. Am J Gastroenterol 2018;113(10):1540–9.
44. Tornblom H, Van Oudenhove L, Sadik R, et al. Colonic transit time and IBS symptoms: what's the link? Am J Gastroenterol 2012;107(5):754–60.
45. Muller-Lissner S, Bassotti G, Coffin B, et al. Opioid-induced constipation and bowel dysfunction: a clinical guideline. Pain Med 2017;18(10):1837–63.
46. Keefer L, Drossman DA, Guthrie E, et al. Centrally mediated disorders of gastrointestinal pain. Gastroenterology 2016;150(6):1408–16.
47. Grunkemeier DM, Cassara JE, Dalton CB, et al. The narcotic bowel syndrome: clinical features, pathophysiology, and management. Clin Gastroenterol Hepatol 2007;5(10):1126–39 [quiz 1121-2].
48. Drossman DA, Morris CB, Edwards H, et al. Diagnosis, characterization, and 3-month outcome after detoxification of 39 patients with narcotic bowel syndrome. Am J Gastroenterol 2012;107(9):1426–40.
49. Harris RE, Napadow V, Huggins JP, et al. Pregabalin rectifies aberrant brain chemistry, connectivity, and functional response in chronic pain patients. Anesthesiology 2013;119(6):1453–64.
50. Lee KJ, Kim JH, Cho SW. Gabapentin reduces rectal mechanosensitivity and increases rectal compliance in patients with diarrhoea-predominant irritable bowel syndrome. Aliment Pharmacol Ther 2005;22(10):981–8.

# Complementary and Alternative Medicine Therapies for Irritable Bowel Syndrome

Jordan M. Shapiro, MD[a],*, Jill K. Deutsch, MD[b]

## KEYWORDS

- Complementary and alternative medicine • Irritable bowel syndrome
- Mind-body medicine • Traditional medicine

## KEY POINTS

- Complementary and alternative medicine (CAM) is commonly used by patients with irritable bowel syndrome.
- There are many factors contributing to providers' challenges in counseling patients on CAM use, including lack of communication about CAM use, poor quality and quantity of evidence, and limited federal regulation of CAM therapies.
- By better understanding the spectrum and limitations of CAM therapy, providers can better counsel patients on use.

## INTRODUCTION

Disorders of gut-brain interaction (DGBIs), such as irritable bowel syndrome (IBS), are some of the most common reasons for patients to visit both pediatric and adult gastroenterologists; yet, only 30% of patients with IBS seek medical care.[1–4] Despite a lack of mortality associated with IBS, patients with IBS suffer tremendous morbidity due to their symptoms, subsequent dietary restriction, mood disturbances, and interference with daily activity.[5,6] Many patients with IBS ultimately seek complementary and/or alternative therapies for symptom relief.[6]

### What Is in a Name? Complementary, Alternative, or Integrative?

For the sake of simplicity, this article uses complementary and alternative medicine (CAM), although the preferred nomenclature has changed over time. Many of the changes in nomenclature have mirrored changes in the name of the National Center

[a] Section of Gastroenterology and Hepatology, Baylor College of Medicine, 7200 Cambridge Street, A8.172, MS:BCM901, Houston, TX 77030, USA; [b] Section of Gastroenterology and Hepatology, Yale New Haven Hospital, 40 Temple Street, Suite 1A, New Haven, CT 06510, USA
* Corresponding author.
E-mail address: jmshapir@bcm.edu
Twitter: @drjshapiro (J.M.S.); @GIJill (J.K.D.)

Gastroenterol Clin N Am 50 (2021) 671–688
https://doi.org/10.1016/j.gtc.2021.03.009
0889-8553/21/© 2021 Elsevier Inc. All rights reserved.

gastro.theclinics.com

for Complementary and Integrative Health (NCCIH), which is 1 of 27 centers within the National Institutes of Health. NCCIH originally was founded in 1991 as the Office of Alternative Medicine. It was renamed the National Center for Complementary and Alternative Medicine in 1998 and then NCCIH in 2014. These name changes arose, in part, to reframe the conversation about CAM therapies around an agreed-upon standard of care, often referred to as *conventional medicine*.[7] **Table 1** provides more detailed description of CAM nomenclature. These definitions are dynamic, and some therapies previously considered CAM now are mainstays of conventional treatment of IBS (eg, hypnotherapy and cognitive behavioral therapy).

## CLASSIFICATION OF COMPLEMENTARY AND ALTERNATIVE MEDICINE THERAPIES

The NCCIH places CAM therapies into 2 groups: natural products, which often are sold as dietary supplements (eg, herbs, vitamins and minerals, and probiotics), and mind-body medicine (eg, hypnotherapy, cognitive behavioral therapy, and yoga).[12] In addition, several therapies fall into traditional/newer systems of medicine (eg, Ayurveda, traditional Chinese medicine, and reiki). Some natural products (eg, turmeric) and mind-body medicine therapies (eg, acupuncture) may be considered part of traditional/newer medicinal systems as well. Examples of therapies in different classes of CAM are listed in **Table 2**.

## CHARACTERISTICS OF COMPLEMENTARY AND ALTERNATIVE MEDICINE USE FOR IRRITABLE BOWEL SYNDROME
### How Common Is Complementary and Alternative Medicine Use in General?

A landmark study highlighting the commonality of CAM use was published by Eisenberg and colleagues[13] in 2003; 1529 patients completed telephone interviews about

**Table 1**
**Nomenclature for complementary and alternative medicine therapies**

| Nomenclature for Medical Therapies | Definitions |
| --- | --- |
| Conventional | The usual methods of healing or treating disease that are taught in Western medical schools.[8]; sometimes referred to as standard of care |
| Alternative | Therapies used in place of conventional therapies. Any therapy or system of healing or treating disease not included in the traditional medical curricula of Western medical schools[9] |
| Complementary | Therapies used in conjunction with conventional therapies; any of the practices of alternative medicine accepted and utilized by mainstream medical practitioners[10] |
| Integrative | An evidence-based use of conventional and complementary therapies; a practice of medicine that reaffirms the importance of the relationships between practitioner and patient, focuses on the whole person, is informed by evidence, and makes use of all appropriate therapeutic approaches, health care professionals, and disciplines to achieve optimal health and healin.[11] |
| Nontraditional vs traditional | Terminology that differs in meaning depending on the perspective. For example, "traditional" may imply ancient systems of medicine or, with a current frame of reference, may refer to conventional medical therapies. |
| Eastern vs Western medicine | Eastern medicine often is used to denote systems of medicine that originated in India (Ayurveda) and China (traditional Chinese medicine). Western medicine, however, the current standard of practice of medicine in the United States and Europe, is considered the standard of care in academic settings in most parts of the world. |

**Table 2**
**Examples of therapies within each class of complementary and alternative medicine**

| Class of Complementary and Alternative Medicine Therapies | Examples |
| --- | --- |
| Natural products | Vitamins/minerals<br>Herbs (eg, turmeric)<br>Peppermint oil<br>Prebiotics and probiotics<br>Fiber<br>STW-5 (Iberogast) |
| Mind-body medicine | Cognitive-behavior therapy<br>Gut-directed hypnotherapy<br>Diaphragmatic breathing<br>Yoga<br>Massage (eg, tuina in traditional Chinese medicine)<br>Chiropractic medicine<br>Osteopathic medicine |
| Medicinal systems | Ayurveda<br>Traditional Chinese medicine<br>Reiki<br>Homeopathy |

their use of what the investigators termed, "unconventional therapy" (ie, CAM therapies). One-third (33.8%) of respondents reported use of at least 1 CAM therapy in the prior year, 72% did not inform their medical doctors of CAM use, and estimates of annual spending on CAM amounted to $13.7 billion. Several follow-up studies also found that patients' use of CAM therapies has increased over time.[14–16]

### How Common is Complementary and Alternative Medicine Use for Irritable Bowel Syndrome?

Multiple international studies on the prevalence of CAM use for IBS report approximately 50% of patients with IBS use CAM (range 21%–73%).[17–21] The US 2012 National Health Interview Study (NHIS), which included 13,505 subjects, found that 42% of participants used CAM in the prior year, 3% of which were for a gastrointestinal (GI) condition.[22] Of individuals who used CAM for a GI condition, 47% used 3 or more CAM therapies. In a prospective study of 1012 patients with DGBIs, 35% reported using CAM in the year prior, at a median annual cost of $200.[23]

### What Types of Complementary and Alternative Medicine Do Patients Use for Irritable Bowel Syndrome?

Several studies have assessed the specific types of CAM therapies used by patients with IBS. One US-based study found that the most common CAM treatments used for DGBIs were ginger, massage therapy, and yoga.[23] In an Italian study, 78% of patients using CAM reported a preference for "biologically based therapy," which included herbs (37%), dietary supplements (26%), and vitamins (15%), whereas 11% preferred mind-body interventions (meditation and art), 6% manipulation (massage), and 5% an alternative medical system (homeopathy).[17] The US 2012 NHIS similarly found that herbs and supplements were the most commonly used CAM (23%), followed by mind-body exercise (11.7%), massage (11.3%), and chiropractic/osteopathic manipulation (11.2%). The most commonly used herbs and supplements were fish oil

(14.3%), other herbs and supplements (5.2%), glucosamine (4.6%), and probiotics or prebiotics (4.3%).[22]

### Why Do Patients Use Complementary and Alternative Medicine for Irritable Bowel Syndrome?

Most Western providers assume that a majority of patients turn to CAM as a consequence of failure of or dissatisfaction with conventional medicine. This assumption is not supported by data from survey research.[14–16] It turns out that many patients are attracted by several real and perceived attributes of CAM therapies, revolving around themes involving natural therapies and wellness/prevention. In 1 study of patients with IBS, the primary reasons for CAM use was reported as follows: 51% stated it was a "more natural approach"; 25% cited "failure of traditional medicine"; and 24% noted a "fear for adverse effects" of conventional medications.[24] In the 2012 NHIS, the most common reasons for CAM use for a GI condition were "general wellness or disease prevention"; "it is natural"; it "can be practiced/done on your own"; and it "treats the causes and not just the symptoms."[22] It is unknown whether or not CAM use differs between patients with IBS who are seen by medical professionals and those who self-manage their IBS symptoms.

### Satisfaction with Complementary and Alternative Medicine Use/Perceived Benefits

Despite patients' enthusiasm for CAM, their satisfaction with the effectiveness of CAM therapies is more subdued. In the aforementioned Italian study, satisfaction with CAM use for IBS was "good" in 16%, "fair" in 65%, and "poor" in 19%.[17] Despite fair or poor satisfaction, 81% of patients were willing to try CAM therapies again. The 2012 NHIS survey found the top perceived benefits for CAM were "improved overall health and feeling better"; "a sense of control over one's health"; "easier to cope with health problems"; and "reduced stress or improved relaxation."[22]

### Communication with Providers About Complementary and Alternative Medicine for Irritable Bowel Syndrome

Whether or not CAM use is discussed during clinical encounters depends on open communication between patients and providers, with providers playing a key role in facilitating discussions about CAM. Patients' communication with their physicians about CAM use for IBS was 70% in 2 studies.[22,24] When patients do not disclose CAM use to their providers, 82% cite physicians not asking about CAM use as the reason.[24] In another study, only 19% of patients using CAM for their IBS received recommendations from their providers to do so.[17] One study found that despite infrequent referrals by physicians to CAM providers, patients were very likely (>75%) to see CAM providers recommended by their physicians for IBS.[23] The study considered dieticians, psychologists/psychiatrists, and naturopaths as CAM providers. Dieticians and clinical psychologists now are widely considered key members of multidisciplinary conventional care for patients with IBS.[25]

### Where Do Patients Get Their Information About Complementary and Alternative Medicine for Irritable Bowel Syndrome?

One-third of patients (34%) in 1 study obtained information about CAM therapies from the media, 24% from the Internet, 16% from friends, 7% from family members, and only 19% from health care providers.[17] Compared with patients with Crohn disease, patients with IBS were significantly more likely to consult a CAM practitioner (41%) if conventional treatment failed.

## SELECTED COMPLEMENTARY AND ALTERNATIVE MEDICINE THERAPIES FOR IRRITABLE BOWEL SYNDROME

Tables 3–5 highlight natural products (ie, herbs and dietary supplements) and mind-body therapies commonly used and/or previously studied for the treatment of IBS (see **Table 3** for herbs, **Table 4** for dietary supplements, and **Table 5** for mind-body medicine therapies). These tables are not all inclusive but highlight background information, proposed mechanisms of action, common dosing (when applicable), outcomes of clinical studies, and safety data for each therapy.

**Table 3**
**Natural products—herbal therapies for the treatment of irritable bowel syndrome**

| Herbal Therapy | Characteristics |
|---|---|
| Aloe<br>*Aloe vera* | Background<br>• The leaves of the succulent *A vera* plant produce a clear gel and yellow latex that have used for purported health benefits for centuries.<br>Mechanism of action<br>• *A vera* acts as a stimulant laxative[26] and has analgesic[27] and anti-inflammatory[28] effects that may be helpful for abdominal pain.<br>Clinical studies<br>• Meta-analysis of 3 RCTs, including 151 patients with IBS, reported significant improvement in IBS symptom scores with *A vera* compared with placebo ($P = .02$)[26]<br>Safety<br>• *A vera* may cause diarrhea and melanosis coli, and a small case series reported reversible acute hepatitis.[29]<br>• In addition, *A vera* may reduce absorption of anticoagulants and glucose-lowering medications. |
| Cannabis<br>*Cannabis sativa*<br>Marijuana | Background<br>• THC and CBD are the most common cannabinoids.[30]<br>• THC is the primary psychoactive constituent.[30]<br>• Phytocannabinoids (plant-derived), endocannabinoids (endogenously produced), and synthetic cannabinoids can bind cannabinoid receptors.[31]<br>Mechanism of action<br>• In the gut, cannabinoids inhibit excitatory nerve transmission, slowing motility from the stomach to the colon; other studies have demonstrated analgesic effects.[32]<br>Clinical studies<br>• No trials have assessed the clinical impact of whole *C sativa* or CBD on IBS symptoms.<br>• Dronabinol (Marinol), a nonselective synthetic cannabinoid receptor agonist, has been studied in patients with IBS-D and IBS-M.[33a]<br>• Effects of dronabinol on colonic motility of patients with IBS-D and IBS-M have been varied, and no studies have demonstrated changes in rectal sensation with use of dronabinol.[33–36]<br>Safety<br>• Higher THC:CBD ratios are associated with more anxiety and hallucinations.[30,32]<br>• Cannabis was the greatest risk factor for IBS-related hospitalizations in a large study using the US National Inpatient Sample database.[37]<br>• Cannabinoid hyperemesis syndrome is a known risk of chronic cannabis use.[38] |

(continued on next page)

**Table 3**
**(continued)**

| Herbal Therapy | Characteristics |
|---|---|
| Peppermint oil<br>*Mentha piperita* | Background<br>• Oil is steam-distilled from leaves of the flowering peppermint plant.[39]<br>• Menthol, the main active ingredient, is absorbed rapidly.[39]<br>• Enteric coated capsules delay release of most of the menthol until the colon.[40]<br>Mechanism of action<br>• Smooth muscle relaxation, modulation of visceral sensitivity, antimicrobial activity, anti-inflammatory effects, and impact on psychosocial distress[39]<br>Recommended dose<br>• 182 mg of small-intestinal-release peppermint oil, 3 times daily, 30 min before meals[41]<br>• IBGard®, 180 mg 1–3 times daily, 30–90 min before meals<br>Clinical studies<br>• Meta-analysis of 12 RCTs with 835 patients found peppermint oil improved global IBS symptoms (NNT 3) and abdominal pain (NNT 4).[42]<br>• A more recent double-blind RCT of 190 patients randomized patients to receive small intestine release peppermint oil, ileocolonic release peppermint oil, or placebo for 8 wk and found no difference in weekly average of worst daily abdominal pain. Peppermint oil did improve secondary outcomes (abdominal pain, discomfort, and IBS severity).[41]<br>Safety<br>• Well tolerated, although can be associated with heartburn (especially nonenteric coated), diarrhea, nausea, vomiting, allergic reactions, asthma exacerbations, and atrial fibrillation[43–45] |
| STW-5 (Iberogast®) | Background<br>• Over-the-counter, fixed combination of 9 herbs (including peppermint) for the treatment of IBS<br>Mechanism of action<br>• Spasmolytic, reduced visceral hyperalgesia[46]<br>Common dose<br>• 1 mL by mouth up to 3 times/d<br>Clinical studies<br>• RCT of 208 patients with IBS receiving STW-5 vs placebo showed reduced composite IBS symptom score at 2 wk and 4 wk compared with placebo.[47]<br>Safety<br>• Several ingredients can cause liver injury, and 1 case required liver transplant.[48,49]<br>• May potentiate sedative and anxiolytic effects of other medications and cause bleeding[50–52] |
| Turmeric<br>*Curcuma longa* | Background<br>• Member of the ginger family of plants[53]<br>• Curcumin is the main active ingredient[53]<br>• Consumed as whole root, dried spice, or a curcumin extract[53,54]<br>Mechanism of action<br>• Antioxidant, antinociceptive, anti-inflammatory properties<br>Common dose<br>• Up to 2 g by mouth daily in divided doses |

*(continued on next page)*

**Table 3**
***(continued)***

| Herbal Therapy | Characteristics |
|---|---|
|  | Clinical studies |
|  | • Systematic review and meta-analysis of 326 patients with IBS in 3 studies found no statistically significant difference in IBS symptoms between curcumin-containing compounds and placebo. The studies were noted to have high risk of bias and heterogeneity, and 3 different formulations containing curcumin with or without other ingredients were used.[55] |
|  | Safety |
|  | • Turmeric has minimal side effects even up to a dose of 12 g daily.[56] |

*Abbreviations:* CBD, cannabidiol; NNT, number needed to treat; THC, delta-9-tetrahydrocannabinol.

[a] FDA approved for nausea and vomiting associated with chemotherapy and for anorexia and weight loss in patients with acquired immunodeficiency syndrome under the trade name, Marinol.

**Table 4**
**Natural products—dietary supplements for the treatment of irritable bowel syndrome**

| Dietary Supplement | Characteristics |
|---|---|
| Glutamine | Background |
|  | • Essential amino acid and energy source for rapidly dividing epithelial cells of the GI tract[57] |
|  | • Glutamine depletion may lead to intestinal permeability.[57] |
|  | Mechanism of action |
|  | • Facilitates restoration of normal intestinal permeability[57] |
|  | Common dose |
|  | • 5 mg by mouth 3 times daily |
|  | Clinical studies |
|  | • RCT of 54 patients with postinfection IBS led to significant improvements in overall and individual IBS symptoms compared with placebo[58] |
|  | Safety |
|  | • Abdominal pain and bloating, although occurred equally between glutamine and placebo groups[58] |
| Melatonin | Background |
|  | • Neurohormone secreted by pineal gland in a circadian pattern in response to decreased light and also is present in enterochromaffin cells of Challenges with Complementary and Alternative the GI tract where it acts in a paracrine manner[59] |
|  | • Abnormal sleep is common in patients with IBS[60–62] |
|  | Mechanism of action |
|  | • Inhibits intestinal contractions, improves sleep, and influence on the microbiome[60–63] |
|  | Common dose |
|  | • 3 mg taken 30–60 min before sleep |

*(continued on next page)*

| Table 4 (continued) | |
|---|---|
| **Dietary Supplement** | **Characteristics** |
| | Clinical studies
• One RCT of 3 mg of melatonin nightly vs placebo showed decreased mean abdominal pain scores but no differences in bloating, stool type or frequency, anxiety, depression, sleep patterns, or polysomnography findings. Two additional studies have found similar findings.[64,65]
Safety
• Daytime drowsiness was similar between melatonin and placebo.[64,65] |
| Vitamin D | Background
• Vitamin D is a fat-soluble vitamin that can be ingested in food or as a supplement or made by exposure to sunlight.[66]
• Vitamin D functions as a steroid hormone and regulates absorption of calcium and phosphate from the gut and bone remodeling.[66]
• Vitamin D deficiency is associated with higher severity of clinical symptoms and lower quality of life in IBS.[67]
Mechanism of action
• Vitamin D deficiency has been associated with increased intestinal permeability, dysbiosis of the gut microbiome, inflammation, depression and anxiety, and reduced quality of life, all of which also are seen in patients with IBS.[66]
Common dose
• 400–800 IU/d (higher doses may be used in deficiency states)
Clinical studies
• RCT trial of 116 patients with IBS found vitamin D supplementation led to significant improvements in IBS-SSS, IBS-QOL, and total symptom scores compared with placebo ($P < .05$).[68] A second RCT of 112 adolescents with IBS and vitamin D deficiency found similar benefits.[69]
• An RCT of 74 IBS patients and vitamin D deficiency found that vitamin D for 9 wk led to significant improvements in IBS-SSS ($P < .01$) and interleukin 6 ($P = .02$) vs placebo.[70]
Safety
• Excess vitamin D from supplementation and cause hypercalciuria and hypercalcemia acutely. Chronic intoxication may cause nephrocalcinosis, bone demineralization, and pain.[71] |

*Abbreviations:* IBS-SSS, IBS severity scoring system; IBS-QOL, IBS quality of life; IU, international.

| Table 5 |
| --- |
| Mind-body medicine for the treatment of irritable bowel syndrome |

| Mind-Body Medicine | Characteristics |
| --- | --- |
| Yoga | Background<br>• The term, *yoga*, comes from the Sanskrit root *yuj*, meaning "to yoke" or "to join."[72]<br>• Ancient practice rooted in Indian philosophy that seeks to unite the mind, body, and spirit using a series of stretching poses (asana), breathing practices (pranayama), and meditation (dhyana).<br>Mechanism of action<br>• May impact gut-brain axis by reducing stress, altering autonomic nervous system function, and improving sleep and quality of life.[73] Unclear if movement and/or breathing have mechanical impacts on the GI tract.<br>Clinical studies<br>• Systematic review of 6 RCTs with 273 patients found yoga reduced bowel symptoms, IBS severity, and anxiety and improved quality of life and physical functioning compared with conventional care.[74] No meta-analysis done due to significant heterogeneity of the studies.<br>• RCT of yoga vs low FODMAP diet for 12 wk found statistically significant within group improvements in IBS-SSS scores but no difference between groups.[75]<br>Safety<br>• No safety data were reported in studies of yoga for IBS.<br>• The broader yoga literature highlights musculoskeletal injuries as the most common injuries. Injuries most likely are with handstands, shoulder stands, and headstands and while practicing without supervision.[76] |
| Acupuncture | Background<br>• Ancient therapy from traditional Chinese medicine using needles to stimulate flow of energy (qi) at points along energetic meridians.<br>Mechanism of action<br>• Unknown<br>Clinical studies<br>• Systematic review and meta-analysis of 17 RCTs with 1806 patients found no difference in IBS symptom severity between acupuncture vs sham acupuncture.[77]<br>• RCT of 233 patients randomized to receive 10 weekly acupuncture sessions in addition to routine care vs routine care alone found a significant improvement in IBS-SSS in the acupuncture group.[78] A follow-up study found persistence of treatment effect at 12 mo but not 24 mo.[79]<br>• Double-blind, sham-controlled study of acupuncture vs sham acupuncture demonstrated no difference in outcomes between groups.[80]<br>Safety<br>• Systematic review of 115 articles (17 case series and 98 case reports), with 479 patients categorized adverse events as traumatic injuries, infectious events, and other adverse events, with traumatic adverse events the most common.[81] |
| Manual therapy | Background<br>• Manual therapies include massage, osteopathy, and chiropractic medicine.<br>• Studies about CAM use for IBS report that patients use manual therapies.[22,23]<br>• There is some evidence supporting the use of massage to treat constipation,[82] but only the traditional tuina therapy—which combined massage, acupressure, myofascial release, and reflexology—has been studied in IBS. |

(*continued on next page*)

| Table 5 (continued) | |
|---|---|
| **Mind-Body Medicine** | **Characteristics** |
| | Mechanism of action |
| | • Unknown |
| | Clinical studies |
| | • Systematic review of 8 studies (5 IBS-D and 3 IBS-C) with 545 patients found tuina with routine care resulted in significant improvement in symptoms compared with routine care alone, but that the effect was no better than routine care when tuina was used alone.[83] |
| | Safety |
| | • No studies of tuina reported safety data. |
| | • Manual therapies generally are safe, although high-amplitude, high-velocity movements used in chiropractic medicine have been associated with greater risks, including vertebral artery dissection.[84] |

*Abbreviations*: FODMAP, fermentable oligosaccharides, disaccharides, monosaccharides, and polyols; IBS-C, IBS with constipation; IBS-D, IBS with diarrhea; IBS-SSS, IBS severity scoring system.

## CHALLENGES WITH COMPLEMENTARY AND ALTERNATIVE MEDICINE THERAPIES
### A Brief History of the Regulation of Dietary Supplements as Food

It is estimated that there are 80,000 dietary supplements for sale over the counter in the United States, with 1000 new supplements introduced each year, with a market value of more than $40 billion.[85] The enormity of the market is daunting not only from a regulatory standpoint but also for health care providers who struggle to stay up to date with the typically scant peer-reviewed literature pertaining to dietary supplements. In addition, the history of regulatory standards for supplements in the United States provides another important vantage point as to why it is so difficult to find, interpret, and give recommendations for or against specific dietary supplements.

Many of the challenges in finding evidence for or against the use of supplements are related directly to the categorization of dietary supplements as food rather than drugs. In 1906, less than a year after the infamous publication of Upton Sinclair's *The Jungle*, Congress passed the Pure Food and Drug Act, which led to the creation of the Bureau of Chemistry (later named the US Food and Drug Administration [FDA], in 1930).[86,87] The Act also put in place regulations to prevent sales of adulterated and misbranded foods, drugs, liquor, and medicine. Per the Act, food included items used for food, drink, confectionary, or condiment by man or animal, whether simple, mixed, or compounded; and drugs were any substances intended to cure, mitigate, or prevent disease of man or animal. The advent of vitamins brought forth challenges with whether to consider supplements as food or drugs. The eventual decision that dietary supplements be classified as foods allowed supplement manufacturers to be subjected to significantly less restrictive regulations compared with drug manufacturers.[86,87]

Since the Pure Food and Drug Act of 1906, several other attempts by Congress to regulate dietary supplements were enacted. The most notable of these was passed by Congress in 1994 and is known as the Dietary Supplement Health and Education Act (DSHEA).[88] DSHEA more formally defined supplements as food rather than drugs. Under DSHEA, the FDA defined specific labeling requirements (ie, "This statement has not been evaluated by the FDA."), regulations for new dietary ingredients marketed after DSHEA were put forth, and requirements for good manufacturing processes created (eg, how a supplement is prepared, packed, and held). DSHEA does not require manufacturers of dietary supplements to obtain premarketing approval or demonstrate efficacy or safety of dietary supplements. For new dietary ingredients, manufacturers need only submit a report highlighting history of use or other evidence of safety establishing that the ingredient used is reasonably expected to be safe within 75 days of marketing a given supplement.[86] This is in contrast to drugs, for which the FDA requires premarket evaluation of safety and efficacy as well as extensive post-marketing surveillance. Despite the FDA's ability to investigate reports of contaminants and/or safety and pull products from the market due to safety concerns, the onus of monitoring and reporting safety concerns to the FDA falls upon supplement companies.[88] Furthermore, there is no centralized list of dietary supplements on the market, which further limits FDA regulatory capacity.

### Relative Lack of Rigorous Research

A Cochrane review on herbal medicines for treatment of IBS included 75 randomized controlled trials (RCTs) involving 7957 participants, with only 3 studies deemed high quality.[89] A more recent systematic review and meta-analysis of CAM therapies for IBS included 66 RCTs (compared with placebo or sham).[90] Herbal therapy (relative risk [RR] 1.57; 95% CI, 1.31–1.88; heterogeneity as indicated by $I^2$ = 77%), dietary supplements (RR 1.95; 95% CI, 1.02–3.73; $I^2$ = 75%), and mind-body therapy (RR 1.67; 95% C,: 1.13–2.49; $I^2$ = 63%) were significantly better than placebo or sham intervention. For abdominal pain, herbal therapy was the only intervention with significant benefit (standard mean difference [SMD] 0.47; 95% CI, 0.20–0.75; $I^2$ = 82%), with mind-body therapy demonstrating borderline statistical significance (SMD 0.29; 95% CI, −0.01–0.59; $I^2$ = 78%). Body-based and energy healing therapies showed no benefit. Overall evidence of included studies was considered low.[90]

### The Breadth of Safety Concerns Related to Complementary and Alternative Medicine Therapies

Many patients and providers believe that natural equates to safe.[24] There often is a general lack of data available, however, to meaningfully counsel patients on the safety of CAM therapies. There are examples of severe adverse events related to CAM therapies, such as hepatotoxicity from Iberogast® (Bayer Australia Limited, New South Wales, Australia) requiring liver transplantation.[48] In addition, many herbs and supplements have potential risks of causing interactions with other medications. When such case reports or case series of adverse events appear in the literature, it can be challenging to know if these are rare and/or idiosyncratic events or if they simply are

---

**Box 1**
**Recommendations for eliciting history of complementary and alternative medicine use in patients with irritable bowel syndrome**

- Ask all patients about use of CAM therapies.
- Ask about specific CAM therapies used for IBS (past, present, and intended).
- Ask about main drivers for use of CAM therapies.
- Ask where patients get their information about CAM therapies.
- Ask about which CAM therapies have helped symptoms.
- Ask about adverse events related to the use of CAM therapies.

---

**Box 2**
**Recommendations for guiding patients on use of complementary and alternative medicine therapies**

1. Define the duration of treatment trials. (eg, a trial of 2–4 wk).

2. Patients' and providers' treatment expectations (eg, set goals) should be aligned.

3. Help the patient understand optimal dose, timing, and frequency of any recommended supplement.

4. Inform patients of potential adverse events and any known drug-supplement interactions.

---

underreported. Risk of underreporting of adverse events also may occur with manual therapies, in which case there may be a disincentive for providers to report their own complications. For example, a systematic review of adverse events related to acupuncture found that only 20% of the case series and reports were published by the practitioners performing the procedure at the time of the adverse event.[91]

Lack of standardized regulations for supplements also poses the threat of being dosed over the recommended or desired amount. For example, 1 study of over-the-counter melatonin supplements found that doses varied from less than 83% to more than 478% of the labeled dose and that 26% contained serotonin.[92] Therefore, even when a suggested dose has reasonable evidence to support it, the potential for overdosing and underdosing patients is significant, again due to lack of standardization.

CAM therapies typically are over the counter, and out-of-pocket expenses can be significant for patients. Americans spent more than $30 billion on CAM therapies in 2016, and that number is thought to be increasing over time.[93] Patients may use CAM therapies in place of well-evidenced, conventional treatments, posing additional risks of harm.

Lastly, physicians receive little to no training in CAM. The Academic Consortium for Integrative Medicine and Health consists of more than 75 academic medicine centers in the United States and abroad and has sought to incorporate medical education on CAM therapies for Western medical trainees and practitioners. There are no widely used, standardized curricula in US medical schools, however in **Box 1** and **Box 2**.

## RECOMMENDATIONS FOR ASKING ABOUT AND COUNSELING PATIENTS ON COMPLEMENTARY AND ALTERNATIVE MEDICINE USE

Despite the limitations of the evidence for many CAM therapies, patients continue to express interest in and make use of CAM therapies. Therefore, it is helpful for providers to develop approaches for both eliciting a history of CAM use (**Box 1**) and counseling patients on use of CAM therapies (**Box 2**). Some guidance, based on the experience of the authors, is provided in **Box 1** and **Box 2**.

## SUMMARY

IBS remains a common and often difficult to manage condition. Despite a growing literature base related to CAM therapies for IBS, significant limitations in study design hinder the evidence-based application of many of these therapies to patients. Nonetheless, patients often use CAM therapies in attempts to alleviate symptoms and improve quality of life; CAM often allows patients to feel in control of their symptoms. Therefore, providers should familiarize themselves with various CAM therapies, identify resources for finding evidence-based CAM literature, and explicitly ask patients about their use of CAM.

## CLINICS CARE POINTS

---

- Providers should ask all patients with IBS about CAM use because CAM use is common, often not due to dissatisfaction with conventional care, and may not be disclosed to providers.

- Many natural products and mind-body medicine therapies have been studied for the treatment of IBS, although the overall evidence for CAM therapies to treat IBS is low quality.

- The evidence for safety of many CAM therapies is lacking, and safety concerns related to CAM therapies include known side effects, many of which are idiosyncratic (eg, hepatotoxicity of Iberogast); unrecognized side effects; interactions with conventional therapies (eg, herb-drug interactions); risks related to forgoing conventional therapies; and cost.

- Dietary supplements are regulated as foods, limiting the ability of the FDA to require demonstration of efficacy or safety prior to marketing of supplements.

- Physicians receive little training in counseling patients on the use of CAM therapies.

- Use of shared decision making for CAM in the treatment of IBS may help providers to better understand which CAM is being used, how patients became interested in using CAM, and what is or is not known about efficacy and safety.

---

## DISCLOSURE

Dr.Shapiro was supported by a T32 training Grant (5T32DK083266-08) and with the use of resources and facilities from the Texas Medical Center Digestive Disease Core (2P30DK056338-16), both funded by the NIH NIDDK. In addition, the project was supported by resources from the Houston VA HSR&D Center for Innovations in Quality, Effectiveness and Safety (CIN13-413). The views expressed are those of the authors and not necessarily those of the NIH, NIDDK, Department of Veterans Affairs, the U.S. government, or Baylor College of Medicine. Dr.Deutsch had no funding sources.

## REFERENCES

1. van Tilburg MA, Hyman PE, Walker L, et al. Prevalence of functional gastrointestinal disorders in infants and toddlers. J Pediatr 2015;166(3):684–9.
2. Lewis ML, Palsson OS, Whitehead WE, et al. Prevalence of functional gastrointestinal disorders in children and adolescents. J Pediatr 2016;177:39–43.e3.
3. Ford AC, Bercik P, Morgan DG, et al. Characteristics of functional bowel disorder patients: a cross-sectional survey using the Rome III criteria. Aliment Pharmacol Ther 2014;39(3):312–21.
4. Chang SYJM. Consulters and nonconsulters in irritable bowel syndrome: what makes an IBS patient? Pract Gastroenterol 2003;6:15–26.
5. Staller K, Olén O, Söderling J, et al. Mortality risk in irritable bowel syndrome: results from a nationwide prospective cohort study. Am J Gastroenterol 2020; 115(5):746–55.
6. Drossman DA, Morris CB, Schneck S, et al. International survey of patients with IBS: symptom features and their severity, health status, treatments, and risk taking to achieve clinical benefit. J Clin Gastroenterol 2009;43(6):541–50.
7. NCCIH Timeline. Available at: https://www.nccih.nih.gov/about/nccih-timeline. Accessed December 3, 2020.

8. Conventional Medicine. Available at: https://www.merriam-webster.com/dictionary/conventional%20medicine. Accessed December 3, 2020.

9. Alternative Medicine. Available at: https://www.merriam-webster.com/dictionary/alternative%20medicine. Accessed December 3, 2020.

10. Complementary Medicine. Available at: https://www.merriam-webster.com/dictionary/complementary%20medicine. Accessed December 3, 2020.

11. Academic Consortium for Integrative Medicine and Health, Introduction. Available at: https://imconsortium.org/about/introduction/. Accessed December 3, 2020.

12. Complementary, Alternative, or Integrative Health: What's In a Name?. Available at: https://www.nccih.nih.gov/health/complementary-alternative-or-integrative-health-whats-in-a-name. Accessed December 3, 2020.

13. Eisenberg DM, Kessler RC, Foster C, et al. Unconventional medicine in the United States. Prevalence, costs, and patterns of use. N Engl J Med 1993; 328(4):246–52.

14. Eisenberg DM, Kessler RC, Van Rompay MI, et al. Perceptions about complementary therapies relative to conventional therapies among adults who use both: results from a national survey. Ann Intern Med 2001;135(5):344–51.

15. Astin JA. Why patients use alternative medicine: results of a national study. JAMA 1998;279(19):1548–53.

16. Eisenberg DM, Davis RB, Ettner SL, et al. Trends in alternative medicine use in the United States, 1990-1997: results of a follow-up national survey. JAMA 1998;280(18):1569–75.

17. Larussa T, Rossi M, Suraci E, et al. Use of complementary and alternative medicine by patients with irritable bowel syndrome according to the Roma IV criteria: a single-center Italian survey. Medicina (Kaunas) 2019;55(2).

18. Kong SC, Hurlstone DP, Pocock CY, et al. The Incidence of self-prescribed oral complementary and alternative medicine use by patients with gastrointestinal diseases. J Clin Gastroenterol 2005;39(2):138–41.

19. Erdogan Z, Kurçer MA. Dietary supplement use in gastrointestinal symptom management and effect on hopelessness levels in patients with irritable bowel syndrome. Holist Nurs Pract 2019;33(3):155–62.

20. Carmona-Sanchez R, Tostado-Fernandez FA. [Prevalence of use of alternative and complementary medicine in patients with irritable bowel syndrome, functional dyspepsia and gastroesophageal reflux disease]. Rev Gastroenterol Mex 2005;70(4):393–8. La prevalencia del uso de medicina alternativa y complementaria en pacientes con sindrome de intestino irritable, dispepsia funcional y enfermedad por reflujo gastroesofagico.

21. Koloski NA, Talley NJ, Huskic SS, et al. Predictors of conventional and alternative health care seeking for irritable bowel syndrome and functional dyspepsia. Aliment Pharmacol Ther 2003;17(6):841–51.

22. Dossett ML, Davis RB, Lembo AJ, et al. Complementary and alternative medicine use by US adults with gastrointestinal conditions: Results from the 2012 National Health Interview Survey. Am J Gastroenterol 2014;109(11):1705–11.

23. van Tilburg MA, Palsson OS, Levy RL, et al. Complementary and alternative medicine use and cost in functional bowel disorders: a six month prospective study in a large HMO. BMC Complement Altern Med 2008;8:46.

24. Hung A, Kang N, Bollom A, et al. Complementary and alternative medicine use is prevalent among patients with gastrointestinal diseases. Dig Dis Sci 2015;60(7): 1883–8.

25. Basnayake C, Kamm MA, Stanley A, et al. Standard gastroenterologist versus multidisciplinary treatment for functional gastrointestinal disorders (MANTRA): an open-label, single-centre, randomised controlled trial. Lancet Gastroenterol Hepatol 2020;5(10):890–9.

26. Hong SW, Chun J, Park S, et al. Aloe vera is effective and safe in short-term treatment of irritable bowel syndrome: a systematic review and meta-analysis. J Neurogastroenterol Motil 2018;24(4):528–35.

27. Eamlamnam K, Patumraj S, Visedopas N, et al. Effects of Aloe vera and sucralfate on gastric microcirculatory changes, cytokine levels and gastric ulcer healing in rats. World J Gastroenterol 2006;12(13):2034–9.

28. Werawatganon D, Rakananurak N, Sallapant S, et al. Aloe vera attenuated gastric injury on indomethacin-induced gastropathy in rats. World J Gastroenterol 2014; 20(48):18330–7.

29. Yang HN, Kim DJ, Kim YM, et al. Aloe-induced toxic hepatitis. J Korean Med Sci 2010;25(3):492–5.

30. Bonini SA, Premoli M, Tambaro S, et al. Cannabis sativa: a comprehensive ethnopharmacological review of a medicinal plant with a long history. J Ethnopharmacol 2018;227:300–15.

31. Sharkey KA, Wiley JW. The role of the endocannabinoid system in the brain-gut axis. Gastroenterology 2016;151(2):252–66.

32. Camilleri M. Cannabinoids and gastrointestinal motility: Pharmacology, clinical effects, and potential therapeutics in humans. Neurogastroenterol Motil 2018;30(9): e13370.

33. Esfandyari T, Camilleri M, Busciglio I, et al. Effects of a cannabinoid receptor agonist on colonic motor and sensory functions in humans: a randomized, placebo-controlled study. Am J Physiol Gastrointest Liver Physiol 2007;293(1): G137–45.

34. Wong BS, Camilleri M, Eckert D, et al. Randomized pharmacodynamic and pharmacogenetic trial of dronabinol effects on colon transit in irritable bowel syndrome-diarrhea. Neurogastroenterol Motil 2012;24(4):358.

35. Klooker TK, Leliefeld KE, Van Den Wijngaard RM, et al. The cannabinoid receptor agonist delta-9-tetrahydrocannabinol does not affect visceral sensitivity to rectal distension in healthy volunteers and IBS patients. Neurogastroenterol Motil 2011; 23(1):30–5.e2.

36. Wong BS, Camilleri M, Busciglio I, et al. Pharmacogenetic trial of a cannabinoid agonist shows reduced fasting colonic motility in patients with nonconstipated irritable bowel syndrome. Gastroenterology 2011;141(5):1638–47, e1-7.

37. Patel RS, Goyal H, Satodiya R, et al. Relationship of Cannabis Use Disorder and Irritable Bowel Syndrome (IBS): an analysis of 6.8 million hospitalizations in the United States. Subst Use Misuse 2019;1–10. https://doi.org/10.1080/10826084. 2019.1664591.

38. Venkatesan T, Levinthal DJ, Li BUK, et al. Role of chronic cannabis use: cyclic vomiting syndrome vs cannabinoid hyperemesis syndrome. Neurogastroenterol Motil 2019;31(Suppl 2):e13606.

39. Chumpitazi BP, Kearns GL, Shulman RJ. Review article: the physiological effects and safety of peppermint oil and its efficacy in irritable bowel syndrome and other functional disorders. Aliment Pharmacol Ther 2018;47(6):738–52.

40. Somerville KW, Richmond CR, Bell GD. Delayed release peppermint oil capsules (Colpermin) for the spastic colon syndrome: a pharmacokinetic study. Br J Clin Pharmacol 1984;18(4):638–40.

41. Weerts ZZRM, Masclee AAM, Witteman BJM, et al. Efficacy and safety of peppermint oil in a randomized, double-blind trial of patients with irritable bowel syndrome. Gastroenterology 2020;158(1):123–36.
42. Alammar N, Wang L, Saberi B, et al. The impact of peppermint oil on the irritable bowel syndrome: a meta-analysis of the pooled clinical data. BMC Complement Altern Med 2019;19(1):21.
43. Wilkinson SM, Beck MH. Allergic contact dermatitis from menthol in peppermint. Contact Dermatitis 1994;30(1):42–3.
44. Spurlock BW, Dailey TM. Shortness of (fresh) breath–toothpaste-induced bronchospasm. N Engl J Med 1990;323(26):1845–6.
45. Nurick S. Atrial fibrillation and peppermint eating. Report of a case. Guys Hosp Rep 1963;112:171–4.
46. Allescher HD, Abdel-Aziz H. Mechanism of action of STW 5 in functional dyspepsia and IBS: the origin of multi-target. Dig Dis 2017;35(Suppl 1):18–24.
47. Madisch A, Holtmann G, Plein K, et al. Treatment of irritable bowel syndrome with herbal preparations: results of a double-blind, randomized, placebo-controlled, multi-centre trial. Aliment Pharmacol Ther 2004;19(3):271–9.
48. Sáez-González E, Conde I, Díaz-Jaime FC, et al. Iberogast-induced severe hepatotoxicity leading to liver transplantation. Am J Gastroenterol 2016;111(9): 1364–5.
49. Benninger J, Schneider HT, Schuppan D, et al. Acute hepatitis induced by greater celandine (Chelidonium majus). Gastroenterology 1999;117(5):1234–7.
50. O'Hara M, Kiefer D, Farrell K, et al. A review of 12 commonly used medicinal herbs. Arch Fam Med 1998;7(6):523–36.
51. Gruenwald JBT, Jaenicke C. PDR for herbal medicines. Montvale, NJ: Medical Economics; 1998.
52. Venkataramanan R, Ramachandran V, Komoroski BJ, et al. Milk thistle, a herbal supplement, decreases the activity of CYP3A4 and uridine diphosphoglucuronosyl transferase in human hepatocyte cultures. Drug Metab Dispos 2000;28(11): 1270–3.
53. Hewlings SJ, Kalman DS. Curcumin: a review of its' effects on human health. Foods 2017;6(10):92.
54. Xu XY, Meng X, Li S, et al. Bioactivity, health benefits, and related molecular mechanisms of curcumin: current progress, challenges, and perspectives. Nutrients 2018;10(10):1553.
55. Ng QX, Soh AYS, Loke W, et al. A meta-analysis of the clinical use of curcumin for irritable bowel syndrome (IBS). J Clin Med 2018;7(10):298.
56. Gupta SC, Patchva S, Aggarwal BB. Therapeutic roles of curcumin: lessons learned from clinical trials. AAPS J 2013;15(1):195–218.
57. Achamrah N, Déchelotte P, Coëffier M. Glutamine and the regulation of intestinal permeability: from bench to bedside. Curr Opin Clin Nutr Metab Care 2017;20(1): 86–91.
58. Zhou Q, Verne ML, Fields JZ, et al. Randomised placebo-controlled trial of dietary glutamine supplements for postinfectious irritable bowel syndrome. Gut 2019; 68(6):996–1002.
59. Chen CQ, Fichna J, Bashashati M, et al. Distribution, function and physiological role of melatonin in the lower gut. World J Gastroenterol 2011;17(34):3888–98.
60. Jarrett M, Heitkemper M, Cain KC, et al. Sleep disturbance influences gastrointestinal symptoms in women with irritable bowel syndrome. Dig Dis Sci 2000; 45(5):952–9.

61. Wong RK, Yang C, Song GH, et al. Melatonin regulation as a possible mechanism for probiotic (VSL#3) in irritable bowel syndrome: a randomized double-blinded placebo study. Dig Dis Sci 2015;60(1):186–94.

62. Fass R, Fullerton S, Tung S, et al. Sleep disturbances in clinic patients with functional bowel disorders. Am J Gastroenterol 2000;95(5):1195–2000.

63. Quastel MR, Rahamimoff R. Effect of melatonin on spontaneous contractions and response to 5-hydroxytryptamine of rat isolated duodenum. Br J Pharmacol Chemother 1965;24:455–61.

64. Lu WZ, Gwee KA, Moochhalla S, et al. Melatonin improves bowel symptoms in female patients with irritable bowel syndrome: a double-blind placebo-controlled study. Aliment Pharmacol Ther 2005;22(10):927–34.

65. Saha L, Malhotra S, Rana S, et al. A preliminary study of melatonin in irritable bowel syndrome. J Clin Gastroenterol 2007;41(1):29–32.

66. Barbalho SM, Goulart RA, Araújo AC, et al. Irritable bowel syndrome: a review of the general aspects and the potential role of vitamin D. Expert Rev Gastroenterol Hepatol 2019;13(4):345–59.

67. Abbasnezhad A, Amani R, Hasanvand A, et al. Association of Serum Vitamin D concentration with clinical symptoms and quality of life in patients with irritable bowel syndrome. J Am Coll Nutr 2019;38(4):327–33.

68. Jalili M, Vahedi H, Poustchi H, et al. Effects of Vitamin D supplementation in patients with irritable bowel syndrome: a randomized, double-blind, placebo-controlled clinical trial. Int J Prev Med 2019;10:16.

69. El Amrousy D, Hassan S, El Ashry H, et al. Vitamin D supplementation in adolescents with irritable bowel syndrome: Is it useful? A randomized controlled trial. Saudi J Gastroenterol 2018;24(2):109–14.

70. Khalighi Sikaroudi M, Mokhtare M, Janani L, et al. Vitamin D3 supplementation in diarrhea-predominant irritable bowel syndrome patients: the effects on symptoms improvement, serum corticotropin-releasing hormone, and interleukin-6 - a randomized clinical trial. Complement Med Res 2020;27(5):302–9.

71. Pludowski P, Holick MF, Grant WB, et al. Vitamin D supplementation guidelines. J Steroid Biochem Mol Biol 2018;175:125–35.

72. Kavuri V, Raghuram N, Malamud A, et al. Irritable bowel syndrome: yoga as remedial therapy. Evid Based Complement Alternat Med 2015;2015:398156.

73. D'Silva A, MacQueen G, Nasser Y, et al. Yoga as a therapy for irritable bowel syndrome. Dig Dis Sci 2020;65(9):2503–14.

74. Schumann D, Anheyer D, Lauche R, et al. Effect of yoga in the therapy of irritable bowel syndrome: a systematic review. Clin Gastroenterol Hepatol 2016;14(12):1720–31.

75. Schumann D, Langhorst J, Dobos G, et al. Randomised clinical trial: yoga vs a low-FODMAP diet in patients with irritable bowel syndrome. Aliment Pharmacol Ther 2018;47(2):203–11.

76. Cramer H, Quinker D, Schumann D, et al. Adverse effects of yoga: a national cross-sectional survey. BMC Complement Altern Med 2019;19(1):190.

77. Manheimer E, Wieland LS, Cheng K, et al. Acupuncture for irritable bowel syndrome: systematic review and meta-analysis. Am J Gastroenterol 2012;107(6):835–47 [quiz 848].

78. MacPherson H, Tilbrook H, Bland JM, et al. Acupuncture for irritable bowel syndrome: primary care based pragmatic randomised controlled trial. BMC Gastroenterol 2012;12:150.

79. MacPherson H, Tilbrook H, Agbedjro D, et al. Acupuncture for irritable bowel syndrome: 2-year follow-up of a randomised controlled trial. Acupunct Med 2017; 35(1):17–23.

80. Lowe C, Aiken A, Day AG, et al. Sham acupuncture is as efficacious as true acupuncture for the treatment of IBS: a randomized placebo controlled trial. Neurogastroenterol Motil 2017;29(7).

81. Zhang J, Shang H, Gao X, et al. Acupuncture-related adverse events: a systematic review of the Chinese literature. Bull World Health Organ 2010;88(12):915–921C.

82. Yıldırım D, Can G, Köknel Talu G. The efficacy of abdominal massage in managing opioid-induced constipation. Eur J Oncol Nurs 2019;41:110–9.

83. Bu FL, Han M, Lu CL, et al. A systematic review of Tuina for irritable bowel syndrome: Recommendations for future trials. Complement Ther Med 2020;52: 102504.

84. Ernst E. Adverse effects of spinal manipulation: a systematic review. J R Soc Med 2007;100(7):330–8.

85. Gottlieb S. Statement from FDA Commissioner Scott Gottlieb, M.D., on the agency's new efforts to strengthen regulation of dietary supplements by modernizing and reforming FDA's oversight. Available at: https://www.fda.gov/news-events/press-announcements/statement-fda-commissioner-scott-gottlieb-md-agencys-new-efforts-strengthen-regulation-dietary. Accessed December 3, 2020.

86. Kennett G. Time for change: stepping up the FDA's regulation of dietary supplements to promote consumer safety and awareness. J Law Health 2019;33(1): 47–78.

87. Swann JP. The history of efforts to regulate dietary supplements in the USA. Drug Test Anal 2016;8(3–4):271–82.

88. Questions and answers on dietary supplements.(2019, July 22). Available at: https://www.fda.gov/food/information-consumers-using-dietary-supplements/questions-and-answers-dietary-supplements. Accessed March 20, 2021.

89. Liu JP, Yang M, Liu YX, et al. Herbal medicines for treatment of irritable bowel syndrome. Cochrane Database Syst Rev 2006;(1):CD004116.

90. Billings W, Mathur K, Craven HJ, et al. Potential benefit with complementary and alternative medicine in irritable bowel syndrome: a systematic review and meta-analysis. Clin Gastroenterol Hepatol 2020 Sep 19;S1542-3565(20):31296-9. https://doi.org/10.1016/j.cgh.2020.09.035.

91. Chan MWC, Wu XY, Wu JCY, et al. Safety of acupuncture: overview of systematic reviews. Sci Rep 2017;7(1):3369.

92. Erland LA, Saxena PK. Melatonin natural health products and supplements: presence of serotonin and significant variability of melatonin content. J Clin Sleep Med 2017;13(2):275–81.

93. Nahin RL, Barnes PM, Stussman BJ. Expenditures on complementary health approaches: United States, 2012. Natl Health Stat Rep 2016;(95):1–11.

# The Dilemma of Persistent Irritable Bowel Syndrome Symptoms in Patients with Quiescent Inflammatory Bowel Disease

Edith Pérez de Arce, MD[a], Rodrigo Quera, MD[b],
Eamonn M.M. Quigley, MD, FRCP, MACG, FRCPI, MWGO[c],*

KEYWORDS

- Irritable bowel syndrome • Inflammatory bowel disease • Crohn's disease
- Ulcerative colitis • Fecal calprotectin • Brain–gut axis • Microbiome

KEY POINTS

- Irritable bowel syndrome symptoms are common in patients with inflammatory bowel disease who are in apparent remission and, if misinterpreted, can lead to inappropriate escalations in therapy.
- The detection of ongoing inflammatory bowel disease activity can be assisted by the use of biomarkers such as fecal calprotectin.
- If deep remission is confirmed and symptoms persist, other diagnoses need to be entertained, including carbohydrate intolerance, small intestinal bacterial overgrowth, PEI, and bile acid malabsorption/diarrhea.
- Noninflammatory complications of inflammatory bowel disease such as strictures and fistula should also be considered.
- Data on the management of those patients with persistent symptoms and truly quiescent inflammatory bowel disease is scanty and high-quality trials are needed.

---

Conflicts of Interest: Drs E. Pérez de Arce and R. Quera report no conflicts. Dr E.M.M. Quigley serves as a consultant to 4D Pharma, Allergan, Atlantia, Biocodex, Ironwood, Novozymes, Precisionbiotics, Salix, and Vibrant and receives research funding from 4D Pharma, Biomerica, Vibrant, and Zealand Pharma.
<sup>a</sup> Department of Medicine, Division of Gastroenterology, Hospital Clínico Universidad de Chile, Dr. Carlos Lorca Tobar 999, Independencia, Región Metropolitana, Santiago, Chile; <sup>b</sup> Division of Gastroenterology, Inflammatory Bowel Disease Program, Clínica Universidad de los Andes, Estoril 450, Las Condes, Región Metropolitana, Santiago, Chile; <sup>c</sup> Division of Gastroenterology and Hepatology, Lynda K and David M Underwood Center for Digestive Disorders, Houston Methodist Hospital, Weill Cornell Medical College, Houston, TX, USA
* Corresponding author. 6550 Fannin Street, SM 1201, Houston, TX 77030.
E-mail address: equigley@houstonmethodist.org

Gastroenterol Clin N Am 50 (2021) 689–711
https://doi.org/10.1016/j.gtc.2021.03.008
gastro.theclinics.com

## INTRODUCTION

With the use of the full armamentarium that is now at our disposal, endoscopic and histologic remission of inflammation in the patient with inflammatory bowel disease (IBD) is commonly achieved; yet, at least one-third of patients with now apparently quiescent IBD complain of persistent symptoms akin to those that typify irritable bowel syndrome (IBS) and suffer a consequential impairment of their quality of life and mental health.[1,2] Because these IBS-like symptoms are nonspecific and can mimic those suggestive of active IBD, they can be confused with IBD disease activity and lead to unnecessary intensification of treatment. It is for this reason that finding the cause of persistent IBS symptoms in patients with quiescent IBD is a clinical challenge worthy of reflection. If these symptoms do not represent subclinical activity of IBD, are they the harbingers of a "true" IBS superimposed on IBD, or do they reflect postinflammatory macroscopic and/or ultrastructural and functional sequela of IBD in remission? Some have even asked the question: Is IBS a milder expression of IBD?

At this point, it is interesting to imagine how disorders that differ so fundamentally in terms of the extent of involvement of, and degree of inflammation in, the intestinal mucosa could be related in the same individual. Despite the profound differences that distinguish IBS from IBD, there are some similarities that go beyond sharing some clinical symptoms (abdominal pain, diarrhea, bloating, urgency), a chronic course, and typically fluctuating pattern of disease activity.

## DIFFERENCES AND SIMILARITIES BETWEEN IRRITABLE BOWEL SYNDROME AND INFLAMMATORY BOWEL DISEASE

From an epidemiologic point of view, IBD and IBS are different. The prevalence of IBD is estimated to be between 130 and 240 per 100,000 population and both its incidence and prevalence are increasing in parallel with the industrialization and urbanization of populations around the world; consequently, although increasing across the globe, prevalence rates remain highest in Western countries.[3] Its peak incidence is between 20 and 30 years of age, with no significant differences by sex.[4] However, IBS seems to be common around the world and in both urban and rural environments, with a prevalence ranging from 12.8% to 15.0% in the general population; it is more common in women and among those between the ages of 30 and 50 years.[5] In relation to the diagnosis of IBD, this is established on the basis of symptoms (abdominal pain, diarrhea, rectal bleeding), combined with endoscopic, histologic, and/or imaging studies that reveal intestinal inflammation.[6] Interactions between the intestinal microbiota, the immune response, and genetic and environmental factors are key contributors to the pathophysiology of IBD.[6,7]

Nowadays, the diagnosis of IBS rests on clinical criteria such as those proposed in the fourth iteration of the Rome process, Rome IV, in which the cardinal feature of IBS is the presence of abdominal pain associated with defecation or a change in bowel habits in a patient without alarm symptoms (fever, weight loss, bleeding, or anemia),[8] the latter being more indicative of IBD than IBS. The pathophysiology of IBS is complex, multifactorial, and likely heterogeneous and involves environmental, host-related, and psychosocial factors that variably lead to alterations in gastrointestinal motility, visceral sensation, intestinal permeability, immune responses, and the gut microbiota, any and all of which may lead to a disruption in communication along the brain–gut axis.[9]

Interestingly, it has been seen that the role of the brain–gut axis is not exclusive to what were previously referred to as the functional digestive disorders, whose most extensively investigated representative is IBS, but is also invoked in IBD.[10] Some data from small observational studies suggest that psychological distress and stressful events could cause an exacerbation of symptoms in patients with IBD and that psychological factors could be associated with relapse of the disease, thereby generating even greater psychological distress.[11–13]

## IRRITABLE BOWEL SYNDROME IN INFLAMMATORY BOWEL DISEASE: MAGNITUDE OF THE PROBLEM

The first report of the interaction between IBS and IBD was made by Isgar and colleagues[1] in 1983, who studied 98 patients with ulcerative colitis (UC) in clinical and endoscopic remission; 33% had symptoms that qualified as representing IBS according to Manning criteria. Subsequent observational studies using different methodologies and criteria for the remission of IBD placed this prevalence in a range of 19% to 45%.[14–19] A systematic review and meta-analysis of observational studies, in which patients with disease activity were also included, estimated the prevalence of IBS symptoms in IBD at 40%.[20]

However, a more recent and rigorous meta-analysis that included 3169 patients from 18 eligible studies found a pooled prevalence of IBS symptoms in quiescent IBD of 32.5%, which was lower when remission was defined at endoscopy (23.5%) or histology (25.8%) in comparison with clinical scales alone (33.6%); the prevalence was also higher for Crohn's disease (CD) than UC (36.6% vs 28.5%).[2] These prevalence rates are far from trivial, given that the presence of IBS symptoms in IBD has been associated with a marked deterioration in quality of life as well as the occurrence of depression and anxiety.[15] Regardless of the remission criteria used, prevalence data for IBS in IBD remain high. Some authors have described an association between the duration of IBD and the presence of IBS symptoms,[16,21] but not with age, the chronic use of anti-inflammatory treatments, or disease extent, in both UC and CD.[21]

Although most studies of IBS in IBD in remission showed a greater prevalence of IBS symptoms in CD than UC,[2,20] none reported on the use of dedicated imaging or video capsule endoscopy to evaluate small bowel involvement where occult inflammation not detectable by ileo-colonoscopy or biomarkers such as fecal calprotectin (FC) (although the usefulness of FC in this clinical setting is questionable), could linger.[22] In contrast, other potential causes of IBS-like symptoms in IBD (small intestinal bacterial overgrowth [SIBO], carbohydrate malabsorption, bile acid diarrhea, and noninflammatory mechanical complications such as strictures or fistulas) were exhaustively excluded in many of the studies discussed in this article. Therefore, it is likely that, with a more rigorous approach, the prevalence of IBS in IBD would be much lower than has been reported to date.

## PATHOPHYSIOLOGY OF IRRITABLE BOWEL SYNDROME AND INFLAMMATORY BOWEL DISEASE: SOME COMMON GROUND?
### Genetic Aspects

Genome-wide association studies have identified more than 240 susceptibility loci in IBD that include intracellular pathways recognizing microbial products (NOD2), autophagy, as well as genes regulating epithelial barrier function and pathways regulating innate and adaptive immunity.[7] Unlike IBD, genetic factors have not been fully established in IBS; however, both CD and IBS have been associated with genes encoding for members of the tumor necrosis factor superfamily (TNFSF). The TNFSF15 gene encodes for TNF-like protein 1A (TL1A) that is involved in defense against pathogens and modulates the interactions between host and intestinal microbiota. The risk allele for

CD, rs423839 G in the TNFSF15 gene, has been associated with an increased risk of IBS[23] and in a manner similar to that seen with other polymorphisms.[24]

### Immune Activation and Disruption of the Epithelial Barrier

The immune system, well-known to be fundamental to the pathophysiology of IBD, may also play a role in IBS. Accordingly, studies in subgroups of patients with IBS have identified changes suggestive of immune activation. Findings have included an increase in number and activation of mast cells, CD3+ T cells[25,26] and plasma cells[26] in colonic biopsies. In addition, an upregulation of Toll-like receptors (TLRs) and of TLR-4 and TLR-5, in particular, in the colon has been described,[27,28] as well as an increase in the proinflammatory cytokines IL-6, IL-8, and TNF-$\alpha$ in the plasma[29,30] and colonic biopsies.[27] Another finding was an increase in the expression of the chemokine CXCL-11 and its CXCR-3 receptor associated with a decrease in IL-10, an anti-inflammatory cytokine.[27]

The presence of persistent microinflammation could contribute to alterations in the permeability of the intestinal epithelial barrier in patients with quiescent IBD with IBS symptoms similar to that observed in patients with classic IBS.[31] In a subgroup of patients with UC with IBS symptoms despite documented deep remission, higher levels of serum cytokines (IL-1b, IL-6, IL-13, IL-10, and IL-8) were found compared with asymptomatic patients with UC in deep remission, in addition to higher levels of anxiety and depression and a greater perception of stress.[17] In this regard, a recent study observed distinctive profiles of systemic inflammatory proteins in patients with UC and IBS, independent of the activity of UC or the presence of IBS-like symptoms in patients with UC in remission, which suggests that the inflammatory mechanisms of these diseases could be different.[32]

A disruption of the intestinal epithelial barrier has been described in both IBD[33] and IBS.[34,35] One study demonstrated an increase in paracellular permeability, and a decrease in the messenger RNA expression of tight junction proteins (zonula occludens-1, $\alpha$-catenin, and occludin) in cecal biopsies from patients with quiescent IBD with IBS symptoms and in patients with IBS in comparison with those with asymptomatic quiescent IBD and controls. Another significant finding was an increase in intraepithelial lymphocytes and TNF-$\alpha$ expression in biopsies of patients with IBD with IBS-like symptoms, a feature not typically seen in patients with IBS.[36] This last finding also suggests a distinction between classic IBS and the form of IBS that occurs in patients with IBD in remission. Other authors also demonstrated increased intestinal permeability in patients with quiescent IBD with IBS symptoms in comparison with quiescent IBD without such symptoms, as well as in controls.[37] Katinios and colleagues,[31] in contrast, observed increased paracellular permeability of the intestinal epithelium in colonic biopsies from patients with inactive UC (clinical and endoscopic remission) and patients with the mixed subtype of IBS, compared with control patients. It should be noted that these patients with UC had been treated within the previous year for relapse of their disease, which could explain the existence of increased intestinal permeability despite remission and contrasts with findings from studies of patients with UC who were in a more prolonged remission.[37,38]

Finally, a recent study that included 35 patients with IBD in deep remission with IBS symptoms reported an increase in the number of eosinophils in the colonic mucosa compared with asymptomatic patients in remission (mean, 421 eosinophils/mm$^2$ in UC vs 397 eosinophils/mm$^2$ in CD and 36 eosinophils/mm$^2$ in controls) that decreased when they were treated with a hypoallergenic diet and oral budesonide, with a favorable clinical response in 67% within 7 to 10 days.[39] These authors went on to suggest that allergenic foods could trigger an immune response in a previously altered mucosa, thereby explaining the development of IBS-type symptoms in some patients with IBD in remission. It needs to be noted that minor increases in eosinophils have also been described previously in active IBD[40,41]; given the current interest in food-related symptoms in IBS and other functional gastrointestinal diseases, these findings suggest that food allergy could play a role in IBS symptoms in patients with IBD through the effects of eosinophils.

## Alterations in Intestinal Microbiota

Although alterations in gut microbiota, in comparison with the normal population, have been described in both IBS and IBD, evidence of a role for gut microbiota in disease pathogenesis is better established for IBD than for IBS. A decrease in bacterial diversity and qualitative and quantitative changes in various microbial populations have been described in both disorders. For example, an increase in bacterial species such as *Fusobacterium* species, *Pasturellaceae, Proteobacteria, Ruminococcus gnavus*, and *Veillonellaceae* has been described in IBD. In contrast, *Bacteroides* species, *Bifidobacterium* species, *Clostridium* clusters XIVa and IV, *Faecalibacterium prausnitzii*, *Roseburia* species, and *Suterella* species have been found to be decreased. These changes in gut microbiota are believed to exert proinflammatory effects and tend to be more unstable over time in CD than in UC.[42] In IBS, a relative abundance of proinflammatory bacteria species (such a Enterobacteriaceae) has been described in some studies, accompanied by a reduction in *Lactobacillus* and *Bifidobacterium*, in addition to changes in the overall *Firmicutes/Bacteroidetes* ratio.[43] It needs to be emphasized that changes in microbiota composition in IBS have not been consistent, no doubt reflecting the heterogeneity of the IBS phenotype and the impact of such confounders as diet, among others. Microbiota studies in IBD also suffer from variability; here again, a variable clinical phenotype coupled with the effects of active inflammation or disease activity undoubtedly contribute.

An interesting study revealed that the presence of IBS symptoms in patients with quiescent IBD was not associated with distinctive alterations in the abundance of individual bacterial taxa or in global bacterial diversity compared with patients with asymptomatic, quiescent IBD (defined as a FC level of <250 μg/g), active IBD and IBD with occult inflammation (ie, asymptomatic patients with IBD with a FC level of >250 μg/g). However, this study did not include either healthy controls or patients with IBS for comparison.[19] Similarly, Boland and colleagues[44] reported a decrease in the diversity of mucosa-associated microbiota in patients with quiescent CD compared with healthy controls; in addition, Chao1 diversity was lower in CD. Interestingly, there was a trend toward a progressively greater disruption in the microbiome among those with residual symptoms, leading the authors to suggest that the altered microbial composition of this subgroup could be associated with the presence of persistent diarrhea.[44]

## Inflammation-Induced Visceral Hypersensitivity

The level of expression of the transient potential vanilloid veceptor 1 (TRPV1), present on the primary afferent neurons that sense painful stimuli, has been correlated with the phenomenon of visceral hypersensitivity that has been described in several functional gastrointestinal disorders.[45,46] TRPV1-mediated visceral hypersensitivity could be involved in the pathogenesis of pain in patients with IBD in remission. A 3.9-fold increase in TRPV1 immunoreactive nerve fibers has been described in quiescent IBD (deep remission) with IBS-like symptoms, compared with controls, and correlated with the severity of abdominal pain.[47] More studies are required to confirm these findings.

## Alterations in Intestinal Motility

The results obtained from colonic motility studies in IBD are inconclusive.[48,49] Some authors have postulated that chronic inflammation could produce changes in activity in the enteric nervous system that persist even after inflammation has resolved, a phenomenon referred to as inflammation-induced neuroplasticity.[50] Other changes in enteric neuromuscular function reported in the context of chronic inflammation in IBD include an impact on ionic conductance[51] and response to neurotransmitters in smooth muscle, as well as an increased availability of serotonin in inflamed regions secondary to changes in mucosal signaling.[52]

On a macroanatomic level, distortions in the structure of the intestinal wall with atrophy of the mucosa, changes in the muscle layers (fibromuscular dysplasia of the muscularis mucosa and muscular propria), and the development of mural fibrosis, in both CD and UC, would lead to stiffness of the intestinal wall, thereby affecting the motility and compliance of the colon and anorectum.[48]

## THE CONCEPT OF IRRITABLE INFLAMMATORY BOWEL DISEASE

Based on the presented and, albeit far from complete, body of available evidence that suggests that there may be some distinctive features of gut biology in those with quiescent IBD who complain of IBS-type symptoms, we suggest that this clinical scenario be referred to as irritable IBD (IIBD). This syndrome seems to result from the convergence of pathophysiologic elements of both IBS and IBD, resulting in the clinical phenotype compatible with IBS superimposed on an inflammatory phenotype that is IBD. Although the clinical features of IIBD may be indistinguishable from those that characterize classic or typical IBS, there seem to be some distinctive alterations in intestinal permeability, cytokine profiles and gut microbiota, among others, that distinguish IIBD from classic IBS, active IBD or asymptomatic, quiescent IBD.

Based on the model of the gut–brain axis, the generation of symptoms in this subgroup of patients with quiescent IBD could be triggered by variable interactions between luminal contents, stressful events, or psychosocial distress; furthermore, these same abdominal symptoms could then, through a positive feedback loop, trigger the generation of greater stress and/or psychological distress and a repeating and ever-reinforcing vicious cycle of IBS symptoms, stress, and psychological distress. One could go further to speculate that this subgroup of patients may share a specific genotype that predisposes them to the development of persistent symptoms after active inflammation has been overcome.

Undoubtedly, more prospective studies with a rigorous definition of IBD remission are needed to clarify and confirm the very existence of this IIBD concept.

## CLINICAL APPROACH OF IRRITABLE BOWEL SYNDROME IN INFLAMMATORY BOWEL DISEASE

In patients with quiescent IBD and persistent IBS symptoms, the first objective is to establish whether these IBS symptoms are a consequence of 1 of these 3 scenarios:

1. Subclinical IBD activity
2. An unrecognized mechanical or other noninflammatory complication of IBD
3. True IBS

### Step 1: Medical History and Physical Examination

A detailed medical history and thorough physical examination can provide some diagnostic clues. Although the presence of alarm symptoms (rectal bleeding, fever, weight loss, nocturnal diarrhea) will certainly point toward the presence of active IBD, a lack of correlation between symptoms and disease activity in IBD, in general, complicates the interpretation of clinical features.[53,54] The level of adherence to IBD therapies, intercurrent gastrointestinal infection, a newly adopted smoking habit, the consumption of nonsteroidal anti-inflammatory drugs, and the use of other concomitant drugs can all impact on intestinal transit and, thereby, on symptom expression. Constipation is common in patients with IBD in remission and often underestimated, although it can be identified by an assessment of bowel habits, as well as the recognition of such features as difficulty with defecation and the necessity to use digital maneuvers to achieve evacuation.

The medical history should also be directed to uncovering the possible contributions of stress, psychiatric comorbidity, and a history of physical, sexual, or other abuse. The use of validated depression and anxiety symptoms and quality-of-life scales as screening tools can prove invaluable in identifying potential triggers of symptoms. Given the dominance of pain in this syndrome, a dependence on opioids should be flagged as early as possible. Needless to say, the physical examination should be directed to the identification of evidence of active inflammation (tachycardia, hypotension, fever, abdominal tenderness, or an inflammatory mass) or any combination of the complications of active IBD. In this regard, the evaluation of the perianal area and a digital rectal examination should not be omitted.

### Step 2: Evaluation of Inflammatory Activity

Biomarkers of disease activity provide relatively noninvasive methods to guide the clinician, including the erythrocyte sedimentation rate, C-reactive protein (CRP), FC, and lactoferrin (not available in several countries). The erythrocyte sedimentation rate, as a marker of inflammation, is highly nonspecific and can be affected by age, tobacco use, anemia, and drugs such as salicylates[55]; it is, therefore, not recommended to investigate changes in inflammatory activity in IBD.[56] CRP, an acute phase protein produced in the liver, increases in a nonspecific manner in response to inflammation. These responses are genetically determined and a number of specific haplotypes and polymorphisms impact on the expression of CRP. As a consequence, up to 20% of the population may fail to mount an increase in the level of CRP, despite the presence of an ongoing inflammatory state. Indeed, CRP has been found to be inferior to FC as a marker of inflammation in IBD.[56,57]

FC, a biomarker of intestinal inflammatory activity, has been widely used in the differential diagnosis of IBD from functional disorders such as IBS. Indeed, an FC value of less than 40 μg/g was shown to predict a less than 1% probability for the presence of IBD.[56] FC correlates well with endoscopic activity (sensitivity of 88%, specificity of 73%) and, overall, performs better in UC than in CD.[58,59] In IBD, a meta-analysis found that using a threshold of 250 μg/g, FC was able to discriminate between endoscopically active and inactive disease with a sensitivity of 80% and a specificity of 82%.[60] Other inverstigators have suggested more stringent criteria. An FC level of less than 40.5 μg/g was a predictor of histologic remission (area under the receiver operating characteristic curve, 0.755; sensitivity, 41%; specificity, 100%).[61] Currently, an FC value of less than 100 μg/g is considered part of the treatment goal of IBD owing to its ability to predict low-level inflammatory activity in UC and has even been proposed as an acceptable substitute for colonoscopy.[62,63]

It is, therefore, reasonable to suggest that FC values of less than 50 μg/g, and even less than 100 μg/g,[63] should rule out subclinical inflammation as a cause of persistent IBS symptoms in patients with IBD in remission. FC values between 100 and 250 μg/g require more careful attention because they could reflect a need to optimize IBD treatment, or, in patients with CD, to resort to more invasive studies such as ileocolo-noscopy and, video capsule endoscopy, enterography, or even balloon enteroscopy, where indicated.

### Step 3: Rule out Alternative Etiologies

Although IBS-like symptoms are nonspecific and shared by several pathologies, there is a greater probability of uncovering one the following in the context of IBD: SIBO, carbohydrate malabsorption, exocrine pancreatic insufficiency, and bile acid diarrhea.

#### Small intestinal bacterial overgrowth

The current definition of SIBO is "a clinical syndrome of gastrointestinal symptoms caused by the presence of excessive numbers of bacteria within the small bowel."[64] Its diagnosis is controversial, because the time-honored gold standard—the quantification of bacteria in a culture of a jejunal aspirate—is invasive and the threshold for the definition of SIBO has been contentious. In clinical practice nowadays the diagnosis of SIBO is usually established based on the results of breath testing, an indirect and noninvasive method. Breath testing measures hydrogen and methane gases in expired air, produced by bacterial fermentation of an ingested substrate (lactulose or glucose). Breath tests are also problematic with the sensitivity of lactulose for the diagnosis of SIBO ranging from 31% to 68% and specificity from 44% to 100%, whereas the sensitivity of the glucose breath testing has ranged from 20% to 93% and specificity from 30% to 86%.[65] Owing to this variability, the definition of a positive test for SIBO remains controversial.[64]

A recent systematic review and meta-analysis found that the prevalence of SIBO in IBD was 35.5% based on breath testing, with the odds ratio (OR) for SIBO in patient with IBD being 3.9 times that of controls. A link between IBS and SIBO has also been proposed; here again, the quality of evidence is low due to heterogeneity between studies as well as variability in test modality and performance.[66]

Nevertheless, it must be conceded that risk factors for SIBO (small bowel strictures, fistulas, resection of the ileocecal valve, hypochlorhydria, immunosuppressive therapy, and dysmotility)[67] are common among patients with IBD and, particularly, in CD. A recent systematic review and meta-analysis, again based on breath tests,[68] estimated an overall prevalence of SIBO of 22.3% in IBD (OR, 9.51). The risk of SIBO was noted to be higher in CD (OR, 10.86) compared with UC (OR, 7.96). Furthermore, in CD, the presence of fibrostenosing disease (OR, 7.47) and a history of prior surgery (OR, 2.38) were identified as risk factors for SIBO.

A study in a group of individuals with quiescent IBD and IBS-like symptoms documented a 57% prevalence of a positive breath test for SIBO; of these, 57% responded to antibiotic treatment.[69] In another study, the treatment of SIBO in CD was shown to decrease the Harvey Bradshaw Index, a well-validated index of clinical activity.[70]

Because of the apparently high prevalence of SIBO documented in patients with IBD, and especially among those with stricturing CD, this diagnosis should be considered in the patient with IBD with persistent IBS symptoms. Although the common practice is to diagnose SIBO by breath testing, empirical antibiotic treatment may also be considered.

#### Carbohydrate intolerance

Carbohydrate maldigestion leading to intolerance is a relatively frequent cause of functional digestive symptoms (bloating, diarrhea, abdominal pain, and flatulence) and is considered to result from the fermentation by intestinal bacteria of undigested and, therefore, unabsorbed carbohydrates.[71] A high prevalence of lactose intolerance has been documented in IBD.[72] However, a recent systematic review concluded that the prevalence of lactose intolerance was no different from that in the general population and proposed that the high prevalence described in prior studies was related to the ethnic origin of the population studied, which contained a high proportion of individuals who were lactase deficient. In addition, mucosal inflammation of the small bowel in CD will compromise lactase bioavailability and thus lead to lactose malabsorption.[73] Other carbohydrate intolerances, such as those that result from sucrase–isomaltase deficiency, have attracted interest as a potential mimic of IBS.[74] Although this enzyme complex could be vulnerable to loss in the inflamed mucosa of a patient with CD, its status in the patient population has yet to be explored though some proinflammatory cytokines have been shown to downregulate sucrase–isomaltase in enterocytes.[75]

## Bile acid malabsorption

Bile acid malabsorption (BAM) results from the interruption of the recirculation of bile acids through the enterohepatic circulation (increased biosynthesis or secretion of bile acids, or malabsorption in the ileum), leading to their excessive loss into the colon where they cause diarrhea by stimulating motility as well as the secretion of electrolytes, fluid, and mucus.

BAM has been described in a subgroup of patients with diarrhea-predominant IBS (IBS-D) and bile acid sequestrant therapy has produced symptomatic improvement in diarrhea.[76,77] Given the location of the ileal bile salt transporter in the distal ileum, patients with CD are predisposed to BAM as a consequence of ileal disease and/or resection.[78,79]

Diagnostic tests for BAM include quantifying fecal bile acid excretion, the [75]selenium homotaurocholic acid retention test and assays for 7 alpha-hydroxy-4-cholesten-3-one and fibroblast growth factor-19 serum.[80] The availability of these tests varies from country to country. For example, in the United States, [75]selenium homotaurocholic acid retention testing is not available. A therapeutic trial of a bile acid sequestrant is a reasonable approach where access to such tests is not possible, although it needs to be remembered that this strategy is not recommended in patients with CD with extensive ileal involvement or with a history of ileal resection in the past,[81] because complete depletion of the bile salt pool may lead to the development of steatorrhea.[82,83] Accordingly, and given that the role of BAM has not been quantified in IIBD, the risk–benefit ratio of such therapy should be assessed on a case-by-case basis.[81]

## Pancreatic insufficiency

Another cause of IBS symptoms in IBD is pancreatic exocrine insufficiency (PEI). The accuracy of the diagnosis of PEI on the basis of fecal elastase measurement is disputed, because levels may be falsely low in patients with watery stools.[84,85] In a prospective cross-sectional study that included 100 patients with UC and 100 patients with CD (both active or quiescent) as well as 110 healthy controls, PEI was detected in approximately 22% of those with UC and 14% of those with CD on the basis of fecal elastase-1 testing with an OR for PEI in IBD of 10.5.[86] However, there are no reports on the prevalence of PEI in patients with quiescent IBD with persistent IBS symptoms and the benefits of pancreatic enzyme supplementation in this population are unknown. Mindful of these limitations, it seems reasonable to at least consider a diagnosis of PEI in the context of IBS symptoms in the patient with IBD.

### Step 4: Consider the Presence of Structural Alterations

The development of fibrosis is common in CD and may lead to significant clinical complications. However, fibrogenesis has also been documented in UC and can be detected even in areas of the rectal mucosa devoid of apparent inflammation.[87] It is not clear if these changes are related to longstanding disease[88] or to the severity and extent of inflammation, because fibrogenesis has been seen to occur after relatively short periods of activity and even over periods of less than 1 year.[89] In a recent study, Gordon and colleagues[90] found that the severity and chronicity of inflammation in UC were linked to a greater degree of fibrosis in and thickening of muscularis mucosae. The clinical consequences of fibrosis in patients with UC include dysmotility and anorectal dysfunction.[87] Although an imaging study may identify fibrotic involvement in CD, the presence of fibrosis in nonstenotic UC may be more difficult to detect.

What role these and other sequelae of inflammation in IBD, such as fistulae in CD, play in the pathogenesis of IBS symptoms in IBD in apparent remission is unknown, but their ability to produce pain, diarrhea, and defecatory dysfunction is undisputed. The possible contribution of postsurgical sequelae such as adhesions or ischemic strictures must not be forgotten. An algorithmic approach to the assessment of these patients is outlined in **Fig. 1**.

### TREATMENT OPTIONS FOR PATIENTS WITH QUIESCENT INFLAMMATORY BOWEL DISEASE AND PERSISTENT IRRITABLE BOWEL SYNDROME SYMPTOMS

Owing to the paucity of studies in this specific population, the treatment of IBS symptoms in patients in quiescent IBD is largely based on strategies developed for IBS, in

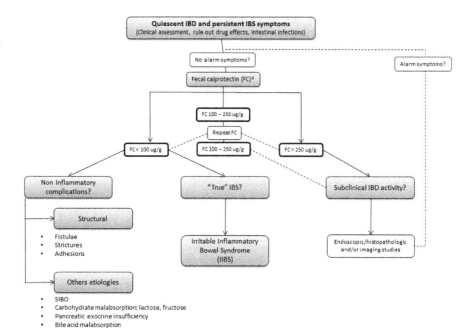

**Fig. 1.** An algorithm that proposes as approach to the assessment of the patent with apparently quiescent IBD but who has persistent IBS-like symptoms. [a] The FC cut off will depend on the clinical setting. These values are applicable in UC.

general. The approach to the patient should be holistic and may call upon dietary modifications, pharmacologic interventions, and psychotherapeutic strategies. The therapeutic plan selection should be based on the predominant symptom(s) and also address any trigger and confounding factors of each individual patient (**Fig. 2**).

## Fiber Supplements

Fiber supplements, especially soluble fiber such as psyllium, have proven useful in the management of IBS.[91] In IBD, data from animal models indicated that fiber consumption promoted the integrity of the intestinal epithelial barrier via short chain fatty acids produced from the bacterial fermentation of fiber; short chain fatty acids constitute a critical fuel for intestinal epithelial cells and also exert immunomodulatory effects[92]

The consumption of fiber in the diet was shown to decrease the frequency of symptomatic flares in a group of patients with quiescent IBD over a 6-month period.[93] However, caution should be exercised in the consumption of insoluble fibers in patients with stenosing CD.

## Antispasmodics

Antispasmodics are widely used in IBS to treat pain in all IBS subtypes and, as a class, proved to be superior to placebo in meta-analyses.[94,95] Current recommendations suggest avoiding the use of certain antispasmodics (hyoscine, hyoscyamine, and dicyclomine) owing to paucity of data supporting their efficacy.[91] The use of antispasmodics in quiescent IBD with IBS symptoms has not been evaluated; however, their use could be considered, based on an extrapolation from the data on IBS in general,

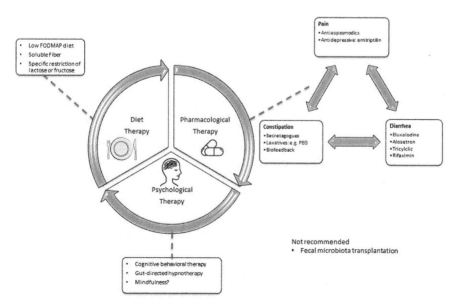

**Fig. 2.** Potential therapeutic solutions for symptoms management in the patient with truly quiescent IBD and persisting IBS-type symptoms. PEG, polyethylene glycol.

as discussed elsewhere in this article. Antispasmodics should be avoided in patients with IBD with stenosis and evidence of disease activity.

### Antidiarrheals

Drugs such as loperamide, a synthetic peripheral μ-opioid receptor agonist, have been used for the management of diarrhea in IBS,[96] owing to their effects on decreasing colonic motility and increasing water and electrolyte absorption. However, based on the available evidence, their use is not currently recommended.[95] In IBD, loperamide has been used for the management of diarrhea in CD and in patients with ileal pouch–anal anastomoses. A placebo-controlled study in a small number of patients[97] demonstrated a decrease in the frequency of stools when using 3 mg of loperamide oxide. A randomized controlled study is currently ongoing to test the effectiveness of loperamide in patients with inactive IBD and symptoms of IBS, among other therapeutic strategies.[98]

Eluxadoline, a mixed opioid agonist/antagonist, has been shown to improve the composite outcome of pain and stool consistency in patients with IBS-D when compared with placebo.[99,100] Serious adverse events associated with eluxadoline include sphincter of Oddi spasm and pancreatitis reported in a small percentage of IBS-D patients without a gallbladder or who were consuming more than 3 alcoholic beverages per day.

Alosetron, a selective serotonin receptor antagonist, has also been used in patients with IBS-D and mixed IBS. A recent meta-analysis that compared the efficacy of alosetron, eluxalodine, ramosetron, and rifaximin in adults with IBS-D and mixed IBS found that alosetron was the most effective in achieving the composite end point of improvement in abdominal pain and stool consistency, as well as on decreasing the global symptoms of IBS and normalizing stool consistency.[101] Adverse effects associated with alosetron include severe constipation and ischemic colitis. There are no data on the efficacy and safety of eluxodine or alosetron in patients with IBD, so their uses should be individualized in patients with quiescent IBD with IBS symptoms, and their potential adverse events considered.

### Treatment of Constipation

There are no clinical trials addressing the treatment of constipation in patients with IBD, so the data presented are based on evidence accumulated in IBS with constipation and chronic constipation.

Polyethylene glycol 3350, an osmotic laxative, demonstrated improvements in stool frequency, stool consistency, and straining, but not abdominal pain or bloating in comparison with placebo in a 4-week study.[102] Its good safety profile makes it an attractive, although untested, candidate for those with quiescent IBD in whom constipation as the predominant symptom.

Secretagogues such as linaclotide, lubiprostone, and plecanatide have shown symptomatic improvement over placebo in IBS with constipation and chronic constipation.[8,95] The use of prokinetic serotonin type 4 receptor agonists such as tegaserod[91] and prucalopride has also been shown to be useful in this subgroup of patients with IBS with constipation and chronic idiopathic constipation, respectively.[8,95]

In the absence of direct evidence on the management of constipation in IBD, an individualized approach to patients is recommended, starting with polyethylene glycol laxatives as a first-line treatment. Future studies are required to validate the use of the newer prescription drugs in IBD. Biofeedback therapy has also shown positive results in patients with IBD with dyssynergic defecation[103]

## Antibiotics

Rifaximin is a nonabsorbable antibiotic, approved by the FDA for the treatment of nonconstipated IBS. Double-blind, placebo-controlled trials demonstrated that treatment with rifaximin for 2 weeks provided significant relief of the IBS symptoms of bloating, abdominal pain and loose or watery stools among patients who had non-constipated IBS.[104] Based on these data and data from a number of other randomized trials, current clinical guidelines recommend the use of rifaximin in patients with IBS-D.[91,95]

The initial studies of rifaximin in IBD showed effectiveness in treating SIBO in patients with inactive ileal CD.[105] Subsequently, Prantera and colleagues[106] demonstrated the induction of remission in patients with moderately active CD after 12 weeks of treatment with rifaximin. However, a recent meta-analysis[107] found that the benefit provided by antibiotics in active CD is modest and may not be clinically meaningful. The effect of antibiotics on maintenance of remission in CD is uncertain.

In patients with quiescent IBD with IBS symptoms, rifaximin could be useful in the treatment of SIBO and diarrhea through its modification of gut microbiota.[108]

## Probiotics

Probiotics are widely used for the management of symptoms in IBS, based on the proposed role attributed to the microbiome in the pathogenesis of the disease. The many different formulations of probiotics available to consumers and heterogeneity of studies have complicated the evaluation of their efficacy. A recent meta-analysis of probiotics in IBS concluded that probiotic studies when pooled and aggregated revealed a significant benefit on IBS symptoms but, owing to the absence of head-to-head comparisons as well as the methodological limitations of many of the studies, could not define superiority for any particular combination, strain, or species of probiotics.[109] In view of the significant heterogeneity between studies, some recent clinical guidelines have gone so far as to recommend against the use of probiotics for the treatment of global symptoms in IBS.[91]

In IBD, a recent systematic review with meta-analysis suggested that probiotics may be as effective as 5-ASA in preventing relapse in quiescent UC.[110] Furthermore, available evidence supports their usefulness in mild to moderate UC and in pouchitis, but not in CD (whether in inducing remission or in preventing relapse of quiescent CD or recurrence after surgery).[110,111]

Future studies are needed to determine whether a specific strain or combination of strains and in what dosage and over what duration of treatment is appropriate for adjunctive or primary therapy in patients with IBD with concomitant IBS symptoms.

## Neuromodulators

Tricyclic antidepressants (TCAs) and selective serotonin reuptake inhibitors commonly used in the management of IBS symptoms have been rebranded from antidepressants to neuromodulators. In general, TCAs have shown better results than serotonin reuptake inhibitors in pain management.[112] The usefulness of TCAs is attributed to their effect on both visceral and central pain owing to their actions on norepinephrine and dopamine receptors, as well as their anticholinergic effects leading to a decrease in abdominal pain and diarrhea. Antidepressant effects could also and simultaneously benefit those with psychological comorbidity. Clinical management guidelines for IBS[91] recommend the use of neuromodulators, and specifically TCAs, to treat global symptoms of IBS; the results of a recent systematic review and meta-analysis support this guidance[112]

The efficacy of antidepressants in IBD is uncertain and limited by the low quality of available evidence.[113] In a small retrospective cohort of quiescent patients with IBD, TCAs achieved moderate improvement in residual gastrointestinal symptoms in almost 60% of patients.[114] In an interesting review based on an approach to gut–brain interactions in IBD, Mikocka-Walus and colleagues[115] postulated that antidepressants could be useful not only in reducing pain, but also in the management of functional symptoms (diarrhea), psychological comorbidities, and sleep disturbance, and even went so far as to propose that they could suppress disease activity through a direct anti-inflammatory effect. If used, it is recommended that one initiate therapy with a low dose (10 mg amitriptyline or 10 mg of desipramine) with gradual upward titration to maximize benefit while minimizing adverse events (dry mouth, insomnia, constipation, flushing, palpitations, and decreased appetite).[91]

### Fecal Microbiota Transplantation

Given the description of alterations in intestinal microbiota in both IBS and IBD, it should come as little surprise that fecal microbiota transplantation (FMT) has emerged as a potential therapeutic option. In IBS, data are still rather limited and conflicting and, although some positive results have been reported, FMT is not currently recommended in clinical guidelines.[91] A systematic review and meta-analysis of FMT in IBD found that FMT seems to be effective in the induction of remission in UC, but the long-term durability of this effect remains unclear.[116] In a recent cross-sectional analysis, IBS symptoms were not associated with distinctive microbiome alterations among patients with IBD; the possible effects of confounding factors could not be excluded.[19] Studies on FMT have not been conducted in patients with quiescent IBD and IBS symptoms, so in the absence of evidence, it is not recommended for now in this subgroup of patients.

### Diet

The benefits of a diet low in fermentable oligosaccharides, disaccharides, monosaccharides and polyols (FODMAPs) in IBS is based on an overall decrease in the severity of symptoms of up to 70%[117]; consequently, its usefulness has been investigated in patients with quiescent IBD.[118–120] In a recent study, 52 patients with quiescent IBD and persistent digestive symptoms were randomized to follow a low FODMAP diet or a control diet for 4 weeks. Those on the low FODMAPs diet achieved a greater degree of relief of specific GI symptoms (bloating and flatulence, but not pain), and a greater improvement in quality of life.[120] These benefits were accompanied by a lower abundance of *Bifidobacterium adolescentis*, *B longum*, and *Faecalibacterium prausnitzii*, but without any changes in markers of inflammation (peripheral T-cell phenotype).[120]

MODULATE, a prospective, long-term study that aims to evaluate the effectiveness of amitriptyline, ondansetron, loperamide and a low-FODMAP diet in patients with quiescent UC with IBS-like symptoms is currently in development.[98]

In recommending a highly restrictive diet to the patient with IBD, its implications for overall nutritional status and psychological well-being as well as microbiome homeostasis must be borne in mind.[121] Ideally, these approaches should be closely monitored by an experienced dietitian with the goal being the gradual reincorporation of as many foods as possible over time.

### Psychological Therapies

Psychosocial factors are often intrinsic to the pathophysiology of IBS, both as triggers and as a perpetuator of symptoms.[122] The prevalence of symptoms of anxiety and anxiety disorder have been reported at 39.1% and 23.0% of patients, respectively, and of symptoms of depression and depressive disorder in 28.8% and 23.3% of patients, respectively.[120] In relation to IBD, depression and anxiety affect up to 25% and 30% of patients, respectively, being more prevalent among those with active disease[123] and 2 to 3 times more common than in the general population.[124] The role of stressors as a trigger for IBD flares remains to be clearly defined.[13]

Several studies have documented higher levels of anxiety and depression,[14,125,126] lower quality of life scores, a higher prevalence of sleep disorders and of the interference of pain in daily activities, and decreased social satisfaction[127] in patients with quiescent IBD with IBS symptoms, in comparison with those who are asymptomatic.

Studies have shown favorable results with the use of neuromodulators (TCAs and serotonin reuptake inhibitors)[112] and of nondrug psychological therapies in IBS.[112,128] With regard to the latter, cognitive behavioral therapy and gut-directed hypnotherapy have the most substantive evidence base.[128] In IBD, the results of psychological therapies are more mixed; however, a recent meta-analysis showed a small, short-term benefit in depression and quality of life scores in patients with quiescent IBD.[129] The effects of psychological therapies on IBS-like symptoms in quiescent IBD are unknown, but their usefulness may be extrapolated from the above-referenced literature from IBS, in general. Mindfulness therapy has been shown to be beneficial in patients with quiescent IBD with IBS symptoms or with high levels of stress in terms of improving quality of life.[130] Sleep quality is also impaired in this subgroup of patients[131] and can be improved with sleep hygiene measures, among others.

## SUMMARY

Although IBS and IBD are distinct entities, some commonalities have been noted of late in terms of pathophysiological mechanisms. The gut–brain axis seems to be influential in both disorders in that psychosocial factors can trigger digestive symptoms and alternately central input can disrupt gut function through interactions with the immune system (leading to immune activation), gut microbiota (disrupting microbial homeostasis), and the intestinal epithelial barrier (enhancing intestinal permeability). IBS symptoms are common in patients with quiescent IBD and determining their cause is critical to successful management. Relatively noninvasive biomarkers such as CRP and FC, in particular, play an important role in detecting ongoing activity of IBD. In the patient with persistent symptoms despite all evidence pointing to true remission, alternative diagnoses should be considered, including SIBO, carbohydrate intolerance, PEI, and BAM. IBS-like symptoms will remain unexplained in most; whether this syndrome of IBS in IBD, so-called IIBD, although supported by some clinical and pathophysiological phenomena, is a distinct entity and different from classical IBS remains speculative. For now, however, and reflecting the current paucity of high-quality clinical trial data, the management of IIBD follows that developed for classic IBS. There is much to do.

## CLINICS CARE POINTS

- IBS-type symptoms are common among patients with IBD who seem to be in clinical remission and require careful assessment.
- Failing to detect low-grade active IBD or, in contrast, assuming disease activity when there is none will lead to inappropriate and potentially harmful decisions regarding treatment.

- Markers of inflammation such as fecal levels of calprotectin or lactoferrin are valuable in detecting evidence of ongoing low-grade activity of IBD.
- Ongoing activity of IBD can be confirmed by endoscopy with biopsy and/or imaging, as appropriate and then treated.
- If there is no evidence of disease activity treatment of IBS-type symptoms in the patient with IBD should follow the same principles as those for IBS in general; however, with the exception of the low-FODMAP diet there is no current evidence to support any therapeutic approach in this population.

## REFERENCES (SYSTEMATIC REVIEWS AND METANALYSES DENOTED BY *)

1. Isgar B, Harman M, Kaye MD, et al. Symptoms of irritable bowel syndrome in ulcerative colitis in remission. Gut 1983;24:190–2.
2. Fairbrass KM, Costantino SJ, Gracie DJ, et al. Prevalence of irritable bowel syndrome-type symptoms in patients with inflammatory bowel disease in remission: a systematic review and meta-analysis. Lancet Gastroenterol Hepatol 2020;5:1053–62 *.
3. Kappelman MD, Rifas-Shiman SL, Kleinman K, et al. The prevalence and geographic distribution of Crohn's disease and ulcerative colitis in the United States. Clin Gastroenterol Hepatol 2007;5:1424–9.
4. Malik TA. Inflammatory bowel disease: historical perspective, epidemiology, and risk factors. Surg Clin North Am 2015;95:1105–22.
5. Lovell RM, Ford AC. Global prevalence of and risk factors for irritable bowel syndrome: a meta-analysis. Clin Gastroenterol Hepatol 2012;10:712–21 *.
6. Kuhnen A. Genetic and environmental considerations for Inflammatory Bowel Disease. Surg Clin North Am 2019;99:1197–207.
7. Chang JT. Pathophysiology of Inflammatory Bowel Diseases. N Engl J Med 2020;383:2652–64.
8. Mearin F, Lacy BE, Chang L, et al. Bowel Disorders. Gastroenterology 2016. [epub ahead of print].
9. Powell N, Walker MM, Talley NJ. The mucosal immune system: master regulator of bidirectional gut-brain communications. Nat Rev Gastroenterol Hepatol 2017; 14:143–59.
10. Gracie DJ, Hamlin PJ, Ford AC. The influence of the brain-gut axis in inflammatory bowel disease and possible implications for treatment. Lancet Gastroenterol Hepatol 2019;4:632–42.
11. Gaines LS, Slaughter JC, Horst SN, et al. Association Between Affective-Cognitive Symptoms of Depression and Exacerbation of Crohn's Disease. Am J Gastroenterol 2016;111:864–70.
12. Bitton A, Sewitch MJ, Peppercorn MA, et al. Psychosocial determinants of relapse in ulcerative colitis: a longitudinal study. Am J Gastroenterol 2003;98: 2203–8.
13. Wintjens DSJ, de Jong MJ, van der Meulen-de Jong AE, et al. Novel perceived stress and life events precede flares of inflammatory bowel disease: a prospective 12-month follow-up study. J Crohns Colitis 2019;13:410–6.
14. Gracie DJ, Williams CJ, Sood R, et al. Negative effects on psychological health and quality of life of genuine irritable bowel syndrome-type symptoms in patients with inflammatory bowel disease. Clin Gastroenterol Hepatol 2017;15: 376–84.e5.

15. Gracie DJ, Hamlin JP, Ford AC. Longitudinal impact of IBS-type symptoms on disease activity, healthcare utilization, psychological health, and quality of life in inflammatory bowel disease. Am J Gastroenterol 2018;113:702–12.
16. Henriksen M, Høivik ML, Jelsness-Jørgensen LP, et al, IBSEN Study Group. Irritable bowel-like symptoms in ulcerative colitis are as common in patients in deep remission as in inflammation: results from a population-based study [the IBSEN Study]. J Crohns Colitis 2018;12:389–93.
17. Jonefjäll B, Öhman L, Simrén M, et al. IBS-like Symptoms in patients with ulcerative colitis in deep remission are associated with increased levels of serum cytokines and poor psychological well-being. Inflamm Bowel Dis 2016;22:2630–40.
18. Jonefjäll B, Strid H, Ohman L, et al. Characterization of IBS-like symptoms in patients with ulcerative colitis in clinical remission. Neurogastroenterol Motil 2013;25:756.e8.
19. Shutkever O, Gracie DJ, Young C, et al. No Significant Association Between the Fecal Microbiome and the Presence of Irritable Bowel Syndrome-type Symptoms in Patients with Quiescent Inflammatory Bowel Disease. Inflamm Bowel Dis 2018;24:1597–605.
20. Halpin SJ, Ford AC. Prevalence of symptoms meeting criteria for irritable bowel syndrome in inflammatory bowel disease: systematic review and meta-analysis. Am J Gastroenterol 2012;107:1474–82 *.
21. Simrén M, Axelsson J, Gillberg R, et al. Quality of life in inflammatory bowel disease in remission: the impact of IBS-like symptoms and associated psychological factors. Am J Gastroenterol 2002;97:389–96.
22. Sipponen T, Haapamäki J, Savilahti E, et al. Fecal calprotectin and S100A12 have low utility in prediction of small bowel Crohn's disease detected by wireless capsule endoscopy. Scand J Gastroenterol 2012;47:778–84.
23. Zucchelli M, Camilleri M, Andreasson AN, et al. Association of TNFSF15 polymorphism with irritable bowel syndrome. Gut 2011;60:1671–7.
24. Swan C, Duroudier NP, Campbell E, et al. Identifying and testing candidate genetic polymorphisms in the irritable bowel syndrome (IBS): association with TNFSF15 and TNFα. Gut 2013;62:985–94.
25. Bashashati M, Moossavi S, Cremon C, et al. Colonic immune cells in irritable bowel syndrome: a systematic review and meta-analysis. Neurogastroenterol Motil 2018;30(1). https://doi.org/10.1111/nmo.13192. *.
26. Burns G, Carroll G, Mathe A, et al. Evidence for local and systemic immune activation in functional dyspepsia and the irritable bowel syndrome: a systematic review. Am J Gastroenterol 2019;114:429–36 *.
27. Shukla R, Ghoshal U, Ranjan P, et al. Expression of Toll-like receptors, pro-, and anti-inflammatory cytokines in relation to gut microbiota in irritable bowel syndrome: the evidence for its micro-organic basis. J Neurogastroenterol Motil 2018;24:628–42.
28. Scully P, McKernan DP, Keohane J, et al. Plasma cytokine profiles in females with irritable bowel syndrome and extra-intestinal co-morbidity. Am J Gastroenterol 2010;105:2235–43.
29. Ohman L, Simrén M. Pathogenesis of IBS: role of inflammation, immunity and neuroimmune interactions. Nat Rev Gastroenterol Hepatol 2010;7:163–73.
30. Dinan TG, Quigley EM, Ahmed SM, et al. Hypothalamic-pituitary-gut axis dysregulation in irritable bowel syndrome: plasma cytokines as a potential biomarker? Gastroenterology 2006;130:304–11.

31. Katinios G, Casado-Bedmar M, Walter SA, et al. Increased colonic epithelial permeability and mucosal eosinophilia in ulcerative colitis in remission compared with irritable bowel syndrome and health. Inflamm Bowel Dis 2020; 26:974–84.

32. Moraes L, Magnusson MK, Mavroudis G, et al. Systemic inflammatory protein profiles distinguish irritable bowel syndrome (IBS) and ulcerative colitis, irrespective of inflammation or IBS-like symptoms. Inflamm Bowel Dis 2020;26: 874–84.

33. Jenkins RT, Ramage JK, Jones DB, et al. Small bowel and colonic permeability to 51Cr-EDTA in patients with active inflammatory bowel disease. Clin Invest Med 1988;11:151–5.

34. Dunlop SP, Hebden J, Campbell E, et al. Abnormal intestinal permeability in subgroups of diarrhea-predominant irritable bowel syndromes. Am J Gastroenterol 2006;101:1288–94.

35. Piche T, Barbara G, Aubert P, et al. Impaired intestinal barrier integrity in the colon of patients with irritable bowel syndrome: involvement of soluble mediators. Gut 2009;58:196–201.

36. Vivinus-Nébot M, Frin-Mathy G, Bzioueche H, et al. Functional bowel symptoms in quiescent inflammatory bowel diseases: role of epithelial barrier disruption and low-grade inflammation. Gut 2014;63:744–52.

37. Chang J, Leong RW, Wasinger VC, et al. Impaired intestinal permeability contributes to ongoing bowel symptoms in patients with inflammatory bowel disease and mucosal healing. Gastroenterology 2017;153:723–31.

38. Wallon C, Persborn M, Jönsson M, et al. Eosinophils express muscarinic receptors and corticotropin-releasing factor to disrupt the mucosal barrier in ulcerative colitis. Gastroenterology 2011;140:1597–607.

39. Tozlu M, Cash B, Younes M, et al. Dilemma in post-IBD patients with IBS-D symptoms: a 2020 overview. Expert Rev Gastroenterol Hepatol 2021;15:5–8.

40. Zezos P, Patsiaoura K, Nakos A, et al. Severe eosinophilic infiltration in colonic biopsies predicts patients with ulcerative colitis not responding to medical therapy. Colorectal Dis 2014;16:O420–30.

41. Bischoff SC, Mayer J, Nguyen QT, et al. Immunohistological assessment of intestinal eosinophil activation in patients with eosinophilic gastroenteritis and inflammatory bowel disease. Am J Gastroenterol 1999;94:3521–9.

42. Glassner KL, Abraham BP, Quigley EMM. The microbiome and inflammatory bowel disease. J Allergy Clin Immunol 2020;145:16–27.

43. Rodiño-Janeiro BK, Vicario M, Alonso-Cotoner C, et al. A review of microbiota and irritable bowel syndrome: future in therapies. Adv Ther 2018;35(3):289–310.

44. Boland K, Bedrani L, Turpin W, et al. Persistent diarrhea in patients with Crohn's disease after mucosal healing is associated with lower diversity of the intestinal microbiome and increased dysbiosis. Clin Gastroenterol Hepatol 2021;19: 296–304.

45. Matthews PJ, Aziz Q, Facer P, et al. Increased capsaicin receptor TRPV1 nerve fibres in the inflamed human oesophagus. Eur J Gastroenterol Hepatol 2004;16: 897–902.

46. Chan CL, Facer P, Davis JB, et al. Sensory fibres expressing capsaicin receptor TRPV1 in patients with rectal hypersensitivity and faecal urgency. Lancet 2003; 361:385–91.

47. Akbar A, Yiangou Y, Facer P, et al. Expression of the TRPV1 receptor differs in quiescent inflammatory bowel disease with or without abdominal pain. Gut 2010;59:767–74.

48. Torres J, Billioud V, Sachar DB, et al. Ulcerative colitis as a progressive disease: the forgotten evidence. Inflamm Bowel Dis 2012;18:1356–63.

49. Bassotti G, Villanacci V, Mazzocchi A, et al. Colonic propulsive and postprandial motor activity in patients with ulcerative colitis in remission. Eur J Gastroenterol Hepatol 2006;18:507–10.

50. Mawe GM. Colitis-induced neuroplasticity disrupts motility in the inflamed and post-inflamed colon. J Clin Invest 2015;125:949–55.

51. Akbarali HI, Hawkins G, Ross GR, et al. Ion channel remodeling in gastrointestinal inflammation. Neurogastroenterol Motil 2010;22:1045–55.

52. Mawe GM, Hoffman JM. Serotonin signaling in the gut–functions, dysfunctions and therapeutic targets. Nat Rev Gastroenterol Hepatol 2013;1:473–86.

53. Gracie DJ, Williams CJ, Sood R, et al. Poor correlation between clinical disease activity and mucosal inflammation, and the role of psychological comorbidity, in inflammatory bowel disease. Am J Gastroenterol 2016;111:541–55.

54. Colombel JF, Keir ME, Scherl A, et al. Discrepancies between patient-reported outcomes, and endoscopic and histological appearance in UC. Gut 2017;66: 2063–8.

55. Litao MK, Kamat D. Erythrocyte sedimentation rate and C-reactive protein: how best to use them in clinical practice. Pediatr Ann 2014;43:417–20. 8.

56. Menees SB, Powell C, Kurlander J, et al. A meta-analysis of the utility of C-reactive protein, erythrocyte sedimentation rate, fecal calprotectin, and fecal lactoferrin to exclude inflammatory bowel disease in adults with IBS. Am J Gastroenterol 2015;110:444–54 *.

57. Ma C, Battat R, Parker CE, et al. Update on C-reactive protein and fecal calprotectin: are they accurate measures of disease activity in Crohn's disease? Expert Rev Gastroenterol Hepatol 2019;13:319–30.

58. D'Haens G, Ferrante M, Vermeire S, et al. Fecal calprotectin is a surrogate marker for endoscopic lesions in inflammatory bowel disease. Inflamm Bowel Dis 2012;18:2218–24.

59. Peyrin-Biroulet L, Sandborn W, Sands BE, et al. Selecting Therapeutic Targets in Inflammatory Bowel Disease (STRIDE): determining therapeutic goals for treat-to-target. Am J Gastroenterol 2015;110:1324–38.

60. Lin JF, Chen JM, Zuo JH, et al. Meta-analysis: fecal calprotectin for assessment of inflammatory bowel disease activity. Inflamm Bowel Dis 2014;20:1407–15 *.

61. Theede K, Holck S, Ibsen P, et al. Fecal calprotectin predicts relapse and histological mucosal healing in ulcerative colitis. Inflamm Bowel Dis 2016;22:1042–8.

62. Jelsness-Jørgensen LP, Bernklev T, Moum B. Calprotectin is a useful tool in distinguishing coexisting irritable bowel-like symptoms from that of occult inflammation among inflammatory bowel disease patients in remission. Gastroenterol Res Pract 2013;2013:620707.

63. Ungaro R, Colombel JF, Lissoos T, et al. A treat-to-target update in ulcerative colitis: a systematic review. Am J Gastroenterol 2019;114:874–83.

64. Pimentel M, Saad RJ, Long MD, et al. ACG clinical guideline: small intestinal bacterial overgrowth. Am J Gastroenterol 2020;115:165–78.

65. Khoshini R, Dai SC, Lezcano S, et al. A systematic review of diagnostic tests for small intestinal bacterial overgrowth. Dig Dis Sci 2008;53:1443–54 *.

66. Shah A, Talley NJ, Jones M, et al. Small intestinal bacterial overgrowth in irritable bowel syndrome: a systematic review and meta-analysis of case-control studies. Am J Gastroenterol 2020;115:190–201 *.

67. Quigley EMM, Murray JA, Pimentel M. AGA clinical practice update on small intestinal bacterial overgrowth: expert review. Gastroenterology 2020;159: 1526–32.

68. Shah A, Morrison M, Burger D, et al. Systematic review with meta-analysis: the prevalence of small intestinal bacterial overgrowth in inflammatory bowel disease. Aliment Pharmacol Ther 2019;49:624–35 *.

69. Gu P, Patel D, Lakhoo K, et al. Breath test gas patterns in inflammatory bowel disease with concomitant irritable bowel syndrome-like symptoms: a controlled large-scale database linkage analysis. Dig Dis Sci 2020;65:2388–96.

70. Cohen-Mekelburg S, Tafesh Z, Coburn E, et al. Testing and treating small intestinal bacterial overgrowth reduces symptoms in patients with inflammatory bowel disease. Dig Dis Sci 2018;63:2439–44.

71. Gibson PR. Use of the low-FODMAP diet in inflammatory bowel disease. J Gastroenterol Hepatol 2017;32(Suppl 1):40–2.

72. Eadala P, Matthews SB, Waud JP, et al. Association of lactose sensitivity with inflammatory bowel disease–demonstrated by analysis of genetic polymorphism, breath gases and symptoms. Aliment Pharmacol Ther 2011;34:735–46.

73. Szilagyi A, Galiatsatos P, Xue X. Systematic review and meta-analysis of lactose digestion, its impact on intolerance and nutritional effects of dairy food restriction in inflammatory bowel diseases. Nutr J 2016;15:67 *.

74. Garcia-Etxebarria K, Zheng T, Bonfiglio F, et al. Increased Prevalence of Rare Sucrase-isomaltase Pathogenic Variants in Irritable Bowel Syndrome Patients. Clin Gastroenterol Hepatol 2018;16:1673–6.

75. Ziambaras T, Rubin DC, Perlmutter DH. Regulation of sucrase-isomaltase gene expression in human intestinal epithelial cells by inflammatory cytokines. J Biol Chem 1996;271:1237–42.

76. Wong BS, Camilleri M, Carlson P, et al. Increased bile acid biosynthesis is associated with irritable bowel syndrome with diarrhea. Clin Gastroenterol Hepatol 2012;10:1009–15.

77. Bajor A, Tornblom H, Rudling M, et al. Increased colonic bile acid exposure: a relevant risk factor for symptoms and treatment in IBS. Gut 2015;64:84–92.

78. Li N, Zhan S, Tian Z, et al. Alterations in Bile Acid Metabolism Associated with Inflammatory Bowel Disease. Inflamm Bowel Dis 2021. https://doi.org/10.1093/ibd/izaa342.

79. Vítek L. Bile acid malabsorption in inflammatory bowel disease. Inflamm Bowel Dis 2015;21:476–83.

80. Vijayvargiya P, Camilleri M, Shin A, et al. Methods for diagnosis of bile acid malabsorption in clinical practice. Clin Gastroenterol Hepatol 2013;11:1232–9.

81. Sadowski DC, Camilleri M, Chey WD, et al. Canadian association of gastroenterology clinical practice guideline on the management of bile acid diarrhea. J Can Assoc Gastroenterol 2020;3:e10–27.

82. Hofmann AF, Poley JR. Role of bile acid malabsorption in pathogenesis of diarrhea and steatorrhea in patients with ileal resection. I. Response to cholestyramine or replacement of dietary long chain triglyceride by medium chain triglyceride. Gastroenterology 1972;62:918–34.

83. Poley JR, Hofmann AF. Role of fat maldigestion in pathogenesis of steatorrhea in ileal resection. Fat digestion after two sequential test meals with and without cholestyramine. Gastroenterology 1976;71:38–44.

84. Fischer B, Hoh S, Wehler M, et al. Faecal elastase-1: lyophilization of stool samples prevents false low results in diarrhoea. Scand J Gastroenterol 2001;36: 771–4.

85. Leeds JS, Oppong K, Sanders DS. The role of fecal elastase-1 in detecting exocrine pancreatic disease. Nat Rev Gastroenterol Hepatol 2011;8:405–15.

86. Maconi G, Dominici R, Molteni M, et al. Prevalence of pancreatic insufficiency in inflammatory bowel diseases. Assessment by fecal elastase-1. Dig Dis Sci 2008;53:262–70.

87. Latella G, Rieder F. Time to look underneath the surface: ulcerative colitis-associated fibrosis. J Crohns Colitis 2015;9:941–2.

88. Mitomi H, Okayasu I, Bronner MP, et al. Comparative histologic assessment of proctocolectomy specimens from Japanese and American patients with ulcerative colitis with or without dysplasia. Int J Surg Pathol 2005;13:259–65.

89. de Bruyn JR, Meijer SL, Wildenberg ME, et al. Development of fibrosis in acute and longstanding ulcerative colitis. J Crohns Colitis 2015;9:966–72.

90. Gordon IO, Agrawal N, Willis E, et al. Fibrosis in ulcerative colitis is directly linked to severity and chronicity of mucosal inflammation. Aliment Pharmacol Ther 2018;47:922–39.

91. Lacy BE, Pimentel M, Brenner DM, et al. ACG clinical guideline: management of irritable bowel syndrome. Am J Gastroenterol 2021;116:17–44.

92. Ogata M, Ogita T, Tari H, et al. Supplemental psyllium fibre regulates the intestinal barrier and inflammation in normal and colitic mice. Br J Nutr 2017;118: 661–72.

93. Brotherton CS, Martin CA, Long MD, et al. Avoidance of fiber is associated with greater risk of Crohn's disease flare in a 6-month period. Clin Gastroenterol Hepatol 2016;14:1130–6.

94. Ford AC, Moayyedi P, Lacy BE, et al. American College of Gastroenterology monograph on the management of irritable bowel syndrome and chronic idiopathic constipation. Am J Gastroenterol 2014;109(Suppl 1):S2–26.

95. Ford AC, Moayyedi P, Chey WD, et al. American College of Gastroenterology monograph on management of irritable bowel syndrome. Am J Gastroenterol 2018;113(Suppl 2):1–18.

96. Efskind PS, Bernklev T, Vatn MH. A double-blind placebo-controlled trial with loperamide in irritable bowel syndrome. Scand J Gastroenterol 1996;31:463–8.

97. van Outryve M, Toussaint J. Loperamide oxide for the treatment of chronic diarrhoea in Crohn's disease. J Int Med Res 1995;23:335–41.

98. ISRCTN.com. MODULATE: a study to evaluate the effectiveness of either amitriptyline, ondansetron, loperamide, or dietary intervention (the low FODMAP diet) against standard dietary advice for the treatment of diarrhoea in patients with stable ulcerative colitis. Available at: http://www.isrctn.com/ISRCTN16086699. Identifier: ISRCTN16086699. Accessed December 17, 2020.

99. Lembo AJ, Lacy BE, Zuckerman MJ, et al. Eluxadoline for Irritable Bowel Syndrome with Diarrhea. N Engl J Med 2016;374:242–53.

100. Brenner DM, Sayuk GS, Gutman CR, et al. Efficacy and safety of eluxadoline in patients with irritable bowel syndrome with diarrhea who report inadequate symptom control with loperamide: RELIEF Phase 4 Study. Am J Gastroenterol 2019;114:1502–11.

101. Black CJ, Burr NE, Camilleri M, et al. Efficacy of pharmacological therapies in patients with IBS with diarrhoea or mixed stool pattern: systematic review and network meta-analysis. Gut 2020;69:74–82 *.

102. Chapman RW, Stanghellini V, Geraint M, et al. Randomized clinical trial: macrogol/PEG 3350 plus electrolytes for treatment of patients with constipation associated with irritable bowel syndrome. Am J Gastroenterol 2013;108:1508–15.

103. Rezaie A, Gu P, Kaplan GG, et al. Dyssynergic defecation in inflammatory bowel disease: a systematic review and meta-analysis. Inflamm Bowel Dis 2018;24: 1065–73 *.

104. Pimentel M, Lembo A, Chey WD, et al. Rifaximin therapy for patients with irritable bowel syndrome without constipation. N Engl J Med 2011;364:22–32.

105. Biancone L, Annese V, Ardizzone S, et al. Safety of treatments for inflammatory bowel disease: clinical practice guidelines of the Italian Group for the Study of Inflammatory Bowel Disease (IG-IBD). Dig Liver Dis 2017;49:338–58.

106. Prantera C, Lochs H, Grimaldi M, et al. Rifaximin-extended intestinal release induces remission in patients with moderately active Crohn's disease. Gastroenterology 2012;142:473–81.

107. Townsend CM, Parker CE, MacDonald JK, et al. Antibiotics for induction and maintenance of remission in Crohn's disease. Cochrane Database Syst Rev 2019;2(2):CD012730.

108. Soldi S, Vasileiadis S, Uggeri F, et al. Modulation of the gut microbiota composition by rifaximin in non-constipated irritable bowel syndrome patients: a molecular approach. Clin Exp Gastroenterol 2015;8:309–25.

109. Ford AC, Harris LA, Lacy BE, et al. Systematic review with meta-analysis: the efficacy of prebiotics, probiotics, synbiotics and antibiotics in irritable bowel syndrome. Aliment Pharmacol Ther 2018;48:1044–60 *.

110. Derwa Y, Gracie DJ, Hamlin PJ, et al. Systematic review with meta-analysis: the efficacy of probiotics in inflammatory bowel disease. Aliment Pharmacol Ther 2017;46:389–400 *.

111. Abraham BP, Quigley EMM. Probiotics in inflammatory bowel disease. Gastroenterol Clin North Am 2017;46:769–82.

112. Ford AC, Lacy BE, Harris LA, et al. Effect of antidepressants and psychological therapies in irritable bowel syndrome: an updated systematic review and meta-analysis. Am J Gastroenterol 2019;114:21–39 *.

113. Mikocka-Walus A, Prady SL, Pollok J, et al. Adjuvant therapy with antidepressants for the management of inflammatory bowel disease. Cochrane Database Syst Rev 2019;4(4):CD012680.

114. Iskandar HN, Cassell B, Kanuri N, et al. Tricyclic antidepressants for management of residual symptoms in inflammatory bowel disease. J Clin Gastroenterol 2014;48:423–9.

115. Mikocka-Walus A, Ford AC, Drossman DA. Antidepressants in inflammatory bowel disease. Nat Rev Gastroenterol Hepatol 2020;17:184–92.

116. Paramsothy S, Paramsothy R, Rubin DT, et al. Faecal microbiota transplantation for inflammatory bowel disease: a systematic review and meta-analysis. J Crohns Colitis 2017;11:1180–99 *.

117. Halmos EP, Power VA, Shepherd SJ, et al. A diet low in FODMAPs reduces symptoms of irritable bowel syndrome. Gastroenterology 2014;146:67–75.e5.

118. Halmos EP, Christophersen CT, Bird AR, et al. Consistent prebiotic effect on gut microbiota with altered FODMAP intake in patients with Crohn's disease: a randomised, controlled cross-over trial of well-defined diets. Clin Transl Gastroenterol 2016;7:e164.

119. Cox SR, Prince AC, Myers CE, et al. Fermentable carbohydrates [FODMAPs] exacerbate functional gastrointestinal symptoms in patients with inflammatory bowel disease: a randomised, double-blind, placebo-controlled, cross-over, re-challenge trial. J Crohns Colitis 2017;11:1420–9.

120. Cox SR, Lindsay JO, Fromentin S, et al. Effects of Low FODMAP diet on symptoms, fecal microbiome, and markers of inflammation in patients with quiescent

inflammatory bowel disease in a randomized trial. Gastroenterology 2020;158:
176–88.e7.

121. Staudacher HM. Nutritional, microbiological and psychosocial implications of
the low FODMAP diet. J Gastroenterol Hepatol 2017;32(Suppl 1):16–9.

122. Zamani M, Alizadeh-Tabari S, Zamani V. Systematic review with meta-analysis:
the prevalence of anxiety and depression in patients with irritable bowel syndrome. Aliment Pharmacol Ther 2019;50:132–43 *.

123. Mikocka-Walus A, Knowles SR, Keefer L, et al. Controversies revisited: a systematic review of the comorbidity of depression and anxiety with inflammatory
bowel diseases. Inflamm Bowel Dis 2016;22:752–62 *.

124. Walker JR, Ediger JP, Graff LA, et al. The Manitoba IBD cohort study: a
population-based study of the prevalence of lifetime and 12-month anxiety
and mood disorders. Am J Gastroenterol 2008;103:1989–97.

125. Perera LP, Radigan M, Guilday C, et al. Presence of irritable bowel syndrome
symptoms in quiescent inflammatory bowel disease is associated with high
rate of anxiety and depression. Dig Dis Sci 2019;64:1923–8.

126. Ozer M, Bengi G, Colak R, et al. Prevalence of irritable bowel syndrome-like
symptoms using Rome IV criteria in patients with inactive inflammatory bowel
disease and relation with quality of life. Medicine (Baltimore) 2020;99:e20067.

127. Abdalla MI, Sandler RS, Kappelman MD, et al. Prevalence and impact of inflammatory bowel disease-irritable bowel syndrome on patient-reported outcomes in
CCFA Partners. Inflamm Bowel Dis 2017;23:325–31.

128. Black CJ, Thakur ER, Houghton LA, et al. Efficacy of psychological therapies for
irritable bowel syndrome: systematic review and network meta-analysis. Gut
2020;69:1441–51 *.

129. Gracie DJ, Irvine AJ, Sood R, et al. Effect of psychological therapy on disease
activity, psychological comorbidity, and quality of life in inflammatory bowel disease: a systematic review and meta-analysis. Lancet Gastroenterol Hepatol
2017;2:189–99 *.

130. Berrill JW, Sadlier M, Hood K, et al. Mindfulness-based therapy for inflammatory
bowel disease patients with functional abdominal symptoms or high perceived
stress levels. J Crohns Colitis 2014;8:945–55.

131. Zargar A, Gooraji SA, Keshavarzi B, et al. Effect of irritable bowel syndrome on
sleep quality and quality of life of inflammatory bowel disease in clinical remission. Int J Prev Med 2019;10:10.

# Integrated Care for Irritable Bowel Syndrome

## The Future Is Now

Sameer K. Berry, MD, MBA[a], William D. Chey, MD, RFF[b],*

### KEYWORDS

- Integrative care • Multidisciplinary care • Pharmacotherapy • Nutrition • Diet
- Behavioral therapy • Psychological therapy • Complimentary alternative therapy

### KEY POINTS

- Although irritable bowel syndrome care delivery has evolved to include dietitians and psychologists (multidisciplinary care), this care still is fragmented because these providers to not work together with the gastroenterologist.
- Prospective research demonstrated significantly improved outcomes when these providers work collaboratively to develop an integrated treatment plan.
- Barriers to scaling integrated care include limited access to gastroenterology-trained ancillary providers, cost, and archaic reimbursement models.
- Potential solutions to these barriers include telehealth platforms, sharing ancillary providers between clinics, and health policy changes.

## INTRODUCTION

Irritable bowel syndrome (IBS) is a common condition that is defined by the presence of recurrent bouts of abdominal pain in association with altered bowel habits.[1] Although this opening sentence seems straightforward enough, like IBS, there is

Funding: None.

Potential Conflicts of Interest—S.K. Berry: Consultant: Oshi Health. W.D. Chey: Consultant: Abbvie, Alfasigma, Allakos, Alnylam, Arena, Bayer, Biomerica, Cosmo, Ironwood, Nestle, Phathom, QOL Medical, Redhill, Salix, Urovant, and Vibrant; Research Funding: Biomerica, Commonwealth Diagnostics International, QOL Medical, Salix, and Vibrant; and Stock Options: GI on Demand, Modify Health, and Ritter.

[a] Division of Gastroenterology, Michigan Medicine, 1500 East Medical Center Drive, 3910Q Taubman Center, Ann Arbor, MI 48109, USA; [b] Digestive Health Integrated Care Program, GI Physiology Laboratory, Michigan Food for Life Kitchen, Michigan Bowel Control Program, Division of Gastroenterology, Michigan Medicine, 1500 East Medical Center Drive, 3912 Taubman Center, Ann Arbor, MI 48109-5362, USA

* Corresponding author.

E-mail address: wchey@med.umich.edu

Twitter: @umfoodoc (W.D.C.)

Gastroenterol Clin N Am 50 (2021) 713–720

https://doi.org/10.1016/j.gtc.2021.04.006

more to it than meets the eye. Just as all birds have feathers, all IBS patients have abdominal pain. That said, although a sparrow and an eagle both are birds, they clearly differ in many important ways. The same analogy can be applied to patients with symptoms suggestive of IBS. Although all patients have pain, the severity, frequency, and quality of pain can differ dramatically among patients. At the same time, some IBS patients have diarrhea, others have constipation, and still others have a mixture of both. The heterogeneity of the clinical phenotype guarantees heterogeneity in the pathogenesis of this condition. Although IBS is a single syndrome, it likely is composed of several different diseases. In the absence of a unifying pathophysiology or the ability to identify the pathophysiologic abnormality responsible for an individual patient's symptoms, it should come as no surprise that different medications are more effective in some patients than others. The literature suggests that effective medications for IBS lead to significant improvement in overall symptoms in fewer than half of patients and offer a modest therapeutic gain of 7% to 15% over placebo.[2,3]

Further adding to the complexity of IBS, the pathophysiology and illness experience are not only heterogeneous but also multifactorial. In other words, different combinations of factors are likely to interplay to cause an IBS patient's illness experience. The biopsychosocial model of IBS provides a construct within which multiple issues, including diet, environment, psychological state, and physiologic and genetic factors, interact to influence not only a patient's symptoms but also how a patient reacts to and copes with their symptoms and, in turn, how their illness has an impact on their quality of life and ability to function (**Fig. 1**).

These principals are at the heart of why so many health care providers dread caring for IBS patients: "IBS patients are all crazy," "IBS patients are all whiners," "They call too often and are too demanding," and "IBS patients never get better." At face value, there is some truth to these claims. IBS patients are more likely to suffer with psychological comorbidity, do consume more health care resources, and, as previously discussed, often do not improve with commonly recommended medications. For the most part, such attributions place responsibility for these negative perceptions and outcomes squarely at the feet of the IBS patient. What if, however, a step back is taken from these preconceived notions and stereotypes to reconsider these issues—not solely as failures of the patient but rather as a series of failures of the systems of

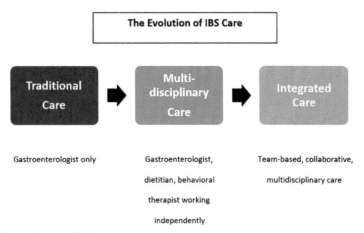

**Fig. 1.** The evolution of IBS care.

care delivery? If doing so, many of these issues offer opportunities to reimagine and modernize the clinical care model. The following paragraphs discuss just that—considering how recent evidence suggests that optimal clinical outcomes and improved patient satisfaction can be achieved best by collaborative, integrated care.

## THE EVOLUTION OF CARE FOR IRRITABLE BOWEL SYNDROME

Patients with IBS typically are managed by their primary care physician (PCP) and only when symptoms are severe are they referred to a gastroenterologist. For many decades, neither group had much to offer IBS patients other than largely un-proved, over-the-counter remedies and reassurance. The description of the first fiberoptic endoscope by Basil Hirschowitz and colleagues at the University of Mich-igan in 1957 ushered in the modern age of gastroenterology.[4] Over the ensuing more than 60 years, gastroenterologists established endoscopy as a reliable means of excluding structural diseases, such as inflammatory bowel disease and cancer. From a treatment perspective, new drug development dominated the management of patients with gastrointestinal disorders/diseases. In situations where an under-standing of aberrant disease–related pathophysiology informed new drug develop-ment, as with biologics for inflammatory bowel disease or antivirals for hepatitis C, the results have been stunning. On the other hand, for conditions where medications have been developed to address symptoms rather than disease-specific abnormal-ities in pathophysiology, the benefits have been more modest and incremental. This may seem an indictment of medications for IBS. It is not so much a criticism of the medications, however, as it is an indictment of the linear approach to treating a nonlinear, multidimensional condition, one that involves a complex web of environ-mental, behavioral, socioeconomic, biological, and genetic factors. Further, it also is important to realize that evidence-based medical treatments for IBS are a relatively recent phenomenon—the first Food and Drug Administration–approved drug for diarrhea predominant IBS with diarrhea was alosetron in 2000 and for constipation predominant IBS was lubiprostone in 2008.

There has been a growing recognition that diet and behavioral interventions are at least as effective as pharmacotherapy, and recent surveys suggest that community gastroenterologists are offering such treatments to their IBS patients.[5,6] Although non-pharmacologic treatments are delivered best by a trained gastroenterology (GI) dieti-tian and/or GI psychologist, other recent surveys of members of the American College of Gastroenterology found that only 40% to 50% had access to a GI dietitian and fewer than 40% had access to a GI psychologist.[6] Aside from access, there are other shortcomings to the nonintegrated, multidisciplinary care model. From a patient's perspective, each service provider (PCP, gastroenterologist, dietician, and psycholo-gist) remains at a stand-alone facility, often leaving the patient to coordinate informa-tion sharing as well as navigate different electronic medical records/patient portals, scheduling processes, travel to appointments, work-related obligations, and billing systems. This provider and system fragmentation and lack of communication increase the likelihood that patients receive conflicting advice and experience uncertainly regarding where to turn when problems or questions arise (**Fig. 2**).

In addition, there are significant differences between a general dietitian or psychol-ogist and a specially trained GI dietitian or GI psychologist. A general dietician must provide counseling to patients with a wide range of diseases. A general psychologist cares for patients with anxiety, depression, posttraumatic stress disorder, insomnia, and other mental health issues. Just as it is unrealistic to expect that a PCP will be as knowledgeable as a gastroenterologist about IBS, so too is it unrealistic to expect

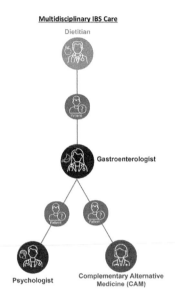

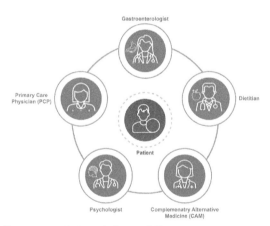

**Fig. 2.** Multidisciplinary versus integrated care delivery.

that a general dietitian or psychologist will be adequately trained to deliver evidence-based diet and behavioral interventions for a patient with IBS. In cases of behavioral therapies, in addition to knowledge gaps, there are fundamental differences in the services provided by a GI psychologist versus a general psychologist. Although the latter often engages in long-term psychotherapy for mental health issues, GI psychologists deliver short-term (6–8 sessions), evidence-based interventions, such as cognitive-behavioral therapy or hypnosis, which are focused on improving a patient's IBS symptoms.[5] These interventions are not necessarily intended to address chronic, general mental health issues. A separate referral to a general psychologist may be needed for IBS patients with significant comorbid mental illness.

Thus, although the dissemination of multidisciplinary care is a step in the right direction, it should be viewed as an intermediary step rather than the destination. On the horizon and gradually moving closer into view is integrated health care, also known as interprofessional health care, which the American Psychological Association defines as "an approach characterized by a high degree of collaboration and communication among health professionals".[7] What makes integrated health care unique is the sharing of information among team members related to patient care and the establishment of a comprehensive treatment plan to address the biological, psychological and social needs of the patient. The interprofessional healthcare team includes a diverse group of members (eg, physicians, nurses, psychologists and other health professionals), depending on the needs of the patient." An ever-increasing number of large GI practices and academic medical centers are developing such collaborative teams to more effectively manage their patients with IBS. Another term that is gaining popularity is integrative medicine. Integrative medicine puts the patient at the center of care and attempts to holistically address physical, emotional, mental, social, spiritual, and environmental/lifestyle influences that affect a person's health. Integrative medicine emphasizes care of the whole person rather than care of a disease. Integrative medicine emphasizes dietary and lifestyle reforms and incorporates modern health care recommendations along with complementary alternative treatments, such as acupuncture, yoga, and massage.[8]

## INTEGRATED CARE BECOMES EVIDENCE BASED

Until recently, integrated care has been more a common-sense aspiration of intuitive reasoning than an evidence-based solution for IBS patients. A recent pragmatic RCT by Basnayake and colleagues[9] for the first time brought to life the benefits of integrated care (n = 123) versus standard care (n = 65) for patients with functional GI disorders, many of whom had IBS. The standard care arm was run by an experienced gastroenterologist who could obtain external referrals to dieticians or psychologists. The integrated care team consisted of gastroenterologists, dietitians, psychiatrists, and behavioral therapists, all working as a team. Patients in the integrated care clinic were more likely to achieve symptom improvement (84% vs 57%, respectively; $P = .001$) and had higher rates of condition-specific improvement, psychological well-being, and quality of life. Approximately 60% of patients in both study arms had IBS, a majority of whom self-reported moderate or severe symptoms. Among those with IBS in the integrated care arm, there was a significant improvement in global symptoms (85% vs 65%, respectively; $P = .04$) and a greater proportion reported a greater than 50-point reduction from baseline IBS–symptom severity score scores (66% vs 38%, respectively; $P = .02$).[9]

The median cost per patient was marginally higher in the integrated clinic versus the control arm ($2485 vs $2421, respectively; $P < .01$), likely because this model concentrates the total cost of caring for these patients upfront through parallel processing as opposed to prolonging care delivery through sequential appointments. Surprisingly, the cost per patient who achieved the primary outcome of global symptom improvement was lower in the integrated care arm versus the standard care arm ($2549 vs $3136, respectively; $P < .01$), mostly due to fewer PCP visits and a reduction in unnecessary endoscopy and blood tests. This cost reduction in patients who achieved symptom improvement is important because further studies may demonstrate that it offsets the upfront cost of setting up an integrated clinic, especially with improvements in enrolling the most appropriate patients.

**Table 1**
**Barriers and solutions to implementing integrated care delivery for irritable bowel syndrome**

| Barriers | Solutions |
|---|---|
| Limited evidence to support the clinical or economic benefits of integrated care | Promising preliminary research requires validation in additional studies. |
| Limited access to dietitians and psychologists with GI-specialized training | Increased training opportunities for dietitians and behavioral therapists with in interest in GI conditions |
| High upfront cost and logistical barriers to developing integrated care clinics within traditional in-person facilities | Telehealth platforms that offer full-stack virtual clinics with all of the elements of integrated care |
| Current fee-for-service reimbursement model that incentivizes procedures instead of cognitive, nonendoscopic interventions | Health policy changes that move from fee-for-service to value-based payments |

It is critical to note that the differences between integrated care and standard care should not be attributed to the various interventions (medications, dietary, and behavioral) but rather to the structure in which these interventions are delivered to patients. More than half of the patients enrolled into this study previously had tried dietary therapy without relief. Both study arms used gastroenterologists who were senior clinicians with experience managing functional GI patients. Therefore, the key driver of symptom improvement and cost reduction appears to have been the organizational structure of an integrated clinic, where these interventions are delivered simultaneously by a team of multidisciplinary expert care providers.

## BARRIERS AND SOLUTIONS TO INTEGRATED CARE

Currently, integrated care for patients with IBS is confined to a small number of highly motivated practices and large, tertiary academic centers. Several explanations underlie this reality (**Table 1**). First, the literature supporting the benefits of nonmedical therapies and integrated care for IBS only recently has become available. As previously discussed, gastroenterologists are neither properly trained nor financially incentivized to provide education regarding diet or behavioral health interventions and a majority of US gastroenterologists do not have access the properly trained GI dietitians or GI psychologists.[6] At present, there is a paucity of formal training programs or accrediting organizations for dieticians and psychologists who are interested in specializing in GI. Education programs like the one offered by Monash University in Australia on the low fermentable oligosaccharides, disaccharides, monosaccharides, and polyols (FODMAP) diet are attempting to fill this void.[10] Michigan Medicine also offers an annual continuing education program on digestive and liver disorders each year.[11] Other programs for GI dietitians and GI psychologists hopefully will become available in the near future to increase the supply of properly trained providers. In the meantime, a lack of properly trained health care professionals leaves a majority of IBS patients without convenient access to even multidisciplinary care, let alone integrated care.

There also are several structural, cultural, and financial barriers to implementing an integrated care model in most practices. For a practice or academic group to be able to justify the substantial costs of hiring their own GI dietitian and/or GI psychologist, it must have a sufficient number of gastroenterologists to generate enough referrals to fill these provider's schedules. For example, at Michigan Medicine, where there have been GI dietitians since 2007 and a fully integrated care model, including GI psychologists since 2015, requires approximately 10 clinical gastroenterologist full-time equivalents' (FTEs) to support 1 GI dietitian FTE and 15 clinical gastroenterologist FTEs to support 1 GI psychologist FTE. These numbers make obvious the challenges facing smaller practices who want to adopt an integrated care model.

The compensation model in the United States still is largely fee for service and rewards procedural interventions more than cognitive services. This reimbursement structure provides significant challenges for both patients and providers. IBS patients may not have adequate coverage for the various services provided in an integrated care model. Even within the same insurance company, there are numerous plans per geography with varying preauthorization requirements and limitations on total number of dietary or behavioral visits. The back-office cost of handling these logistics make it difficult for traditional GI practices, who rely largely on endoscopy revenue, to adopt this model of care. Larger academic systems may be more likely to absorb these costs but still require stakeholder buy-in from administrators who are operating on increasingly narrow margins. Other cultural issues and institutional priorities around issues, such as nonmedical providers working *with* as opposed to *for* the gastroenterologist and dedication of precious work space to nonmedical providers are additional issues that need to be considered carefully, discussed with administration, and navigated.

There are some possible remedies to the substantial headwinds that confront the widespread adoption of integrated care. It might be possible for several smaller practices to share a GI dietitian and/or GI psychologist through telehealth. These remote integrated care options are starting to become available. Such systems allow any provider or group to access integrated care services without having to navigate the practical difficulties and financial outlays necessary to convert a traditional GI practice to integrated care. There also are novel care delivery platforms that house all the providers required to provide integrated IBS care direct-to-patient in a virtual format, known as full-stack virtual clinics, that create the possibility of providing leapfrog opportunities in accessing integrated IBS care. From a financial perspective, it is hoped that the shift in health policy toward value-based payments might better align financial incentives with the benefits offered by integrated care.

## SUMMARY

It is clear that not all IBS patients are created equally. The multidimensional nature of this pathophysiologically and clinically diverse condition should make clear the need for interdisciplinary solutions. One size does not fit all when it comes to treatment plans for IBS patients. Although the move from traditional care to multidisciplinary care will bring solutions to a larger proportion of IBS patients, this care model fails to break down the silos that impede communication and collaboration between providers as well as the very practical issues that follow multiple visits to multiple providers in multiple locations. Integrated care offers the possibility of breaking down these silos and providing solutions to many of the shortcomings of siloed multidisciplinary care. Although integrated care is an aspirational goal, its widespread adoption will require solutions to a range of structural, cultural, and financial issues.

## CLINICS CARE POINTS

- Medications and dietary and behavioral interventions all are evidence-based treatment options for IBS patients.

- Most gastroenterologists do not have access to dietitians or psychologists with the necessary GI training to care for IBS patients.
- Even when these patients have access to GI-trained dietitians/psychologists, if they are not working alongside the gastroenterologist, outcomes are not optimized.

## REFERENCES

1. Chey WD, Kurlander J, Eswaran S. Irritable bowel syndrome: a clinical review. JAMA 2015;313(9):949–58.
2. Lacy BE, Pimentel M, Brenner DM, et al. ACG clinical guideline: management of irritable bowel syndrome. Am J Gastroenterol 2021;116(1):17–44.
3. Ford AC, Moayyedi P, Chey WD, et al. American college of gastroenterology monograph on management of irritable bowel syndrome. Am J Gastroenterol 2018;113(S2):1–18.
4. Bossuyt P, Vermeire S, Bisschops R. Scoring endoscopic disease activity in IBD: artificial intelligence sees more and better than we do. Gut 2020;69(4):788–9.
5. Chey WD, Keefer L, Whelan K, et al. Behavioral and diet therapies in integrated care for patients with irritable bowel syndrome. Gastroenterology 2021;160(1):47–62.
6. Lenhart A, Ferch C, Shaw M, et al. Use of dietary management in irritable bowel syndrome: results of a survey of over 1500 United States gastroenterologists. J Neurogastroenterol Motil 2018;24(3):437–51.
7. Integrated Health Care. Available at: https://www.apa.org/health/integrated-health-care. Accessed February 19, 2021.
8. Definition of integrative medicine - NCI Dictionary of Cancer Terms - National Cancer Institute. Available at: https://www.cancer.gov/publications/dictionaries/cancer-terms/def/integrative-medicine. Accessed February 19, 2021.
9. Basnayake C, Kamm MA, Stanley A, et al. Standard gastroenterologist versus multidisciplinary treatment for functional gastrointestinal disorders (MANTRA): an open-label, single-centre, randomised controlled trial. Lancet Gastroenterol Hepatol 2020;5(10):890–9.
10. Take online FODMAP training | Monash FODMAP - Monash Fodmap. Available at: https://www.monashfodmap.com/online-training/dietitian-course//. Accessed February 19, 2021.
11. CME | Internal Medicine | Michigan Medicine | University of Michigan. Available at: https://medicine.umich.edu/dept/intmed/education-training/cme. Accessed February 19, 2021.

# Moving?

## Make sure your subscription moves with you!

To notify us of your new address, find your **Clinics Account Number** (located on your mailing label above your name), and contact customer service at:

**Email: journalscustomerservice-usa@elsevier.com**

**800-654-2452** (subscribers in the U.S. & Canada)
**314-447-8871** (subscribers outside of the U.S. & Canada)

**Fax number: 314-447-8029**

**Elsevier Health Sciences Division**
**Subscription Customer Service**
**3251 Riverport Lane**
**Maryland Heights, MO 63043**

*To ensure uninterrupted delivery of your subscription, please notify us at least 4 weeks in advance of move.